International Practice Development in Health and Social Care

International Practice Development in Health and Social Care

Second Edition

Edited by

Kim Manley
Valerie Wilson
Christine Øye

WILEY Blackwell

This second edition first published 2021

Registered Offices
John Wiley & Sons, Inc., 111 River Street, Hoboken, NJ 07030, USA
John Wiley & Sons Ltd, The Atrium, Southern Gate, Chichester, West Sussex, PO19 8SQ, UK

Editorial Office
9600 Garsington Road, Oxford, OX4 2DQ, UK

For details of our global editorial offices, customer services, and more information about Wiley products visit us at www.wiley.com.

Wiley also publishes its books in a variety of electronic formats and by print-on-demand. Some content that appears in standard print versions of this book may not be available in other formats.

Library of Congress Cataloging-in-Publication Data

Names: Manley, Kim (Lecturer in nursing), editor. | Wilson, Val (Valerie), 1961– editor. | Øye, Christine, editor.
Title: International practice development in health and social care / edited by Kim Manley, Valerie J. Wilson, Christine Øye.
Other titles: International practice development in nursing and healthcare
Description: Second edition. | Hoboken, NJ : Wiley-Blackwell, 2021. | Preceded by International practice development in nursing and healthcare / edited by Kim Manley, Brendan McCormack, Val Wilson. 1st edition. 2008. | Includes bibliographical references and index.
Identifiers: LCCN 2020051121 (print) | LCCN 2020051122 (ebook) | ISBN 9781119698357 (paperback) | ISBN 9781119698494 (adobe pdf) | ISBN 9781119698500 (epub)
Subjects: MESH: Evidence-Based Nursing–methods | Patient-Centered Care–methods | International Cooperation | Leadership
Classification: LCC RT41 (print) | LCC RT41 (ebook) | NLM WY 100.7 | DDC 610.73–dc23
LC record available at https://lccn.loc.gov/2020051121
LC ebook record available at https://lccn.loc.gov/2020051122

Cover Design: Wiley
Cover Images: © KTSDESIGN/SCIENCE PHOTO LIBRARY/Getty Images

Set in 9.5/11.5pt Palatino by Spi Global, Pondicherry, India
Printed and bound by CPI Group (UK) Ltd, Croydon, CR0 4YY

C9781119698357_260321

Contents

List of contributors *xi*
Foreword by Cheryl Atherfold *xv*
Foreword by Michael West *xvi*
Acknowledgements *xviii*

1. **Transforming Health and Social Care Using Practice Development** **1**
Kim Manley, Valerie Wilson, and Christine Øye
Setting the scene at this time of high challenge 1
Practice development: its relevance to contemporary health and social care and crisis 2
Practice development: growing scope and impact from interprofessional collaboration and working with shared values 3
Developments since 2008 international edition 4
Living our values as editors and authors 7
The key concepts and structure of the book 8
Conclusion 10
References 10

2. **Shaping Health Services Through True Collaboration Between Professional Providers and Service Users** **14**
Kristin Ådnøy Eriksen, Julia Kittscha, and Greg Fairbrother
Introduction 14
Examples of collaborative approaches 15
Discussion 21
Conclusion 23
References 24

3. **Turning Point: Curious Novice to Committed Advocate** **26**
Catherine Adams, Ciaran Crowe, Crystal McLeod, and Giselle Coromandel
Inclusivity, relatability, effectiveness – Ciaran's Eureka 27
Building contextual readiness – Cathy's nemesis and enlightenment 29
Engagement 30
Facilitation – Crystal's unrecognised talent 31
Co-production – collective ownership 33

Giselle's experience with co-production 34
Conclusion 35
References 36

4. **Sustainable Person-Centred Communities Design and Practice** **39**
Sharon Lee, Mayur Vibhuti, and Tobba Therkildsen Sudmann
Introduction 39
The litmus test – what are sustainable person-centred communities? 45
Facilitating creative and brave practitioners – critical appreciation of sustainable person-centred communities' design and practice 47
Concluding remarks 48
References 49

5. **Promoting Person-Centred Care for Older People** **52**
Victoria Traynor, Hui-Chen (Rita) Chang, Andreas Büscher, and Duncan McKellar
Introduction 52
Illustrating the application of claims, concerns and issues 53
Case studies 53
International, cross-setting and interdisciplinary learning 60
Conclusion and implications for undertaken practice development in aged care services 62
References 62

6. **Education Models Embedding PD Philosophy, Values and Impact – Using the Workplace as the Main Resource for Learning, Developing and Improving** **65**
Rebekkah Middleton, Tracey Moroney, Carolyn Jackson, and Ruth Germaine
Introduction 65
Case study 1: The value of integrating a person-centred curriculum 66
Case study 2: Place-based learning 69
Measuring the impact of CPD in the workplace 73
Summary and conclusion 83
References 83

7. **Critical Ethnography: A Method for Improving Healthcare Cultures in Practice Development and Embedded Research** **86**
Christine Øye, Claudia Green, Katherine Kirk, Cecilia Vindrola-Padros, and Greg Fairbrother
Introduction 86
Critical ethnographer as an embedded researcher 87
Introducing two case studies 88
Critical ethnography: a method for discovering 'hidden' practices and an avenue for practice development 94
Conclusion 97
References 97

8. A Global Manifesto for Practice Development: Revisiting Core Principles **99**
Sally Hardy, Simone Clarke, Irena Anna Frei, Claire Morley, Jo Odell, Chris White, and Valerie Wilson

Introduction 99
Revising the PD principles through a stakeholder review process 100
Emergent themes 104
Comparing the 2008 PD principles with the revised 2020 PD \ principles 110
Conclusion 115
References 116

9. Theorising Practice Development **118**
Emma Radbron, Clint Douglas, and Cheryl Atherfold

Introduction 119
Theoretical origins 119
Working with the 'critical' in critical reflection 120
Connecting through crisis: critical social science and person-centredness in PD research 122
Theory in action: a bicultural perspective 124
Reflecting on the future of theory and practice development 127
Invited commentary – Dr Deborah Baldie 128
References 129

10. Unpacking and Developing Facilitation **131**
Rebekkah Middleton, Margaret Kelly, Caroline Dickson, Valerie Wilson, Famke van Lieshout, Kathrin Hirter, and Christine Boomer

Introduction 131
Unpacking facilitation – an overview 131
Facilitator development – developing person-centred facilitators 136
Facilitator development – moving to advanced facilitation 140
Conclusion 144
References 145

11. Re-Imagining Participation in Processes of Facilitation: a Case for 'Humble Assertiveness' **147**
Gudmund Ågotnes, Karen Tuqiri, and Kristin Ådnøy Eriksen

Introduction 147
The process of facilitation – case examples 149
The complexity of facilitation – achieving meaningful participation 152
A commonality: culture 153
A commonality: participation 155
An approach towards facilitation: humble assertiveness 156
References 157

12. **Leadership Relationships** **159**
Rebekkah Middleton, Shaun Cardiff, Kim Manley, and Belinda Dewar
Introduction 159
Relational leadership 160
Guiding lights of leadership 164
Leadership development strategies that enable effective workplace cultures 167
Conclusion 170
References 171

13. **From Fractured to Flourishing: Developing Clinical Leadership for Frontline Culture Change** **173**
Duncan McKellar, Helen Stanley, Kim Manley, Selena Moore, Tyler Lloyd, Clare Hardwick, and Julia Ronder
Introduction 173
Background 173
The case studies 175
Discussion 182
Conclusion 184
References 184

14. **Systems Leadership Enablement of Collaborative Healthcare Practices** **187**
Annette Solman, Kim Manley, and Jane Christie
Introduction 187
Developing systems leadership and management capability using facilitated learning 187
Keeping people focused with increasingly complex healthcare systems 190
Systems leadership and workforce factors influencing transformation 191
The role of facilitative leadership in improving care for older people across the system 196
Conclusion 197
References 198
References 204

15. **Recognising and Developing Effective Workplace Cultures Across Health and Social Care that are Also Good Places to Work** **205**
Kate Sanders, Jonathan Webster, Kim Manley, and Shaun Cardiff
What is workplace culture and why is it important? 205
Background to collaborative inquiry 206
Developing 'guiding lights' through collaborative inquiry 207
Conclusion 216
References 217

16. **Wellbeing at Work** **220**
Tristi Brownett, Valerie Wilson, and Alera Bowden
Introduction 220
What is wellbeing? 220
Flourishing 221
Why wellbeing matters at work 222
Dissemination and sustainability 225
Key moments on the journey 229
Launching the Wellbeing Strategy 229
Recognising the person and celebrating their achievements 229
Knowing what matters 230
Enhanced communication opportunities 231
Access to education 231
Living our values 231
Key insights 232
Conclusion 233
References 234

17. **Flourishing People, Families and Communities** **237**
Carolyn Jackson, Valerie Wilson, Tanya McCance, and Albara Alomari
What is community flourishing? 237
Facilitating community engagement and development using practice development principles 240
Empowering citizens and communities to flourish through participatory research methods 241
Conclusion 247
References 248

18. **Practice Development – Towards Co-Creation, Innovation and Systems Transformation to Foster Person-Centred Care** **251**
By Christine Øye, Valerie Wilson, and Kim Manley
Introduction 251
Societal challenges for a new decade 252
Practice development and person-centred care 252
Practice development and user involvement through co-creation 254
Practice development and innovation 255
Practice development and system approaches 256
PD: enabling through leadership and facilitation 257
Practice development beyond methods and a new global manifesto for PD 258
New directions through the International Practice Development Collaborative (IPDC) 259
Q1 Who are the up-and-coming practice developers in your area? 259

Q2 What professions (and consumers) do you currently engage in PD work? 260
Q3 What areas of PD should we be focusing on in the coming years? 260
Q4 What is one thing you would like to celebrate in relation to PD? 261
Conclusion 261
References 262

Index 265

List of contributors

Catherine Adams, Clinical Midwifery Consultant, NNSWLHD, Australia

Kristin Ådnøy Eriksen, Associate Professor, Western Norway University of Applied Sciences, Norway

Gudmund Ågotnes, Associate Professor, Western Norway University of Applied Sciences, Norway

Albara Alomari, Lecturer, Western Sydney University, Australia

Cheryl Atherfold, Deputy Chief Nurse Waikato District Health Board, New Zealand

Christine Boomer, Research Fellow, Nursing research and practice development, University of Ulster, Northern Ireland

Alera Bowden, Clinical Nurse Consultant ISLHD/University of Wollongong Australia

Tristi Brownett, Senior Lecturer, Health Promotion and Public Health, Canterbury Christ Church University, England

Andreas Büscher, Professor of Nursing Science, Osnabrück University of Applied Sciences, Germany

Shaun Cardiff, Senior Lecturer, Fontys University of Applied Sciences, Einthoven, The Netherlands

Hui Chen (Rita) Chang, Senior Lecturer, University of Wollongong, Australia

Jane Christie, Senior Development Manager, West Lothian Health and Social Care Partnership, Scotland. Honorary Associate Lecturer, Queen Margaret University, Edinburgh. Fellow of the International Institute of Practice Transformation

Simone Clarke, Registered Nurse (Bachelor of Applied Science Nursing). Essentials of Care Program Manager, Children's Hospital Westmead, Sydney Children's Hospitals Network. Australia

Giselle Coromandel, Consumer advocate and President of Better Births Illawarra (a not for profit advocacy group), Australia

Ciaran Crowe, Consultant Obstetrician and Gynaecologist, Clinical Associate DME. EKHUFT, England

Belinda Dewar, RN (Adult). Registered Nurse Teacher, Diploma (Life Sciences), BSc (Hons), MSc, PhD, Director – Wee Culture, Scotland

Caroline Dickson, Senior Lecturer, Queen Margaret University, Edinburgh, Scotland

Clint Douglas, Conjoint Professor and Nursing Chair, QUT School of Nursing and Metro North Hospital and Health Service, Brisbane, Australia

Greg Fairbrother, Nurse Consultant, Patient and Family-centred Care Research, Sydney Local Health District. Adjunct Associate Professor, University of Sydney Faculty of Medicine and Health, Australia

Irena Anna Frei, Lead Facilitator, Practice Development School. Former Head Practice Development Unit Nursing, Basle Switzerland

Ruth Germaine, Systems Transformation Fellow, Primary Care Networks East Kent Training Hub, England

Claudia Green, Organisational Development Consultant, Organisational Development and Learning – People and Culture, Western Sydney Local Health District, Australia

Clare Hardwick, Head of Inpatient Therapy Services, East Kent Hospitals University NHS Foundation Trust (EKHUFT), England

Sally Hardy, Dean, School of Health Sciences, Faulty of Medicine and Health Sciences, University of East Anglia, Norwich

Kathrin Hirter, Clinical Nurse Specialist, Basle, Switzerland

Carolyn Jackson, Director, ImPACT Research Group, University of East Anglia, Norwich, England

Margaret Kelly, Implementation Manager, Leading better Value Care, ACI, NSW, Australia

Katherine Kirk, Research Fellow, Health Services Management Centre, University of Birmingham

Julia Kittscha, Clinical Nurse Consultant, Stomal Therapy, ISLHD/ University of Wollongong, Australia

Sharon Lee, Primary Care Workforce Programme Manager/Queens Nurse, Kent and Medway Primary Care Training Hub, England

Famke van Lieshout, Associate Professor, Fontys University of Applied Sciences, Einthoven, The Netherlands

Tyler Lloyd, Head Biomedical Scientist, EKHUFT, England

Kim Manley, Professor of Practice Development and Co-Director, ImPACT Centre, University of East Anglia, Norwich, England. Emeritus Professor, Canterbury Christ Church University, England. Visiting Professor, Wollongong University, Australia

Tanya McCance, Mona Grey Professor of Nursing, R&D, University of Ulster, Belfast, Northern Ireland

Duncan McKellar, Head of Unit, Older Persons' Mental Health Service, Northern Adelaide Local Health Network, Australia

Crystal McLeod, Improvement and Transformation Manager, Programme Lead for Maternity Transformation, EKHUFT, England

Rebekkah Middleton, Senior Lecturer, Wollongong University, Australia

Selena Moore, Ward Manager, Kings D, William Harvey Hospital, EKHUFT, England

Claire Morley, Statewide Nursing Director, Nursing and Midwifery Excellence, Tasmanian Health Service, Australia

Tracey Moroney, Head, School of Nursing and Deputy Dean, Faculty of Science, Medicine and Health, University of Wollongong, Australia

Jo Odell, Practice Development Facilitator, Foundation of Nursing Studies, London, England

Christine Øye, Professor of Health and Social care Service Research, Western Norway University of Applied Sciences. Center of Care Research

Emma Radbron, Nurse Manager - iMPAKT Study ISLHD/University of Wollongong, Australia

Julia Ronder, Consultant in Child and Adolescent Psychiatry. Consultant in Community Paediatrics (ADHD), EKHUFT, England

Kate Sanders, Practice Development Facilitator, Foundation of Nursing Studies, London, England

Annette Solman, Chief Executive, Health Education and Training Institute NSW Health, Australia

Helen Stanley, Associate Tutor, University of Surrey. Associate Consultant, Royal College of Nursing. Doctoral student, Canterbury Christ Church University, England

Tobba Therkildsen Sudmann, Physiotherapist. Social Scientist Sociology, PhD. Professor, Western Norway University of Applied Sciences, Norway

Victoria Traynor, Professor of Aged and Dementia Care, University of Wollongong, Australia

Karen Tuqiri, Director of Nursing, Prince of Wales Hospital, Sydney, Australia

Mayur Vibhuti, GP and Visiting Reader in Medical Leadership Canterbury Christ Church University, England

Cecilia Vindrola-Padros, Co-Director, Rapid Research Evaluation and Appraisal Lab (RREAL), UCL, London UK

Jonathan Webster, Professor of Practice Development and Co-Director, ImPACT, University of East Anglia, Norwich, England. Associate Facilitator, Foundation of Nursing Studies

Chris White, Practice Development Education Nurse Manager, Sydney Children's Hospitals Network, Australia

Valerie Wilson, Professor of Nursing, Illawarra Shoalhaven Local Health District, Prince of Wales Hospital, Sydney and University of Wollongong, Australia. Visiting Professor University of Ulster, Northern Ireland

Foreword

Navigating contemporary health and social care

As I reflect on this unprecedented time in history that we are experiencing with the global COVID-19 pandemic, I observe that the strength and creativity required of healthcare teams everywhere have been challenged and are to be celebrated. This edition of *International Practice Development in Health and Social Care* has transpired during this season. The chapters unfold as authentic 'word portraits' from the contributors' practice to form a collage of the ways that healthcare responds in myriad contexts.

Within its pages, application of practice development across the life span and care continuum advocates for the voice of vulnerable members of our communities. Theory and courage merge to provide frameworks and approaches that align with individual practitioners' values, and identity and indigenous knowledge are honoured as foundations of person centredness for individuals, teams and organisations.

Growing a workforce that thrives as it meets the needs of the people it serves requires vision, leadership and a relational participatory culture that is agile and can respond to increasing demands and complexity at all levels. Skilled facilitation enables growth to be cultivated and fractured aspects of team culture to be resolved, providing an environment of wellbeing and self-care.

This edition is a compelling narrative of experience and theory within a global context, woven together to provide a pathway towards a values-based journey of flourishing for healthcare recipients, practitioners, teams and organisations.

Cheryl Atherfold
Deputy Chief Nurse, Waikato District Health Board,
Percival Flats, Hamilton, New Zealand

Foreword

Compassionate leadership, teamworking and reflection in practice development

The pandemic has triggered global tragedy, pain, fear, anxiety and darkness. Yet, at the darkest times there is an opportunity for the light of learning to stream in. I believe that the three key areas of learning from this crisis are compassionate leadership, teamworking and reflection.

Compassion is the core value of our healthcare system and it is the most potent healthcare intervention. The challenge is for us to create cultures in our organisations where staff are both encouraged and enabled to deliver high-quality, compassionate care. Leaders must embody compassion in the way they lead by attending to those they lead ('listening with fascination'); seeking a shared understanding via dialogue of the challenges those they lead face; being emotionally intelligent and empathising; and finally helping those they lead to deliver high-quality, compassionate, patient-centred care. This theme is powerfully developed in the leadership chapters in this volume.

Effective teamwork is fundamental to healthcare, practice development and the flourishing of staff. It is teams that innovate through collaboration, cooperation and co-design. Our teamworking skills are probably more important than our technical skills for practice development. Team members must have the courage to eliminate the blockages caused by hierarchy and professional boundaries. Team members must genuinely value diversity, be it professional, opinion or demographic, so that we use the knowledge, skills, abilities and experience of all for practice development. Effective teamworking is core to practice development, to high-quality care, to innovation and to the mental health of staff. This volume effectively reinforces those messages through both evidence and experience.

The third theme that is exemplified in every one of the contributions in this volume is the importance of our taking time to be still, to reflect and to learn. Leaders, teams and organisations are more productive, effective and innovative when they take time out to pause and reflect. Such times of stillness are associated with wellbeing, but also with productivity and innovation. Busy health and care teams which take time out on a regular basis, to stop, to debrief, to review, are on average between 35 and 40 per cent more productive than teams that simply keep reacting to chronic excessive workload.

These three themes are fundamental to practice development, as they were to helping us during the dark times of this pandemic. Above all, for genuine practice development, we must build belonging and trust, and develop cultures of compassion. We must come to see ourselves, the people we work with, those we care for and the people we lead as fundamentally more caring, cooperative and compassionate if we are to create a brighter future. This volume helps us to do precisely that.

Michael West is Senior Visiting Fellow at The King's Fund and Professor of Organisational Psychology at Lancaster University.

Acknowledgements

We would like to thank everyone who has contributed to chapters in this book and shared their time and expertise so freely. You have all been an inspiration. We would also like to recognise the unconditional support of family and friends in this endeavour as we constantly worked to achieve deadlines. We would especially like to thank Maree Parker, who so diligently worked with our manuscripts to ensure everything was in place and correctly presented.

1. *Transforming Health and Social Care Using Practice Development*

Kim Manley, Valerie Wilson, and Christine Øye

Setting the scene at this time of high challenge

As we write this chapter, we are in the middle of a global pandemic that is testing the resilience and values of people, communities, health and social care systems everywhere. Practice development (PD) offers practical strategies for how these challenges can be addressed founded on values-based ways of working that are compassionate, person-centred, safe and effective.

Despite the often unpredictable challenges faced when providing care, of which the current pandemic is an extreme example, practice guided by the values outlined above will be recognised in the workplace by the priority given to well-being, how teams manage challenges, and ways of working that involve everyone through collaboration, inclusion and participation to enable empowerment. The multiple perspectives and expertise resulting from this approach when applied to systematic learning and improvement that questions assumptions will enable positive and sustainable change to occur.

Regardless of setting, PD involves creating the conditions in which practitioners individually and collectively flourish. These conditions are associated with positive benefit for those who both provide and experience health and social care (West 2016; Braithwaite et al. 2017).

This introductory chapter aims to explain the relevance of PD and its potential to support health and social care at every level through focusing on what matters to people. Additionally, the chapter will outline developments since the first edition in 2008 and highlight how PD principles have driven the content of chapters and the ways in which the authors have worked together to bring you this latest edition.

International Practice Development in Health and Social Care, Second Edition.
Edited by Kim Manley, Valerie Wilson, and Christine Øye.

Practice development: its relevance to contemporary health and social care and crisis

PD is about our individual and collective practice as health and social care practitioners in any setting. Our purpose based on what matters to people has at its heart relationships with individuals, people and communities based on a shared set of values and visions about how we work together and with those experiencing care.

However, most health and social care is provided in teams and increasingly across complex systems, where workplace culture and contexts are recognised as powerful influencers on how care is experienced by both recipients and providers. Social norms reflect the values considered to be important (either implicitly or explicitly) and through the culture experienced impact how we work and learn together.

Workplace culture influences whether assumptions are challenged, learning and shared goals are implemented, aspirations are fulfilled, and subsequently whether valued staff are retained and health outcomes achieved.

Prerequisites to achieving good workplace cultures include leadership and facilitation expertise anchored in the values that enable collective approaches built on shared direction and purpose. These prerequisites are integral to PD and for this reason, a collaborative PD journey often begins by exploring and agreeing key values *'up front'*.

A growing evidence base through PD research together with a commitment to knowledge translation has helped us to understand not just what strategies work, why they work and for whom they work (Wilson and McCormack 2006), but also how to engage people and how to embed and sustain learning and evaluation in the workplace (Dewing 2010).

The knowledge base derived from practice-based research with people in different contexts is particularly important as frontline practitioners across all settings (individual homes, care homes, communities and hospitals) are risking their lives in relation to COVID-19 to provide care that is not just safe but that courageously keeps people at the heart of care, both recipients and team colleagues.

The pandemic has tested the key values and person-centred approaches championed and facilitated through PD about how we communicate. The use of protective clothing inevitably dehumanises our *humanness* through detracting from showing that the person we are communicating with is a unique person. Because of muffled verbal and non-verbal communication, the message that the person is at the heart of our purpose can be lost. We have all been heartened by the innovative ways and sheer persistence in overcoming these physical barriers when committed to human values by those who care. This recognises the tremendous burden on practitioners and carers and the need for practitioners to be supported and treated in a person-centred way too.

The notable cohesion and interprofessional teamwork that have resulted from a shared purpose and direction during the pandemic have also required total community collaboration. Powerful impact is demonstrated when people genuinely work together, breaking down the professional silos and barriers that often hinder effective collaboration.

Teams which have already learned to work together with shared values and visions will be more prepared for crisis situations, such as COVID-19, to find effective person-centred ways of working despite challenges experienced and *'top-down'* instructions. Practice developers in teams work with contextual barriers to find promising ways despite challenges, by co-creating ways of working for innovative solutions.

The pandemic has generated a crisis in how we work together. PD theory draws on the work of Bryan Fay (1987) to understand the nature of crisis informed through critical social science to explain how such challenges can lead to creative innovations that inform both future systems and ways of working. Fay's theory itself has been revised to capture the creativity generated through PD research (McCormack and Titchen 2006).

Creativity in response to crisis has already resulted in dramatic increases in virtual ways of working and communication supported by technology. With family members not able to be at the bedside of seriously ill relatives, technology has connected people to those important to them. Telemedicine is replacing the resource-intensive provision of outpatient follow-up clinics; previously perceived barriers are being recognised as assumptions, enabling them to be dismantled to free up more people-orientated ways of working. Different teams and partners are connecting virtually to enable prompt decision-making and action, with seismic shifts in genuine interprofessional working and learning. COVID-19 has freed us from the taken-for-granted assumptions around innovations, to cut through red tape and implement new policies, procedures and practices.

It is timely to recognise in this pandemic year that it is also the year of the nurse and midwife, and that nursing has upheld the values of person-centred, compassionate care and safety over the past century. This has particularly come to the fore in the current crisis, where it has been recognised widely and publicly that these values are important to society.

Practice development: growing scope and impact from interprofessional collaboration and working with shared values

PD as a formal methodology has been driven by nursing and midwifery across all its specialisms, but is increasingly embraced by other health and social care professionals. One of the eight revised principles of PD emphasises its increasing relevance to all:

PD is fundamentally about person-centred practice that promotes safe and effective workplace culture where all can flourish.

Chapter 8 discusses this principle together with seven others underpinning PD methodology.

This edition of the book marks a groundswell of involvement in PD, with many other professions globally experiencing its relevance. The *International Practice Development Journal*, a peer-review publication launched in 2011, has been instrumental in championing the uptake of PD concepts by different professional groups, further enabling interprofessional practice, and also disseminating its growing evidence base.

Contributions have embraced interdisciplinary and medical leadership programmes to support transformation (Akhtar et al. 2016), physiotherapists using person-centred frameworks when caring for people with long-term conditions (Dukhu et al. 2018), a biomedical scientist focusing on their own learning (Jackson 2013), an obstetrician and maternity team preparing for maternity transformation (Crowe and Manley 2019), a United Church minister reflecting on learning about self (Eldridge 2011), a physiotherapist reflecting on transformative learning (Owen 2016), an anaesthetist reflecting on transforming self as a leader (Adegoke 2017), an intensivist exploring the relevance of PD to quality improvement (Lavery 2016), allied health professionals drawing on PD principles (Bradd et al. 2017), therapists supporting mental health and family wellbeing (Karlsson et al. 2013), and social workers in the care of older people (Cronqvist and Sundh 2013).

Interprofessional practice is a much stronger focus of publications, with the journal publishing special issues from a range of professions that critically examine concepts relevant for the tradition of PD, for example a Special Issue on Person, Care and Aging (Øye et al. 2020).

Whilst PD has become more interprofessional, it has also experienced expansion on other fronts endorsed by its growing theoretical insights and research, with increasing numbers of postgraduate students undertaking research into PD and person-centred practice, applied to a changing world. For example, PD has influenced system-wide approaches, providing the foundation for 1) the statewide Essentials of Care programme across New South Wales, now embedded in practice (NSW 2014), and 2) state strategy for education and training (see Chapter 14). In the UK, PD methodology combined with action-orientated research approaches and realist evaluation (with which it has a strong affinity) has informed systems thinking for workforce transformation and systems leadership (Manley et al. 2016; Manley and Jackson 2020), insights into the development of safety culture (Manley et al. 2019), and multiprofessional continuous professional development (Manley et al. 2018).

Developments since 2008 international edition

Areas of expansion over the past decade have included:

- a growing focus around person-centredness research;
- systems-level working;
- integration of facilitation of learning, development and improvement;
- growing recognition of workplace culture and how key values of person-centredness, effectiveness and holistic safety are embedded through both leadership and facilitation; and
- a growing continuum of knowledge and research activity embracing knowledge translation, evaluation and the birth of the *'embedded researcher'*.

Person-centredness is a central concept of PD informing its purpose.

It has been more than a decade since Brendan McCormack and Tanya McCance published their seminal person-centred textbook (McCormack and McCance 2010), which has gone on to inform the work of a growing international community of practice and forms the basis of a significant number of doctoral theses. There is an expanding body of evidence around the theory that informs person-centred practice (McCormack and McCance 2016), the factors that impact on developing person-centred cultures as well as the facilitation that enables it (Kelly et al. 2018) and the measures that can provide feedback on its achievement (Slater et al. 2017; McCance et al. 2020). Recent emphasis is on the need to develop person-centred practices and cultures, noting that these are most influential if person-centredness is to be experienced by all (Edgar et al. 2020). See Chapter 17 for a case study which outlines research being undertaken on measuring person-centredness.

Integrated whole-systems working was the focus of a dedicated chapter in the 2008 edition (McCormack et al. 2008), and has always influenced PD thinking, guiding the formulation and shape of person-centredness. The role of whole systems approaches and their importance are acknowledged by the World Health Organization in its strategy for developing people-centred systems (WHO 2015), recognising that all components of the healthcare system are interdependent. The global pandemic shows this clearly, where what happens in one part of the system impacts on other parts – for example, what happens in public health or community settings dramatically influences demand on intensive care beds, resident mortality in residential homes, and staff as well as citizen wellbeing across countries and continents.

PD, building on whole systems approaches, has been used to understand local health systems through drawing on key values, enablers and skills needed to develop the workforce for sustainable person-centred transformation (Manley and Jackson 2020). Insights embrace an appreciation of the complexity and uniqueness of different contexts, recognising the strategies that work within and across different contexts, appreciatively framing what matters to people in different contexts informed by research perspectives that share similar philosophical underpinnings. The role of systems leadership in complex situations has become recognised as an enabler of collective endeavour (Dreier et al. 2019), particularly practitioner-led approaches (Manley and Jackson 2020) (Chapter 14).

Facilitation has, since PD's inception, been at its heart, through enabling others to become person and relationship centred and person-centred leaders. The skills required are embedded in active learning and structured reflection as well as creativity and curiosity and are increasingly recognised as extending across a continuum of complexity in terms of scope and purpose (Martin and Manley 2017). This scope and purpose overlap with relationship-based approaches to leadership as well as quality and service improvement. Whilst the focus of facilitation is on learning in and about practice and creating learning cultures that prioritise this, there is an increasing recognition that learning, developing and improving are interrelated with knowledge translation, inquiry and innovation. Since the previous edition, the international PD community has pioneered advanced facilitation approaches that embrace all these purposes (see Chapters 10 and 11). Such developments further emphasise how PD can complement other activities such as quality improvement, leadership development, systems transformation and innovation processes at every level of health and social care in a way that prioritises the workplace as a key resource for learning.

Growing recognition of the role of positive workplace cultures and how key values about person-centredness, ways of working and continuing effectiveness are integrated and embedded through both leadership and facilitation at all levels (Manley et al. 2019). Workplace cultures are being recognised more extensively as discrete from organisational cultures in that they directly focus on the interface where care/services are provided and experienced – the microsystems/team level (see Chapters 11, 15 and 18). The relationship with organisational and systems enablers in optimising team leadership is also becoming clearer.

Therefore there is a need for a strong focus on workplace culture as a precursor to achieving better service user experiences, better health outcomes, and good places to work that provide better staff experiences, staff wellbeing and retention (West 2016) (see Chapter 13).

A growing continuum of knowledge and research activity now positively pervades PD. The original PD concept analysis (Garbett and McCormack 2002) built on a broad situational analysis of its potential role and explained how it could add to the body of knowledge based on critical social science (McCormack et al. 1999; Manley and McCormack 2003). Prior to this time, PD was aligned with activities achieving local improvement, but not sustained because it was not embedded in research, policy or commissioning directions. The latter remains a key challenge (although there are examples such as the Essentials of Care programme cited earlier), despite international and national policies that increasingly encourage health and social care professionals and researchers to involve stakeholders and to co-create knowledge for health improvement and innovation. Nevertheless, there is still considerable potential for practice developers and others in health and social care to work in a bottom-up way for sustainable change and add to the body of knowledge. Context-based and participatory research approaches associated with action in the workplace that are practitioner-led have expanded greatly, with examples in this book that illustrate this (see Chapters 16 and 17).

In tandem, but also linked to PD research, has been the continued focus on knowledge translation previously given a high profile in PD methodology because so much research was never used in practice. Knowledge translation research informed the early focus of PD through implementing care that was evidence based and by assumption therefore effective. Knowledge translation has grown into a global movement of its own but continues to share many of the underpinning concepts with PD, such as culture, context, leadership, facilitation, evidence in all its forms, and evaluation. These shared concepts influence not only research implementation but also the implementation of shared values, learning, policy and strategic intent. PD has therefore developed eclectic approaches to using knowledge, blending knowledge and generating knowledge collaboratively in partnership in practice.

PD has excelled in its focus on stakeholder involvement and evaluation informed by the pioneering qualitative researchers Guba and Lincoln (1989) in their *Fourth Generation Evaluation* approach built on three earlier generations of measurement, description and judgement. They argued that working with stakeholder *claims, concerns and issues* should be central to evaluation if empowerment, ownership and implementation are to be achieved. This ethos marries well with PD's principle: collaboration, inclusion and participation. Subsequently, PD has developed its own evaluation approaches such as the *'Praxis model'* (Hardy et al. 2011) and *'Good Enough Evaluation'* (Wilson and McCance 2015), but has also engaged extensively with realist evaluation and critical realist approaches (Wilson and McCormack 2006; McCormack et al. 2007). Realist evaluation shares with PD a focus on contexts, acknowledging their complexity and also theorising from this an understanding about what works, why it works and for whom (termed programme theories), combined with appreciative approaches that remain action orientated and participatory in nature, echoing similarities with the action hypothesis discussed in the previous PD text (Manley et al. 2013).

More recently, the *'embedded research'* concept has emerged, a term that can easily describe the systematic role of PD embedded in practice continuously facilitating improvement but also adding to the body of knowledge about what works through participatory, context-specific research approaches.

In 2008 we argued that PD had come of age:

> *'With its focus on person-centred and evidence-based workplaces and enabling human-flourishing, it offers a coherent approach to unravelling the complexity of workplaces and enabling person-centredness to be realised' (Manley et al. 2008, p. xix).*

So what has changed? Whilst there is much more evidence for the impact of PD on people, their transformation, their teams, users' experiences, its potential to influence systems more widely is still underutilised. Often managerial cultures or single top-down methodological approaches ignore the importance of people or are out of synchrony with contemporary approaches to collective leadership where practitioners have an important voice and their expertise is drawn on as a source of social capital.

Independent evidence is now accruing from more traditional research programmes of the impact of compassionate, caring cultures and teams on quality, people's experiences, staff wellbeing (see Chapter 16) and health outcomes (Dawson 2014, 2018). However, what is not acknowledged in other programmes are the knowledge (both theoretical and practical), the skills and know-how about how to develop and sustain flourishing cultures in complex health and social care settings. The emphasis on person-centred care, cultures and systems remains our focus, as does working with complexity and researching practice *'with* people' rather than *'on* people'. The ultimate purpose at the forefront of our work remains the development of health and social care cultures where people flourish.

Living our values as editors and authors

The first edition of *International Practice Development in Nursing and Health* identified for the first time the principles of PD, distilled from its methodology, methods and key concepts over twenty years.

One of the founding principles of PD first formalised in a realist synthesis of PD methods (McCormack et al. 2007) was ways of working that embrace collaboration, inclusion and participation – termed the 'CIP' principle. Whilst previous PD books have enabled multiple authors to work together across countries, this is the first time that the editors have intentionally and explicitly employed the CIP principles to writing chapters, where authors from eight countries across both hemispheres have been invited to co-create their chapters collaboratively using these principles.

The role of editors over and above the usual focus has been one of facilitation, enabling content to flow and be refashioned through mutual learning, appreciation, critical companionship, connecting through virtual forums and support in enhancing writing skills. For example, two lead authors, senior practitioners, had never written or contributed to a chapter before (in common with many other contributors), but with peer and editor support an effective writing team for each chapter was established, mirroring the support and challenges of the practice world.

PD is about health and social care practice and it is a privilege for the editors to work with so many gifted frontline staff across different settings, most of whom are practitioners, supporting practitioners or are in clinical academic roles as embedded researchers (see Chapter 7).

All contributors have therefore worked to a shared purpose and values but applied these in various chapters to different levels of health and social care and different client groups across life's spectrum, from birth until older age and end of life.

The person's/citizen's voice, in keeping with the values of PD, is strengthened in this edition, so the first chapters following this introduction focus on what matters to people and what involves people working together, co-creation between those who experience and those who provide care to meet people's needs as they themselves see them.

The key concepts and structure of the book

We have radically changed the structure of this book compared with its first edition, reversing the theory and practice examples. We start the book with a strong focus on practice and then in the second part look at how theory links to practice. We have reversed this focus because people are inspired by practice-related stories that demonstrate the impact that PD has. We hope the stories stimulate a deepening interest in the reasons that account for how transformation happens in practice, demystifying the way forward through exploring the key concepts necessary for understanding and use.

The first section, comprising six chapters, describes PD principles in action, either with different client groups or in different settings and system levels. We commence with a focus on the voice of people with stomas and mental health challenges, and how these voices are heard and acted upon in relation to a dedicated health service (Chapter 2). Chapter 4 in contrast focuses on whole communities and what needs to be considered when developing and designing sustainable person-centred communities and integrated person-centred systems.

Chapters 3 and 5 focus on people and their experiences across the life span, from the time surrounding birth and the needs of women and their partners through this transformative experience, moving then to the other end of life to focus on what matters to older people experiencing care in various settings.

As alluded to earlier, PD integrates active learning in and from practice with improving and developing, and also research and inquiry. Chapter 6 focuses on the practical use of educational models that embed PD values in practice, exploring the impact of these and how the workplace is a powerful resource for these activities. Chapter 7 concludes with examples of embedded research using critical ethnography, an approach commonly used in PD to understand the culture of the workplace collaboratively.

The second part of the book explores PD insights and concepts under four broad interdependent themes:

- theoretical perspectives;
- facilitation;
- leadership;
- flourishing cultures.

Developments in our theoretical understanding start with Chapter 8 revising the principles of PD originally developed in the 2008 edition. Based on experiences of people across all countries involved in the International Practice Development Collaborative, the revision enables greater clarity about the key purposes and processes of PD, making it more accessible to not just practitioners and those facilitating them but also commissioners and managers who may be better able to employ the distinct and original support PD can provide towards transformation of services and systems.

Much of PD has been based on the theoretical perspective of critical theory from social science. Chapter 9 revisits this theory to provide contemporary insights about its use and value.

Chapter 10 demystifies facilitation. Facilitation enables others to live their values, learn, and become more person-centred and compassionate, as well as effective, through self-awareness from reflection and helping people to understand the impact they have on others. Chapter 11 focuses on the multiple purpose of facilitation at different levels in the system.

Three chapters on leadership follow, whereas there was only one in the 2008 edition. This is because leadership in tandem with facilitation is a critical enabler to culture change at every level of health and social care. Everyone can be a leader on something and often we become followers and leaders to each other at different times in different contexts. Chapter 12 focuses on relationship-based leadership approaches; Chapter 13 on team leadership to develop flourishing cultures informed by a multiprofessional clinical leadership programme underpinned by PD principles; and Chapter 14 on systems leadership.

The remaining theme, flourishing cultures, includes the latest research (Chapter 15), staff wellbeing at work (Chapter 16), and the concept of flourishing in the context of people, families and communities experiencing health and social care (Chapter 17).

Chapter 18 concludes with a position for the future in relation to the role of PD in continuing inquiry and innovation, capturing the celebrations and aspirations of the International Practice Development Collaborative.

Conclusion

This introductory chapter has set the scene in relation to our current global context, showing the relevance of PD to practitioners individually, collectively and interprofessionally as well as health and social care systems globally. The preceding 13 years have seen much expansion in its evidence base and growing impact, with consistent focus on its values and key concepts. The chapters that follow illustrate how PD achieves its impact, the concepts vital to its methodology and the theoretical insights that account for this.

References

Adegoke, K.A.A. (2017). Novice to transformational leader – a personal critical reflection. *International Practice Development Journal* 7 (1) [10]. https://doi.org/10.19043/ipdj.71.010

Akhtar, M., Casha, J.N., Ronder, J. et al. (2016). Leading the health service into the future: transforming the NHS through transforming ourselves. *International Practice Development Journal* 6 (2) [5]. https://doi.org/10.19043/ipdj.62.005

Bradd, P., Travaglia, J. and Hayen, A. (2017). Practice development and allied health – a review of the literature. *International Practice Development Journal* 7 (2) [7]. https://doi.org/10.19043/ipdj.72.007

Braithwaite, J., Herkes, J., Ludlow, K. et al. (2017). Association between organisational and workplace cultures, and patient outcomes: systematic review. *BMJ Open* 7. https://doi: 10.1136/bmjopen-2017-017708

Cronqvist, A. and Sundh, K. (2013). On collaboration between nurses and social workers in the service of older people living at home. *International Practice Development Journal* 3 (2) [6]. https://www.fons.org/library/journal/volume3-issue2/article6

Crowe, C. and Manley, K. (2019). Assessing contextual readiness: the first step towards maternity transformation. *International Practice Development Journal* 9 (2) [6]. https://doi.org/10.19043/ipdj.92.006

Dawson, J. (2014). Staff experience and patient outcomes: what do we know? A report commissioned by NHS employers on behalf of NHS England. https://www.nhsemployers.org/-/media/Employers/Publications/Research-report-Staff-experience-and-patient-outcomes.pdf

Dawson, J. (2018). Links between NHS staff experience and patient satisfaction: analysis of surveys from 2014 and 2015. Workforce Race Equality Standard (WRES) Team

NHS England. https://www.england.nhs.uk/wp-content/uploads/2018/02/links-between-nhs-staff-experience-and-patient-satisfaction-1.pdf

Dewing, J. (2010). Moments of movement: active learning and practice development. *Nurse Education in Practice* 10 (1): 22–26.

Dreier, L., Nabarro, D. and Nelson, J. (2019). Systems leadership for sustainable development: strategies for achieving systemic change. Harvard Kennedy School. https://www.hks.harvard.edu/sites/default/files/centers/mrcbg/files/Systems%20Leadership.pdf

Dukhu, S., Purcell, C. and Bulley, C. (2018). Person-centred care in the physiotherapeutic management of long-term conditions: a critical review of components, barriers and facilitators. *International Practice Development Journal* 8 (2). https://doi.org/10.19043/ipdj.82.002

Edgar, D., Wilson, V. and Moroney, T. (2020). Which is it, person-centred culture, practice or care? It matters. *International Practice Development Journal* 10 (1). https://doi.org/10.19043/ipdj.101.008

Eldridge, P. (2011). Reflections on a journey to knowing self. *International Practice Development Journal* 1 (1). https://www.fons.org/library/journal/volume1-issue1/article5

Fay, B. (1987). *Critical Social Science*. Cambridge: Polity Press.

Garbett, R. and McCormack, B. (2002). A concept analysis of practice development. *Journal of Research in Nursing* 7 (2). https://doi.org/10.1177/136140960200700203

Guba, E. and Lincoln, Y. (1989). *Fourth Generation Evaluation*. Newbury Park, CA: Sage Publications.

Hardy, S., Wilson, V. and Brown, B. (2011). Exploring the utility of a 'PRAXIS' evaluation framework in capturing transformation: a tool for all seasons? *International Practice Development Journal* 1 (2). https://www.fons.org/library/journal/volume1-issue2/article2

Jackson, A. (2013). A technician's journey through practice development to enlightenment. *International Practice Development Journal* 3 (Conference Supplement Article 2). https://www.fons.org/library/journal/volume3-conferencesupplement/article2

Karlsson, B., Borg, M., Revheim, T. et al. (2013). 'To see each other more like human beings... from both sides.' Patients and therapists going to a study course together. *International Practice Development Journal* 3 (1). https://www.fons.org/library/journal/volume3-issue1/article1

Kelly, R., Brown, D., McCance, T. et al. (2018). The experience of person-centred practice in a 100% single-room environment in acute care settings – a narrative literature review. *Journal of Clinical Nursing* 28 (13-14): 2369–2385.

Lavery, G. (2016). Quality improvement – rival or ally of practice development? *International Practice Development Journal* 6 (1). https://www.fons.org/library/journal/volume6-issue1/article15

Manley, K. and Jackson, C. (2020). The Venus model for integrating practitioner-led workforce transformation and complex change across the health care system. *Journal of Evaluation in Clinical Practice* 26 (2): 622–634.

Manley, K., Jackson, C. and McKenzie, C. (2019). Microsystems culture change – a refined theory for developing person-centred, safe and effective workplaces based on strategies that embed a safety culture. *International Practice Development Journal* 9 (2). https://doi.org/10.19043/ipdj.92.004

Manley, K., Martin, A., Jackson, C. et al. (2016). Using systems thinking to identify workforce enablers for a whole systems approach to urgent and emergency care delivery: a multiple case study. *BMC Health Services Research* 16 (368). https://doi.org/10.1186/s12913-016-1616-y

Manley, K., Martin, A., Jackson, C. et al. (2018). A realist synthesis of effective continuing professional development (CPD): a case study of healthcare practitioners' CPD. *Nurse Education Today* 69: 134–141.

Manley, K. and McCormack, B. (2003). Practice development: purpose, methodology, facilitation and evaluation. *Nursing in Critical Care* 8 (1): 22–29.

Manley, K., McCormack, B. and Wilson, V. (2008). *International Practice Development in Nursing and Healthcare*. Oxford: Blackwell Publishing.

Manley, K., Parlour, R. and Yalden, J. (2013). The use of action hypothesis to demonstrate practice development strategies in action. In: *Practice Development in Nursing and Healthcare (2nd ed)* (eds. B. McCormack, K. Manley and A. Titchen), 252–274. Chichester: Wiley-Blackwell.

Martin, A. and Manley, K. (2017). Developing standards for an integrated approach to workplace facilitation for interprofessional teams in health and social care contexts: a Delphi study. *Journal of Interprofessional Care* 32 (1): 41–51.

McCance, T., Lynch, B., Boomer, C. et al. (2020). Implementing and measuring person-centredness using an APP for knowledge transfer: the iMPAKT app. *International Journal for Quality in Health Care* 32 (4): 251–258.

McCormack, B., Manley, K., Kitson, A. et al. (1999). Towards practice development – a vision in reality or a reality without vision? *Journal of Nursing Management* 7: 255–264.

McCormack, B., Manley, K. and Walsh, K. (2008). Person-centred systems and processes. In: *International Practice Development in Nursing and Healthcare* (eds. K. Manley, B. McCormack and V. Wilson), 17–58. Oxford: Blackwell Publishing.

McCormack, B. and McCance, T. (2010). *Person-Centred Nursing: Theory and Practice*. Chichester: John Wiley & Sons Ltd.

McCormack, B. and McCance, T. eds. (2016). *Person-centred Practice in Nursing and Healthcare*. Oxford: John Wiley & Sons Ltd.

McCormack, B. and Titchen, A. (2006). Critical creativity: melding, exploding, blending. *Educational Action Research* 14 (2): 239–266.

McCormack, B., Wright, J., Dewar, B. et al. (2007). A realist synthesis of the evidence relating to practice development: findings from the literature analysis. *Practice Development in Health Care* 6 (1): 25–55.

New South Wales [NSW] (2014). Essentials of Care: working with the Essentials of Care program. A resource for facilitators. 2nd Edition January 2014. NSW Ministry of Health. https://www.health.nsw.gov.au/nursing/culture/Documents/eoc-facilitation-resources.pdf (accessed 24 June 2020).

Owen, L. (2016). Emerging from physiotherapy practice, masters-level education and returning to practice: a critical reflection based on Mezirow's transformative learning theory. *International Practice Development Journal* 6 (2). https://doi.org/10.19043/ipdj.62.011

Øye, C., Thorkildsen, K.M. and Oddgeir Synnes, O. (2020). Critical perspectives on person, care and ageing: unmasking their interconnections. *International Practice Development Journal* 10 (Suppl, introductory article). https://doi.org/10.19043/ipdj.10Suppl.001

Slater, P., McCormack, B. and McCance, T. (2017). The development and testing of the Person-centred Practice Inventory – Staff (PCPI-S). *International Journal for Quality in Health Care* 29 (4): 541–547.

West, M. (2016). Creating a workplace where NHS staff can flourish. https://www.kingsfund.org.uk/blog/2016/01/creating-workplace-where-staff-can-flourish (accessed 15 June 2020).

Wilson, V. and McCance, T. (2015). Good enough evaluation. *International Practice Development Journal* 5 (Special Issue on person-centredness, Article 10). DOI: 10.19043/ipdj.5SP.012

Wilson, V. and McCormack, B. (2006). Critical realism as emancipatory action: the case for realistic evaluation in practice development. *Nursing Philosophy* 7 (1): 45–57.

World Health Organization [WHO] (2015). *WHO global strategy on people-centred and integrated health services. Interim report*. Geneva, Switzerland: World Health Organization. http://apps.who.int/iris/bitstream/10665/155002/1/WHO_HIS_SDS_2015.6_eng.pdf (accessed 20 January 2020).

2. *Shaping Health Services Through True Collaboration Between Professional Providers and Service Users*

Kristin Ådnøy Eriksen, Julia Kittscha, and Greg Fairbrother

Introduction

In this chapter we present two different examples of true collaboration between health service providers and health service users (consumers). The notion of authentic partnership between healthcare users and service-providing professionals has been promoted by both stakeholder groups for some time now. This partnership goal represents a paradigm shift from prior paternalistic approaches which tended to distance patients and providers under the 'medical model', which prized examination and observation at the expense of relationality and wholism (Barbour 1995). Research findings increasingly support the efficacy of such a shift, in clinical outcome, patient satisfaction and cost terms (WHO 2015). Its essential collaborative drive favours closer and more genuine partnership relationships between providers and consumers. Collaboration represents 'evolving processes whereby two or more social entities actively and reciprocally engage in joint activities aimed at achieving at least one shared goal' (Bedwell et al. 2012, p. 130). True collaboration between professional providers and service users mean striving for reciprocity and requires active, mutual engagement from the involved parties. One party dictating or controlling another party cannot be considered collaboration. This type of engagement would better be described as delegation or coercion (Bedwell et al. 2012).

The drive towards greater collaboration naturally implicates healthcare and community/advocacy organisations, as well as clinicians and individual consumers themselves. People who have chronic conditions have more contact

International Practice Development in Health and Social Care, Second Edition.
Edited by Kim Manley, Valerie Wilson, and Christine Øye.

with providers and systems, often carry a prolonged quality of life burden, and are natural protagonists in the development of forward-leaning groupings and actions which promote better partnerships.

Key concerns of contemporary patient/provider partnership models relate to: i) practice development (PD) and service improvement (how can this be driven in a more consumer-centred way?) (Hall et al. 2018); ii) clinician education (how can consumers be productively involved in this?) (Olasij et al. 2019); iii) clinical policy (how can consumer input be fostered?) (Nilsen et al. 2006; Ocloo and Matthews 2016); and iv) research (how can consumers be brought in to the healthcare research community on an equal footing, as investigators?) (Gray-Burrows et al. 2018). Re-balancing power relations and promoting empowerment are key action areas proposed today. Barriers to such progress in our health systems have been identified. These include tokenism, stigmatising, inadequate information, professional gatekeeping and financial barriers to involvement. Enablers of progress located in Ocloo and Matthews' narrative review (2016) include improving access (or ways into) the workings of healthcare organisations, providing patient support which is confidence building, offering different forms of involvement, resourcing outreach efforts, working on health literacy and working on communication practices more generally. Making high-quality, condition-specific information accessible to consumers in multiple forms and contexts (particularly by supporting the growth of strong information-sharing peer networks) is increasingly understood to be vital in driving progress (Ramsey et al. 2017). Information is the essential seed from which knowledge and knowledge sharing can grow. A specific kind of information, patient feedback/perception data, is a further area which is gaining increasing attention in person-centred care modelling. Better and more partnered approaches to this have been shown to yield benefits to both patients and providers, as the tools used become more relevant, and trust is built and acted upon across the patient–provider divide (Hall et al. 2018; Renedo et al. 2015).

Today's drive towards more inclusive approaches to healthcare delivery is understood to be essential to progress in health organisations. People (particularly those with chronic and long-term conditions) need and wish to take responsibility for their conditions and share in decision-making about their treatment and management (Smith and Dransfield 2019). New and innovative models of care which prize partnership and peer networking are emerging. Models informed by PD principles are prominent among these (Heggdal 2015; Collier 2016). Existing studies of new models have yielded positive results for both patients and systems, but further studies which describe modelled approaches and the results arising from these are needed (Hall et al. 2018).

Examples of collaborative approaches

The two case studies presented in this chapter seek to illustrate such inclusive approaches. In both cases, people with long-term conditions are provided with group-based and informational support structures which offer them opportunities to 'set the agenda' around how the programmes run and, more generally, around the ongoing management of their condition. A key goal is that by being together with others in similar situations, participants can be supported to take responsibility for their health. The first example concerns an information group run by two regional Australian hospitals, supporting people living with a stoma, or people who are close to an ostomate. The second concerns a recovery course run by Norwegian municipal mental health services to provide opportunities for development and learning for persons with mental health or substance abuse problems. The common factors between the two examples are that the services provide frames and structures for inclusion (time, place, routine, professional commitment) and the founding values are person-centred. In each case, there is a focus on acknowledging and including everybody who attends. At the same time, the agenda (e.g. topics and whose voices are given space) is decided together with the participants. There is awareness that knowledge based on lived experience is as valuable as the professional knowledge which the supporting professionals bring to the group-based programmes.

Case 1 Illawarra Ostomy Information Group

Illawarra Ostomy Information Group (IOIG) is an example of service providers and end users working seamlessly together. The approach involves both flexibility and collaboration. Gumuchian et al. (2019) found that people with a chronic illness attend support groups for more than the giving/receiving of support from those with a similar experience or condition. People also attend to receive education and information and to enjoy opportunities to share their knowledge with other members. They also prefer the group to be facilitated by someone suitably trained (Gumuchian et al. 2019). A key goal of the IOIG is to keep the individual healthy whilst optimising use of the service provider's time. Group members often self-manage queries between each other. By sharing experiences, they can sometimes eliminate the need for intervention from the health professional. Such self-management does not involve diagnosis or treatment, but it does involve learning, psycho-emotional support and knowledge development. There is much for this group of people to learn from each other in relation to psychosocial adjustment, and the day-to-day complexities and challenges associated with living with a stoma.

The group has been running for 15 years and meets every second month for two hours in an education room in a private rehabilitation facility. On average, 25 people attend each session. Some people have been coming since the group's inception, others come once or twice a year. New ostomates regularly join. The group is facilitated by two stoma nurses who serve the district, one from the public hospital and one from the private.

All new stoma patients are encouraged to attend and bring a partner or close friend. The value of the support person is not underestimated as they too need to receive support from others in a similar situation. People are told about the group either pre- or post-operatively, depending on the circumstances. There have been times when a meeting has coincided just prior to a person's surgery. In such situations, they have been able to attend and meet others with a stoma as part of their pre-operative preparation and decision-making.

Knowledge building/sharing within the group

The facilitators share news with the group relating to professional development activities they may have attended or participated in, such as conference and research activity. If there are any service provision-related changes that may affect the group, these are also canvassed.

The facilitators organise guest speakers to present to the group on a topic basis. Speakers have included psychologists, exercise physiologists, legal aid practitioners and fellow ostomates who might share their story or particular experiences. The group is encouraged to contribute ideas for topics, during a yearly planning session.

Group members can also contribute by asking questions and by sharing experiences, for example about how they manage a particular problem or situation. This open-forum style facilitates others to ask questions. Some members function as a resource for members with a new stoma during conversation and social chat which typically follows the forum. The social chat is also an opportunity for participants to talk to the facilitators, ask questions individually and make clinic appointments if needed. The facilitators actively connect those seeking information with others who have knowledge and experience which may help.

Sharing knowledge beyond the group

When knowledge that is transferable to other ostomates is shared within the group, members are encouraged to share this more widely by writing for a magazine that is mailed to all ostomates Australia-wide. Examples of topics that group members have written about are 'Managing overnight bag drainage: A self-developed technique' and 'Travelling with a stoma'. The latter article provided advice for camping, cruising and flying. Information about navigating customs in relation to body scanners was found to be particularly useful. Another member designed and made stoma bag covers, including a shower cap-style cover. This member donates the profits from the sales to the local ostomy association.

During every second year the Stomal Therapy Nurses (STNs) facilitate a community study day, which more than 80 community members have attended. Consumers are involved in the planning of the study day and contribute with presentations, manning the registration desk or serving refreshments.

Contributing to professional education

Members have participated in nurse education sessions conducted among non-specialist nurses who work in Illawarra inpatient facilities. This involves attending and sitting with small groups of nurses and answering questions. The idea is to help nurses gain a better understanding of what it is like to live with a stoma and to know more about how to help the patient in hospital who has a stoma.

Facilitating nurses in having conversations with people who have a stoma has significantly improved the nurse education programme. Feedback from staff about this aspect of the education programme suggests that it promotes empathy and increased confidence in looking after someone with a stoma. For nurses who are active in the busy climate we work in, it is not often they have time to sit and listen to their patients outside of the care contract.

From the perspective of the patients who attend these sessions, they also gain from the experience. They may bring a stoma bag to show the staff and explain how they manage. Others prepare information ahead of time that they think will be useful for the nurses. Such material is distributed in handout form. It is clear they want to be heard, as this kind of participation is offered, not requested. Ostomates who have done this voluntary work report great satisfaction in having the opportunity to share their story with interested nurses. Nurses can be seen leaning in, nodding and engaging in active listening. The room is usually abuzz with conversation and learning.

Feedback from ostomates about being involved in the group

Qualitative evaluation has been conducted among IOIG participants. Key areas repeatedly voiced by group participants in response to questioning about their experience of the group and whether/how it helped relate to:

1. The *relational* aspects – connecting with fellow ostomates:
   'It is just so nice to connect with others going through the same journey and struggle.'
   'Talking to others helped me realise I wasn't alone and some issues I had they also had.'

2. The *informational* aspects:
   'I get tips on managing my stoma... this is so helpful.'
   'I've learned different methods of dealing with my bag.'

The following statement from a long-standing group participant offers a sense of what involvement has meant for many who participate:

> *'I have found group to be so very helpful. In my early days it was just really nice to know that I wasn't alone and I was a little surprised as to the amount of people and the varied reasons for their ostomy. Talking with the other members has given me an insight as to what to expect in my new life. An example of this is swimming . . . others said they go every day and that when I finally took the plunge – I would look back and wonder why I was so worried. I took the plunge and they were absolutely right! Another is travelling. I have listened to others talking about how they travel with their ostomy. I have yet to travel overseas but have done a few nights away now, so I'm getting a bit more confident. Just going to the meetings has given me more confidence, and I now feel that I am ready to talk about my experiences and help any newcomer to the group.'*

Case 2 Recovery courses in municipalities in western Norway

The course 'My life, my choices' was developed in partnership between people with lived experience of mental health problems and/or substance abuse and people with professional experience of working in mental health and substance abuse services. The principles for course development were taken from Recovery Colleges (Cameron et al. 2018; King and Meddings 2019). All activities are co-produced by participants and professionals. Course participants are understood to be participants rather than patients, and each person chooses what he or she wants to learn (Perkins et al. 2012, p. 4).

The model challenges the traditional understanding of it being the professionals who have the most important knowledge and competence. The professionals and the people with lived experience learn and create together, valuing lived experience equally with professional experience. The model also challenges established understandings of roles. Professionals and service users are all participants, and all participants contribute. Thus, the privilege of being of help to others is also experienced by persons who traditionally would be receivers of support (Eriksen and Storesund 2019).

The course

'My life, my choices' runs over five weeks, with one theme covered each week, and meets for two days a week. The facilitators (course leaders) are one person with lived experience of mental health problems and one health professional. The participants are service users in the municipal mental health services and healthcare workers in the same services. It is voluntary to take part.

The participants write individual goals at the start of the course and have the opportunity to work with these throughout the course. The 'homework' from week to week may be to do something or reflect on something relevant to a goal and then share this with the group in the following session if they wish. Each week, the groups focus on one theme taken from the conceptual framework of recovery (Leamy et al. 2011): connectedness; hope and optimism about the future; identity; meaning in life; and empowerment (CHIME). Groups explore the themes using methods like brainstorming, drawing, film, evoke cards, sharing experiences, etc., and relate what they share to their own goals and everyday lives.

The courses are planned ahead and the facilitators have a plan for each group session. At the same time, the participants are given the opportunity to shape the course. The participants start the course by agreeing 'house rules' and slowly become responsible for the processes of learning during the course. Taking part in co-creational processes makes it possible to learn based on information and experiences from all those present in the group.

Data from focus groups (on the last course day) indicates that the course is useful to both professionals and service users. Participants learn more about themselves and become aware of areas for development in their own lives. This may be related to the themes: 'The themes in the course are important, they are about life' (Group 5). At the same time, they are perceived as challenging:

'It has been good and bad – I've been exhausted after a session. But I believe the strain is part of moving on' (Group 5).

Participants' experiences

The facilitators strive to create a learning environment that is safe, supportive and non-judgemental. They pay careful attention to how they can make everybody feel welcome and have tools that make it easier for all participants to become involved. On the last day of the course one participant said: 'I feel safe, people are open, inclusive and understanding' (Group 5). It is always a choice to speak in the group. However, experiences show that all participants contribute in the group even if the person may hesitate in the beginning. A woman (aged 40 plus) who was very active in the group said: 'I haven't dared to talk in a group before. . . I have always been shy from my seventh school year until now' (Group 2).

The Evoke cards were useful: 'Using pictures was brilliant. . . It's easier to recognise oneself in the images' (Group 3); 'They make it easier to speak' (Group 4). Each person's contribution is appreciated and there are no right or wrong answers. One participant felt included: 'I was told to feel free to say whatever I liked, nothing was too silly or weird' (Group 3). Participants learn from each other: 'I have been challenged by what others have shared and have learned a lot from listening' (Group 5). The groups seem to represent a different way of being in a social setting: 'I come as I am, I do not worry about details about how I'm dressed' (Group 5); 'This group is different' (Group 1); 'There is an acceptance of problems and challenges as a resource, a sense that everybody is vulnerable, and we all need each other. We meet and talk about things without the wrapping' (Group 2).

The participants appreciated that the professionals participated at the same level as the service users. One participant (a service user) said: 'I realised I know as much as the professionals' (Group 5). Some of the participants experienced being of help to others and this contributed to a more positive view of oneself: 'Think in a new way – being good enough – an experience of being good enough' (Group 1).

Facilitators' experiences

The health professionals who co-facilitated courses were expected to participate in the group by drawing on their own lived life rather than re-stating theoretical definitions and prescriptions about what would be good for other people (Eriksen and Storesund 2019). One facilitator explained: 'The participants define the concepts, not the professionals' (Group 2). This was perceived as positive: 'What is shared is helpful for everyone, both facilitators and participants' (Group 3). Thus, being a facilitator contributed to personal growth: 'It led to extended understanding about myself' (Group 1). Another facilitator reflected: 'To experience that all of us are at the same level – we are equal – is fantastic!' (Group 5). At the same time, it was different to what they were used to and this represented a challenge: 'It is demanding to share and give of yourself. . . and it must be real' (Group 5). 'Everything is turned upside down – it is not defined' (Group 2). Not having the answer and letting the group decide was unusual for some: 'It's hard not to be in control – not knowing what will happen next' (Group 1).

At the same time, the facilitators (both health workers and persons with lived experience) needed professional skills, as good group facilitation requires a sound facilitation skillset. Acknowledgement and adaption to each person in the group, listening skills and situational awareness were all crucial. They strived to find a balance between giving each person room to share what they wanted and at the same time making sure all participants had time to speak. It has been a great advantage in the courses that many of the facilitators had a lot of experience with working with people. They understood the importance of trustworthiness, being a model, building relationships, and had experience in leading different kinds of groups and courses in the health services. The conscious stance of drawing back and letting the participants support and help each other was something they found very rewarding. Sometimes the group facilitated themselves: 'It is good to see how the participants become responsible – they correct each other and give each other their opinions about what is not ok' (Group 5).

A key theme identified in evaluating the programme was that being useful gives meaning in life. This can help to present oneself with a strong identity and help with awareness of one's strengths (empowerment) and feeling of belonging in a group (connectedness).

Discussion

The aims of PD work can be to enhance clinical services, such as to increase quality and safety in healthcare within a unit, to develop shared values and service priorities, and to improve communication within a healthcare team (Bradd et al. 2017). The cases presented in this chapter do not focus on the professionals in a service. However, both cases share other aims and use methodology that are similar to those developed in the PD tradition. The most obvious similarity is that aims relate to enabling human flourishing and enhancing learning and transformative change (Bradd et al. 2017) (see Chapter 8). An important element at play in both cases is also that the facilitators aim to engage authentically with the group members to 'blend personal qualities and creative imagination' (Bradd et al. 2017, p. 2) (see Chapters 10 and 11). PD seeks to rebalance traditional power hierarchies in the health services. In the cases, the rebalancing is about valuing and building on experience-based knowledge (as well as on professionals' knowledge). The facilitators sought to address imbalances in the groups due to experiences in people's lives – like stigmatisation, and lack of opportunity to contribute in society.

In both cases, the importance of facilitation skill as a kind of 'glue' which accommodated the complexity and promoted positive change and growth was heavily apparent. Whilst consumer empowerment was a key target for both groups, it was never a possibility that the group interventions could be run without the presence of a skilled professional or professionals. It's important here to recognise that by 'skilled' is meant skilled as both a clinician and a facilitator. Professional involvement affords safety and also reliable engagement with knowledge sets at play.

In both case studies, the professionals sought to enter into true partnership with patients and service users by striving to 'level out' the value of their knowledge with the knowledge that persons have from their lived experience. Such an approach entails focusing on acknowledging all knowledge (both professional and lived). In this kind of partnership, the professional may realise that the experiences people have from living with a stoma or mental health problems represent knowledge that the professionals need to incorporate and work with if they want to provide optimal services. Professionals may also become more aware of the resources each of their patients have and allow more space for the patient in the caring relationship.

This shift means blending what clinicians have learned in school with what they learn from people living with health problems – valuing that input, being moved by it and changing their views based on it. There is great potential to develop new knowledge in such a true collaboration. Together they will have an array of solutions, advice and examples of how issues can be understood and handled. The groups represent a forum of persons that are open and interested in the same issues. Ideas are valued and developed further, and participants may become more hopeful as they have the opportunity to speak about challenges and expect that others may have experienced the same things (rather than getting stuck with something).

Being in a partnership and learning from each other produces opportunities to take on new roles. The patients are no longer passive recipients of care and support – they are also someone who is of help to others and someone who is learning and developing based on their own motivation and interest. As a patient participant in the stoma group, listening to a narrative about how someone handles travelling with a stoma may not make it possible for that participant to travel, but it may give them hope of expanding from where they are at now. Professionals may have travel-related advice, but the knowledge the group have together about this issue (both academically and experientially) is probably extensive. For some participants in both groups studied, their involvement represented a move away from an established pattern – and the change gave hope and may have altered the way the person thought about themselves. The experience of being someone who knows something that is useful to others is empowering, and providing support to others gives meaning to life.

In both case studies, the agenda in the group was set in the partnership – what is relevant is answered not only from the professional's perspective but from what is relevant for the participants' lives. New knowledge arising from research and new knowledge-based processes in health services is relevant – but so are narratives from people's everyday lives. The groups define what is relevant – for example what is relevant for persons living with stoma to know, and how hope can play a role in a person's recovery in mental health issues. The professional may have a definition for hope and may have knowledge about the role hope can play in a person's life. Defining hope in the group may extend this and make it possible for participants to relate hope to their own everyday life. Definitions are often closed, whilst narratives are open, and the person can choose to relate to it, leave it or expand the meaning.

The longevity of the stoma care group evidences the success of the partnered approach, and the proliferation of the mental health/drug health group across western Norway equally evidences such success. Even though the Norwegian example was to some extent 'boundaried' (as a course, not as an ongoing group), it has been an increasingly common experience that these groups continue to meet after the course has finished. Such a phenomenon is a very powerful indicator of programme success.

Besides the outcome, growth and flourishing related benefits discussed above, partnership models contribute to service quality and service efficiency. In case 1, the existence of an STN-facilitated group provided a way for ostomates to access an informal service without requiring a formalised clinic appointment. One system-related effect of this has been the freeing up of scarce appointment time for clinical matters. Further, the group can also function as a means of screening with consumers as to whether a clinic appointment may be of some benefit. Whilst it's unlikely that such efficiency savings could (or should) result in a lower service presence overall, they certainly contribute to the conduct of an optimised engagement schedule between consumer and professional, and likely impact positively on hospitalisation and other health service utilisation rates. This is equally the case for the recovery course. With positively evaluated courses continuing to meet post completion, it's reasonable to expect that illness-related service utilisation may be reduced among group members over time.

Conclusion

True collaboration between professional providers and service users can be seen as a paradigm shift. In the examples, the providers were facilitators as well as learners, and the service users were both providers and participants. Fundamental issues from PD, such as the use of creative approaches and principles of collaboration, inclusion and participation, can support the services in moving towards more collaborative practices. PD's emphasis on facilitation as a skill to be developed and something that requires reflection is also very helpful in expanding the understanding of the role of healthcare workers in person-centred services.

When professionals work alongside consumers in partnership, there is learning and sharing of knowledge between health professional and consumer, between consumer and consumer, and between health professional and health professional. Within the ostomy information group this collaborative approach evolved to offer STNs a vehicle to empower patients to build a solid knowledge base which can help them become more self-sufficient in managing their life with a stoma.

From the STN perspective, the group members also provide support to their role through supporting each other, being involved in nurse education and fundraising for the ostomy association. Such efforts contribute to nurse scholarships aiming to train more STNs.

The recovery courses change the perspective by being educationally informed rather than therapeutically informed (Perkins et al. 2012, p. 3). The processes of co-production and co-facilitation by those with professional and lived experience, together with the creation of a supportive but challenging culture and environment, provide participants with opportunities for involvement. And maybe even more importantly, with opportunities to be someone that makes a difference. The professionals and persons with lived experience learn together and also share in the privilege of caring for others.

Professionals alone cannot define an illness, know what good treatment is or what the best solution to a person's challenges in everyday life are. The person-centred care movement has opened our eyes to the question: 'What ought to be the starting point when providing services – the health system's prescriptions or each individual patient's needs?' The extent of the benefits for patients and service users in taking part in collaborative approaches to health service (as illustrated in this chapter) promotes a further question: 'Do societies that support people to live empowered lives ultimately need fewer health services?' This question has yet to be answered scientifically but is surely now on the knowledge agenda as we move forward. Sharing the privilege of being of help to other people is satisfying for professionals, and democratisation can and does work for people and service users too.

References

Barbour, A. (1995). *Caring for Patients: A Critique of the Medical Model*. Stanford, CA: Stanford University Press.

Bedwell, W., Wildman, J., Diaz Granados, D. et al. (2012). Collaboration at work: an integrative multilevel conceptualization. *Human Resource Management Review* 22 (2): 128–145.

Bradd, P., Travaglia, J. and Hayen, A. (2017). Practice development and allied health – a review of the literature. *International Practice Development Journal* 7 (2): 1–25.

Cameron, J., Hart, A., Brooker, S., Neale, P. et al. (2018). Collaboration in the design and delivery of a mental health Recovery College course: experiences of students and tutors. *Journal of Mental Health* 27 (4): 374–381.

Collier, A. (2016). Practice development using video-reflexive ethnography: promoting safe space(s) towards the end of life in hospital. *International Practice Development Journal* 6 (1): 1–16.

Eriksen, K.Å. and Storesund, C.V. (2019). Nøkkelen er likeverd – Recoverykursleiarar sine erfaringar med samskaping. *Tidsskrift for psykisk helsearbeid* 16 (4): 237–247.

Gray-Burrows, K., Willis, T., Foy, R. et al. (2018). Role of patient and public involvement in implementation research: a consensus study. *BMJ Quality and Safety* 27 (10): 858–864.

Gumuchian, S.T., Delisle, V.C., Kwakkenbos, L. et al. (2019). Reasons for attending support groups and organizational preferences: the European scleroderma support group members survey. *Disability and Rehabilitation* 41 (8): 974–982.

Hall, A., Bryant, J., Sanson-Fisher, R. et al. (2018). Consumer input into health care: time for a new, active and comprehensive model for consumer involvement. *Health Expectations* 21 (4): 707–713.

Heggdal, K. (2015). 'We experienced a lack of tools for strengthening coping and health in encounters with patients with chronic illness': bridging theory and practice through formative research. *International Practice Development Journal* 5 (2): 1–16.

King, T. and Meddings, S. (2019). Survey identifying commonality across international Recovery Colleges. *Mental Health and Social Inclusion* 23 (3): 121–128.

Leamy, M., Bird, V., Le Boutillier, C. et al. (2011). Conceptual framework for personal recovery in mental health: systematic review and narrative synthesis. *The British Journal of Psychiatry* 199 (6): 445–452.

Nilsen, E.S., Myrhaug, H.T., Johansen, M. et al. (2006). Methods of consumer involvement in developing healthcare policy and research, clinical practice guidelines and patient information material. *Cochrane Database of Systematic Reviews* 3. https://doi.org/10.1002/14651858.CD004563.pub2

Ocloo, J. and Matthews, R. (2016). From tokenism to empowerment: progressing patient and public involvement in healthcare improvement. *BMJ Quality and Safety* 25 (8): 626–632.

Olasij, M., Cross, W., Reed, F. et al. (2019). Mental health nurses' attitudes towards consumer involvement in nursing handover pre and post an educational implementation. *International Journal of Mental Health Nursing* 28 (5): 1198–1208.

Perkins, R., Repper, J., Rinaldi, M. et al. (2012). *Recovery colleges. Implementing recovery through organisational change*. London: Centre for Mental Health. https://www.merseycare.nhs.uk/media/1208/1recovery-colleges.pdf

Ramsey, I., Corsini, N., Peters, M. et al. (2017). A rapid review of consumer health information needs and preferences. *Patient Education and Counselling* 100: 1634–1642.

Renedo, A., Marston, C., Spyridonidis, D. et al. (2015). Patient and public involvement in healthcare quality improvement: how organisations can help patients and professionals to collaborate. *Public Management Review* 17 (1): 17–34.

Smith, J. and Dransfield, A. (2019). Patient and carer involvement in healthcare education, service delivery and research: avoiding tokenism. *Evidence Based Nursing* 22 (3): 65–66.

World Health Organization. (2015). *WHO global strategy on people-centred and integrated health services Interim Report*. Geneva: World Health Organization.

3. *Turning Point: Curious Novice to Committed Advocate*

Catherine Adams, Ciaran Crowe, Crystal McLeod, and Giselle Coromandel

Best practice in maternity care can be defined by the quality triad of safety, effectiveness and person-centredness (Berwick 2013; Royal College of Obstetricians and Gynaecologists 2016; Department of Health and Social Care 2016; Royal College of Midwives 2014). However, despite clarity about what constitutes best practice, national and international crises in relation to maternity care continue to recur. Most notably these include Portlaoise (Ireland) (Health Information and Quality Authority 2015), Djerriwarrh Health Services (Australia) (Wallace 2015) and the Morecombe Bay investigation in England (Kirkup 2015).

Despite having access to both national and international guidelines and policies and awareness of what high-quality maternity care looks like, the biggest challenge facing maternity services is enabling what is already known (i.e. the evidence base) to be implemented and used in clinical practice. The second challenge is understanding why some maternity providers have managed to successfully implement improvements in the quality triad whilst others have not despite the same evidence base being used (Liberati et al. 2019).

Practice development (PD), whilst not a panacea for all issues in healthcare, can be a feasible and effective solution to these two challenges. Contextual readiness of your healthcare setting can be assessed for translating evidence into your practice or to evaluate your workplace culture through analysing the factors that positively influence the quality triad. As the triad is underpinned by learning (Crowe and Manley 2019) and PD has a particular focus on active learning, you could use its tools to evaluate yourself, your service or your team through each of these lenses.

International Practice Development in Health and Social Care, Second Edition.
Edited by Kim Manley, Valerie Wilson, and Christine Øye.

PD is focused on collaboration, inclusivity and a participative approach to developing person-centred, safe and effective cultures (Manley et al. 2008). These principles were found to be lacking in international inquiries into maternity care. Therefore, PD is a useful method to facilitate improvement and transform care.

PD, with its focus on bottom-up change, aims to align change ideas with people's values and generate greater buy-in, which in turn can lead to sustaining workplace transformation.

In this chapter we will describe the experience of transformation within maternity services, drawing from four different contributors in hospital settings across different countries. Transformational PD, person-centred, safe and effective approaches were used to facilitate effective workplace cultures to flourish. An unexpected and positive consequence of the authors' involvement was a turning point in their awareness of the effectiveness of this methodology. The critical recognition that PD could transcend boundaries of countries, health services, professional disciplines and positions was pivotal to the authors' commitment to this methodology in the quest for improving maternity care.

Inclusivity, relatability, effectiveness – Ciaran's Eureka

My experience of PD is relatively recent; however, the impact it has had on my practice as a consultant obstetrician has been enormous.

With an interest in multiprofessional learning, team training and human factors, the only context in which I had heard PD mentioned was in training and development. This was further confined to something that nurses and midwives do whilst medics do medical education.

A desire to provide the best care for women and families led me to understand that I needed to gain knowledge and skills in human factors, ergonomics and quality improvement. At the time I felt like a lone nut. A physician who preached that to prevent harm we needed to have more than excellent technical skills such as operating. I was promoting evidence that non-technical skills were equally, if not more important in reducing the risk of harm ever occurring. Along the way I questioned two things which may resonate with many of you:

1. Why was implementing the research evidence into practice in some maternity units so challenging?
2. Why were some units outstanding, some poor and others eager to improve but just could not convert the successes of others into their local setting?

I sought formal training in clinical leadership and management, something that most of my peers and all my seniors declared was the fluffy stuff and I should stick to developing excellent technical skills. In a bid to help myself and them to identify with the benefits of my experiences, although different from theirs, I tried to demonstrate that both collectively aimed to improve outcomes. You will be familiar either as a clinical doctor yourself or as a non-medic that doctors are an inquisitive, suspicious and highly competitive bunch. They require evidence that is robust and they are difficult to change unless the evidence is clear or there is an opportunity for professional development. Therefore, breaking boundaries and discussing measurement that did not mention a p-value was challenging to say the least.

Although to this day there is no consensus definition of quality improvement, the 'science' of it made me as a medic identify with its merit. I was familiar with the struggles in language that colleagues had with translating human factors and ergonomics evidence from the nuclear and airline industries, so I was prepared for the same conversation converting the lessons from manufacturing to healthcare (Plsek 2014). The important thing for now was that I had something to put a name to, that was generating significant momentum in healthcare and to which I could speak a common technical language to convince medics of its benefits. This language was more familiar and defined by evidence; it was a language that did not frighten them and one which they could engage with.

I had experience through quality improvement (QI) projects of common and special cause variation generated by the systems within which humans live, experience and provide. I became increasingly interested in understanding more about this human element and how much it influenced sustained improvement.

Through human factors training I was acutely aware of how multiprofessional team training improved teamworking and clinical outcomes. I was keen to ensure that the training and development team in my workplace were united and that the staff identified the team by a common language. The midwives were called the PD team, whilst the obstetrician, me, was called the medical education lead. I suggested we needed an inclusive collective name and we agreed upon Faculty of Multiprofessional Learning in Maternity. The success of this strategy was not in the name but in the lived values of inclusivity, collaboration and engagement through the name (see PD principles Chapter 8).

I continued to explore the origins of PD and found myself identifying with it not on a training level but from an angle of improvement. Continuous learning within the workplace at a grassroots level building up small incremental changes refined through naturally occurring PD cycles without staff even knowing the term. I realised that the principles of PD, steeped in science, identified naturally with staff in a way that many had struggled to identify with the technical aspects of other improvement methods. My Eureka moment came as the worlds of human factors, safety science and improvement science came together.

This turning point led me to understand that PD was the key to unlocking why converting evidence into practice remains challenging and why some units have struggled to implement improvement. Without identifying with the inert values and beliefs of people, sustained change is challenging. This was just like my doctor colleagues who struggled to identify with my beliefs in human factors and improvement science all those years ago. Sound familiar?

I used PD tools to align the masses in a shared purpose, recognising that it is a method of continuous improvement that utilises the workplace as a continuous learning source. All improvement requires tremendous determination and all methods have their nuances. No one method is right in all circumstances. I believe in using the right skills and tools for the context within which they will work best.

Sometimes measurement, statistical process control charts and hard QI measurement data speak well. However, I have found the greatest benefit of PD is its diversity in application and relatability to the values of women and frontline staff. A combination which if successful leads to sustained improvement and quality maternity services.

I have used PD to assess the cultural (safety, effectiveness, evaluative) context of a maternity setting: how ready is your service to implement change, best practice and research evidence? Without first understanding this readiness and addressing these contextual factors, implementing and sustaining transformational change is near on impossible. Once you have assessed your service contextual readiness you are in a position to use PD to co-produce workplace transformation with staff. This requires facilitators who are familiar with PD methodology and tools (see Chapters 10 and 11 for more on facilitation).

Building contextual readiness – Cathy's nemesis and enlightenment

It is understood that the principles, tools and methodological processes of PD can be implemented successfully in varied and diverse environments. However, it is essential that all approaches are contextually sensitive to place and person. What is described as an enabler in one setting may be seen very differently in another; what is acceptable, desirable and a priority in one setting may be met with indifference in another.

The context and the characteristics of teams in terms of assumptions, values and beliefs are organic, developed and sustained by the people within the organisation. One observed consequence of these characteristics is clinical variation in outcomes in maternity care where the variations cannot be explained by the characteristics or demographics of the women alone (Lee et al. 2013; Women's Healthcare Australasia 2014). The relationships between care providers, collaborative approaches to care and aspects of team dynamics can influence clinical outcomes (Hastie and Fahy 2011; Downe et al. 2009; Raab et al. 2013). Understanding the significance of context in a change process is crucial to maximise effectiveness. Lack of recognition or understanding of the influence of context has been described as the root cause of mediocre success of programmes regardless of the integrity of, or evidence for, the change (Glasgow et al. 2013; Krein et al. 2010; Taylor et al. 2011).

Contextual factors that influence readiness for change can be described broadly as the collective capability and motivation of the individuals within the organisation for change (Lau et al. 2016; Krein et al. 2010). Organisational attributes such as strong and supportive leadership, participant trust of each other and the organisation with opportunity for engagement, value for the specific change as well as there being an adaptable environment for change will have a positive influence on change implementation (Ovretveit 2011; Taylor et al. 2011; Lavoie-Tremblay et al. 2015; Guerrero and Kim 2013). A triangle of performance has already been described whereby culture, leadership and systems can influence the agility and resilience of the people within the organisation and can directly affect the rate and quality of change strategies. Where strong and positive leadership is evident that promotes a culture of shared status and safety amongst clinicians (Nembhard and Edmondson 2006), there is more likely to be a willingness and effective ability to influence and sustain change.

Implementation of change initiatives is described as mediated and shaped by the organisational culture (Latta 2009) and therefore the focus of assessing effective change should be on *why* or *how* the change occurred rather than *what* the change was, which could provide insights for evaluation and replication (Krein et al. 2010). A targeted assessment of contextual readiness could facilitate the uptake of evidenced-based practice change.

My introduction to PD was accidental and occurred because of a significant omission in a change management process. That was the lack of assessment of contextual readiness to change. It became apparent in the early phase of my PhD study (Adams 2017) that the organisation was not ready for the proposed change, and the remainder of the study was occupied with revealing and measuring the reshaping capabilities to increase readiness for the change.

The maternity teams in the study identified that although there were collegial relationships, the effectiveness of the approach to care was more rhetoric than reality. I captured stories from the clinicians who generously and honestly shared their perceptions of their workplace. There was an overwhelming desire to have a different workplace, to have greater teamwork and collaboration, which was tempered with a strong sense of not knowing how to make a change. This uncertainty led to a sense of inertia, with the easier solution being to maintain the status quo. These stories marked my turning point in recognising the vital component of contextual readiness regardless of the project or the approach to change. Assessment of readiness takes time, motivation, the appropriate tool/method and energy. However, without this investment, engagement and authentic participation can be threatened.

The study continued with a different approach, one that harnessed the energy of the clinicians and their unrecognised or unstated desire to implement change. All clinicians were invited to nominate an obstetric and midwifery peer who they believed had the attributes to be an effective project collaborator. A collaborative approach to recruitment had positive consequences greater than I imagined, which further facilitated engagement and participation. The nominated participants were different from those who may have been nominated normally by the organisation or who normally would have volunteered. The nominated participants felt more visible than ever previously experienced, which increased their willingness to engage and the value of the participation process, which resulted in a more productive and effective contribution (Adams et al. 2016).

Engagement

A facilitator of PD can benefit from having many tools available to support the process. One of these tools, the SCARF© model (Rock 2009), describes how the activation of a person's approach (reward) response can increase engagement, collaboration, cooperation and productivity in a change process. The neuroscience behind this model is not as new as the acronym. SCARF© provides a language to explain and describe the neuroscience of the physical responses to actual or potential barriers to change. The social domains to be considered are status, certainty, autonomy, relatedness and fairness (Rock 2009). By isolating the social domain that is being, or could be, threatened can facilitate the development of strategies by the facilitator to reduce stress responses and create conditions conducive to greater collaboration, cooperation and productivity.

Recognising the social domains assists in understanding that a change process is likely to threaten these domains. Therefore, it is important to increase opportunities to maximise reward responses in the easiest manner possible. For example, a PD project that encouraged a degree of autonomy in design, with a team who developed shared goals to increase relatedness and fairness, would be more likely to engage the team and decrease threat responses.

Strategies that maximise the opportunity for the social domains of participants to be orientated to an approach (reward) response rather than an avoid (threat) response can lead to a culture that embraces change. Investment in the development of facilitators skilled in techniques to predict and recognise potential and actual threats to social domains, and the ability to regulate reactive behaviour, will be crucial. Using social cognitive neuroscience to influence change has not been a conventional methodology in health services, but this may provide an opportunity for organisational shift from system inertia.

Facilitation – Crystal's unrecognised talent

We can see from Cathy's account that facilitation is a key component of PD implementation in any setting. The evidence for a practice improvement or service redesign, the opportunity for the change and the organisational readiness are significant enablers of the process. Their success, however, will be influenced by sound facilitation skills of the transformational leaders engaged in supporting participants through the process. These leaders will have a focus on building relationships that identify and utilise the skills of the many and encourage curiosity and creativity in the process (see Chapters 12 and 13 for more on this). The facilitators themselves can benefit from being active learners and examining their own practice, beliefs and values to move to developing others in the same process. My experience demonstrates the journey from clinical midwife to committed, experienced and authentic PD facilitator (see Chapters 10 and 11 for more on facilitation development).

After many years working as a clinical midwife, I was drawn into the world of improvement through an invitation to implement the Productive Ward programme: 'Releasing Time to Care'. This programme encouraged teams to look at waste within existing ward processes and make changes to improve safety, effectiveness and person-centredness. This was the first time that I experienced the power of the patient voice; of using qualitative as well as quantitative measures of improvement. It was also the first time that I felt that a true board to ward approach to change was embraced and evaluated.

My transformation came from being tasked with delivering this programme, but without the training, tools or methodologies to draw from. I knew *what* needed to be delivered and was left to define the *why* and *how* with the teams and individuals in the programme. Working with colleagues we embarked on this privileged journey of embedding sustainable change but also learning about self and others. We implemented the programme successfully across 52 diverse clinical areas. One participant stated:

> *'Being part of the Productive Ward programme has made me look at everything differently and inspired me to get involved in supporting greater change and share the skills I've learnt with others.' (ITU nurse)*

Active work-based learning facilitated my transformation and was my turning point, where I truly recognised and understood transformational PD facilitation. I had developed skills in this methodology which I could now underpin with a name, formal training and tools which further validated what I had been doing. I had been transformed to think, do and be different, which in turn enhanced my confidence in my ability to facilitate.

I recognised that a shared purpose that draws teams together in a common direction is a vital starting point for effective change and improved workplace cultures. I learned that listening with intent provides a sense of authenticity and an appreciation by the participant that they are truly being heard. I learned that asking enabling questions and supporting teams and individuals to reflect and explore their own ideas and solutions leads to greater engagement and therefore sustainable change. I found that in leading and facilitating high-challenge conversations and ways of working combined with high support I could enable people to challenge ways of working and behaviours, and free them to explore new ideas. The importance of giving feedback in a constructive way promoted creative thinking and how to receive feedback without feeling defensive. These active learning skills laid the foundation of my facilitation practice going forward.

Enabling effective workplace cultures through role modelling and facilitating active work-based learning has been core to our maternity transformation programme. This work was the starting point for establishing trusting relationships with staff in which they were freed to share their existing ways of working and future change ideas. The values clarification contributions were drawn into a conceptual framework, identifying both the ultimate purpose and how the community midwifery team could focus on improvement areas of work by thematically analysing comments into enablers, inhibitors and consequences of best practice services.

Presenting these findings to the leadership team was heralded as 'true transformation'. Some change ideas were approved immediately, including the required equipment that midwives said was essential for them to carry out their roles effectively. The staff appreciated this different approach where their feedback was valued, and that they had been empowered to implement grassroots improvement. This was the start of developing a positive workplace culture. Simple but powerful tools that you could apply to your own workplace that have lasting impacts and bring something magical. The contributions from this foundational piece of work informed development of the full maternity Transformation Programme that can be traced back to the original thematic analysis of participants' comments; this demonstrated true authenticity.

Understanding our own staff, women and organisational demands and priorities for improvement and aligning these to the national direction was key to ensure engagement and ownership (National Maternity Review 2016). Working with and supporting staff to lead on areas of transformation using the workplace as the main source of learning was key to building the programme and enabling change to progress.

In the ideal world, PD methodology would be implemented and embedded in usual workplace business throughout hospitals and maternity teams. Role modelling and visibility of the principles of PD actioned in clinical practice settings can produce change over time. The core improvement team on this programme continue to live and role model the PD principles, facilitating workplace learning and co-production events with women and our maternity partners at every opportunity. They promote change that is aligned to a shared vision and purpose and aim to grow the critical mass of people with PD facilitation skills.

I hope that my experience has shown that PD can comfortably sit together amongst other methodologies that you may be using, but will add something truly transformational through supporting the development of effective workplace cultures that are person-centred and safe.

Co-production – collective ownership

Co-production is advocated as an effective and efficient method of service improvement. It can help with problem-solving, resource utilisation, decision-making and improving relationships between those who use services and those who provide them. There are many examples of its use from across the spectrum of health and social care with great success. The principles of PD explicitly lean towards making co-production a success.

We have used the facilitation tools described above to host a number of collaborative co-production events bringing together two expert groups, providers and recipients of care who learn and co-create together (Realpe and Wallace 2010), leading to the development of effective partnerships. We solved wicked problems such as smoking cessation in pregnancy through to undertaking a full-service evaluation via the lens of women, families and staff. Sense checking our governance systems, what we think we are doing well and where we think we need to improve and align that with where women and frontline staff feel these priorities lie. This approach has led to several simple but effective quality improvement measures, which improved feedback from staff and women. For example, ear plugs for partners to get a good night's sleep through to myth busting about women not wanting to engage with video consultation when in fact we found they were enthusiastic about it. This change in resource utilisation led to a reduction in waiting times in our diabetic clinics.

Staff told us that they felt empowered by actively evaluating and making changes to improve their service. Those in managerial and formal leadership positions also benefited as they explicitly enabled staff to make changes, which resulted in them practising with a collaborative, transformative leadership style.

PD facilitates us to keep a critical eye on how co-productive we are during every interaction and decision made which, directly or indirectly, affects patients. The clinical experience should be an act of active co-production, an opportunity for the two expert groups to make sense of the words used and to bridge the gaps between their thinking. This collaborative effort can help them reach a joint understanding and creates appreciation on both sides for possible or desirable future action: a co-produced care plan or new service pathway. PD tools can support us to do this all the time.

It requires users to be experts in their own circumstances and capable of making decisions, whilst as professionals we must move from being fixers to facilitators. To be truly transformative, co-production requires a relocation of power towards service users. This necessitates new relationships with us as frontline professionals who through training in PD can use the tools to be empowered to take on these new roles. Here we describe how you can overcome the many challenges of generating system-level change from the ground up.

Giselle's experience with co-production

I am an innovation specialist for a large manufacturing company where I problem-solve with customers through co-creation and co-design. I am also a mother of two children and had two empowering natural birthing experiences through the Midwifery Group Practice (MGP) at my local hospital. Through my connections with women in my community I realised that not all women had experiences like mine. They had a terrible spiel around interventions in the birth, how they were not involved in decisions about the birth and how they did not have access to midwifery-led continuity of care. I became impassioned by the inequity in these stories and set out on a journey as a consumer advocate to re-shape the birthing landscape for women in my area. The advocacy group Better Births Illawarra was born.

Elements of this journey that I believe were key to successful change were accurate evidence, robust engagement, commitment to the cause and seizing opportunity. We identified anecdotally that women were not gaining access to the MGP programme due to limited availability, which we believed impacted on their birth experience. We knew we needed evidence that this was an issue, so we conducted a survey of women in the area, which received overwhelming support. We reviewed the evidence in the Cochrane Library, which strengthened our argument. I thought: 'Ok, cool, so the research tells us this is the safest, most cost-effective model, the community wants it, there's clearly a demand, this should be really easy, right? Maybe someone's just overlooked this and once they see the facts, this will be sorted in less than a year.' It would take us a further three years and persistent determination for Better Births Illawarra to achieve one of our goals.

Through an opportunistic encounter with a midwife I was encouraged to speak up. This midwife said midwives often felt powerless to voice their concerns in the system. We sought other women's voices who wanted to 'direct their energy into something that they believe in'. An engaged and committed group of women gathered and it felt like women stepping up to protect and support other women – future mothers. Well prepared with the focus of significant change, we presented to the maternity executive decision-makers. We called for an expansion of the MGP in line with community demand and a refurbishment of the birth suites. We were not talking about a colour scheme change. What we wanted was the use of the BUDset tool (Foureur et al. 2010) to audit the current space and to make scientific decisions on how it could be improved to facilitate normal birth.

Our group opportunistically connected and engaged with a midwifery PhD candidate who facilitated the collation of evidence, a midwifery academic to advise on birth unit redesign, and a journalism student who published an article in the local paper titled 'Seven out of ten miss out'. This article would be the game changer, the turning point that opened doors for our group and gained us a seat at the table as advocates for health reform. A valuable position of influence but a complex one as well; we walked a tightrope trying to build a relationship (with staff) and have a voice, to be taken seriously and to be heard. Staff were not used to working with advocates; three years later we are still working out how to effectively collaborate.

The birth unit design was completed in July 2020 after funding was provided, and Better Births Illawarra remains at the table to provide the voice for birthing women.

Conclusion

All four authors have described a turning point with engagement in the methodology and philosophy of PD. We accidently or inadvertently fell upon PD when we were in search of answers to how we could improve the quality and safety of maternity care. We are now committed advocates of the process and believe in the crucial adoption of PD for supporting effective change. Our experiences were not limited by clinical discipline or professional position, by health service or boundaries of nations. This fact convinced us that with the right tools, contextual readiness, authentic willingness to engage in the process and seizing available opportunity, PD could be used in any setting and be effective for any change process regardless of the specifics of the change.

We were curious novices who had a desire to implement change that could embed evidence into practice that could make a measurable difference to maternity outcomes that could engage the intrinsic motivation of teams that would sustain improvements over time and would create a culture of continuous inquiry. We found this in PD, and we encourage you to explore this for yourself.

You may not yet be familiar with the methodology of PD. What you may have is recognition of opportunities for improvement in clinical practices, you may have some specific concerns with teamwork or organisational practices and don't know what to do or where to go, or you may be curious about other ways of working or being. We encourage you to have the courage to explore PD as a way of transforming the here and now. PD has been the turning point in our transformation, and it could be for you; are you ready for the challenge?

'We often set out to make a difference in the lives of others only to discover we have made a difference to our own' (Ellie Braun-Haley, Canadian author)

References

Adams, C. (2017). *Assessing 'readiness for change' in organisational culture: a descriptive study using a sequential explanatory mixed method design*. PhD. University of Technology Sydney.

Adams, C., Dawson, A. and Foureur, M. (2016). Exploring a peer nomination process, attributes, and responses of health professionals nominated to facilitate interprofessional collaboration. *International Journal of Childbirth* 6 (4): 234–245.

Berwick, D. (2013). *Improving the Safety of Patients in England: a promise to learn – a commitment to act*. London, UK: National Advisory Group on the Safety of Patients in England. https://assets.publishing.service.gov.uk/government/uploads/system/uploads/attachment_data/file/226703/Berwick_Report.pdf (accessed 22 July 2020).

Crowe, C. and Manley, K. (2019). Assessing contextual readiness: the first step towards maternity transformation. *International Practice Development Journal* 9 (2). https://doi.org/10.19043/ipdj.92.006

Department of Health and Social Care (2016). *Safer maternity care: next steps towards the national maternity ambition*. London: Department of Health and Social Care. https://assets.publishing.service.gov.uk/government/uploads/system/uploads/attachment_data/file/560491/Safer_Maternity_Care_action_plan.pdf (accessed 22 July 2020).

Downe, S., Byrom, S., Finlayson, K. et al. (2009). *East Lancashire Childbirth Choices Project: choice, safety and collaboration*. Lancashire, United Kingdom: UCLan Research in Childbirth and Health (ReaCH) Research Group, University of Central Lancashire.

Foureur, M., Leap, N., Davis, D. et al. (2010). Developing the Birth Unit Design Spatial Evaluation Tool (BUDSET) in Australia: a qualitative study. *Health Environments Research and Design* 3 (4): 43–57.

Glasgow, J.M., Yano, E.M. and Kaboli, P.J. (2013). Impacts of organizational context on quality improvement. *American Journal of Medical Quality* 28 (3): 196–205.

Guerrero, E.G. and Kim, A. (2013). Organizational structure, leadership and readiness for change and the implementation of organizational cultural competence in addiction health services. *Evaluation and Program Planning* 40: 74–81.

Hastie, C. and Fahy, K. (2011). Inter-professional collaboration in delivery suite: a qualitative study. *Women and Birth* 24 (2): 72–79.

Health Information and Quality Authority (2015). *Report of the Investigation into the Safety, Quality and Standards of Services Provided by the Health Service Executive to Patients in the Midland Regional Hospital.* Portlaoise, Dublin: Health Information and Quality Authority. tinyurl.com/HIQA-portlaoise (accessed 1 May 2018).

Kirkup, B. (2015). *The Report of the Morecombe Bay Investigation.* London: Department of Health and Social Care. tinyurl.com/Kirkup-MB (accessed 1 April 2018).

Krein, S.L., Damschroder, L.J., Kowalski, C.P. et al. (2010). The influence of organizational context on quality improvement and patient safety efforts in infection prevention: a multi-center qualitative study. *Social Science & Medicine* 71 (9): 1692–1701.

Latta, G.F. (2009). A process model of organizational change in cultural context (OC3 model): the impact of organizational culture on leading change. *Journal of Leadership & Organizational Studies* 16 (1): 19–37.

Lau, R., Stevenson, F., Ong, B.N. et al. (2016). Achieving change in primary care – causes of the evidence to practice gap: systematic reviews of reviews. *Implementation Science* 11 (40). https://doi.org/10.1186/s13012-016-0396-4

Lavoie-Tremblay, M., O'Connor, P., Lavigne, G.L. et al. (2015). Effective strategies to spread redesigning care processes among healthcare teams. *Journal of Nursing Scholarship* 47 (4): 328–337.

Lee, Y., Roberts, C., Patterson, J. et al. (2013). Unexplained variation in hospital caesarean section rates. *The Medical Journal of Australia* 199 (5): 348–353.

Liberati, E.G., Tarrant, C., Willars, J. et al. (2019). How to be a very safe maternity unit: an ethnographic study. *Social Science and Medicine* 223: 64–72. https://doi.org/10.1016/j.socscimed.2019.01.035

Manley, K., McCormack, B. and Wilson, V. (2008). Introduction. In: *International Practice Development in Nursing and Healthcare* (eds. K. Manley, B. McCormack and V. Wilson), 1–16. Oxford: Blackwell.

National Maternity Review (2016). *Better Births: improving outcomes of maternity services in England – a five year forward view for maternity care.* London: National Health Service.

Nembhard, I.M. and Edmondson, A.C. (2006). Making it safe: the effects of leader inclusiveness and professional status on psychological safety and improvement efforts in health care teams. *Journal of Organizational Behavior* 27 (7): 941–966.

Ovretveit, J. (2011). Understanding the conditions for improvement: research to discover which context influences affect improvement success. *BMJ Quality & Safety* 20 (Suppl 1): i18–i23.

Plsek, P. (2014). *Accelerating Healthcare Transformation with Lean and Innovation: The Virginia Mason Experience.* Boca Raton, FL: CRC Press, Taylor & Francis Group.

Raab, C., Will, S., Richards, S. et al. (2013). The effect of collaboration on obstetric patient safety in three academic facilities. *JOGNN: Journal of Obstetric, Gynecologic and Neonatal Nursing* 42 (5): 606–616.

Realpe, A. and Wallace, L.M. (2010). *What is co-production?* London: The Health Foundation. https://qi.elft.nhs.uk/wp-content/uploads/2017/01/what_is_co-production.pdf

Rock, D. (2009). Managing with the brain in mind. *Oxford Leadership Journal* 1 (1): 1–10.

Royal College of Midwives (2014). *High Quality Midwifery Care*. London: RCM.

Royal College of Obstetricians and Gynaecologists (2016). *Maternity Standards*. London: RCOG.

Taylor, S., Dy, S., Foy, R. et al. (2011). What context features might be important determinants of the effectiveness of patient safety practice interventions? *BMJ Quality & Safety*, 20 (7): 611–617.

Wallace, E. (2015). *Executive Summary: Report of an Investigation into Perinatal Outcomes at Djerriwarrh Health Services*. Victoria: Victoria Department of Health and Human Services.

Women's Healthcare Australasia, Canberra, Australia (2014). Benchmarking Maternity Care Individual Report 2012/13.

4. Sustainable Person-Centred Communities Design and Practice

Sharon Lee, Mayur Vibhuti, and Tobba Therkildsen Sudmann

Introduction

Person-centred care is a philosophy that views the individuals using health and social care as equal and collaborative partners in planning, design, co-creation and accomplishment of care to ensure their needs are met (Fix et al. 2018; Paparella 2016; Rubashkin et al. 2018; The Health Foundation 2016). Articulating what it means to be person-centred and how to develop and support the workforce to work in this way, therefore, is key. Defining person-centred care also brings up to date similarities, distinctions and disparities between different philosophies and work processes. For instance, when considering delivery of a person-centred ethos across a community, the collective human, material, fiscal and social performances must be coordinated and directed towards these aims within their cultural context. Furthermore, practitioners, service recipients, users or consumers need a shared understanding of what and how person-centred care can be created, recognized and delineated from alternative forms of care and professional communities. In this chapter, this recognisable distinct ethos and collective practice will be referred to as 'sustainable person-centred communities'.

This chapter explores how sustainable person-centred communities and care emerge, and the key enablers and barriers to support their implementation and maintenance. It also considers implications for policy development within commissioning teams, commissioners, educators and individual service users to support the sustainability of communities of person-centred care.

International Practice Development in Health and Social Care, Second Edition.
Edited by Kim Manley, Valerie Wilson, and Christine Øye.

Person-centred care can be demonstrated in several ways. It can be experienced as a therapeutic relationship between the professional and the individual (Gluyas 2015; Thille et al. 2020). Similarly, it can be understood as a culture that is supported by strong leaders with a desire to change the way in which care is delivered (Greenfield and Marshall 2013), or it can be demonstrated through the drive to improve outcomes of care by commissioning person-centred services. NHS England's (2016) implementation of the Cancer Taskforce Recommendations is a clear example; its aim was to meet the needs of individuals affected by cancer to ensure that people's physical, emotional and social needs were met in a timely and appropriate way and not driven by system targets.

Person-centred care therefore moves away from a paternalistic approach where the healthcare professional is deemed to know what's best for the individual service user (Barnes 1999; Barry and Edgman-Levitan 2012). It is considered a beneficial approach, not only to the citizen but also to healthcare organisations (Kim and Park 2017; Rubashkin et al. 2018). This is partly because it is argued that by putting people at the centre of their care it will not only improve the quality of care but also empower individuals to take control over their own health, and by association reduce some of the demands on health and social care. However, the flip side of this is that persons in need of care need to be conscious about their wants and needs and have knowledge about how their personal aims can be reached. When care recipients in the roles as patients, clients, consumers or partners are invited to take initiative in defining a problem and identifying aims, we implicitly expect them to share our beliefs held about person-centred care. Our expectations probably emerge from a naïve point of departure, that all patients have the knowledge or other resources to be able to exercise agency to reach these aims. A last element of the dark side of person-centred care is that for some, the obligation to take initiative, to be a partner or to participate in defining care is a new burden (Cooke and Kothari 2001; Penderis 2012).

A key enabler for health and social care provision is the available workforce and the model of care used (Gilburt 2016). Without the right skills in the right place at the right time, the person's/citizen's journey through the system may not achieve the desired outcomes of person-centred care. The challenge for person-centred care, however, is ensuring that organisational systems and processes such as time constraints, and sceptical attitudes from professionals who may perceive that they do not have the capacity to adopt the approach fully, do not inhibit the development of person-centred interventions (Moore et al. 2017).

Person-centredness is described by McCormack and McCance (2006) as a method of delivery founded on beneficial affiliations between care providers, citizens and others important to the individual. If person-centredness is to be embedded and justified as a particular ethics of care (Gheaus 2018; Kittay 1999; Munthe et al. 2012), and in the fiscal, cultural and structural organisation of the health and care sector, we can extrapolate an argument for community-based ethics and practice of care. Gheaus (2018) argues that an ethics of care emerges from what she calls *relationship goods*. These goods of constitutive (as well as, often, instrumental) value accrue to individuals by virtue of them being in relationships with other people, something that could not be enjoyed outside relationships (ibid.). Expanding on this, Kittay explains the ethics of care as follows:

'To each according to his or her need for care, from each according to his or her capacity for care, and such support from social institutions as to make available resources and opportunities to those providing care, so that all will be adequately attended in relations that are sustaining.' (Kittay 1999, p. 113)

Gheaus and Kittay remind us that person-centredness and person-centred care is a precarious and sometimes an ephemeral phenomenon, making and maintaining sustainable communities of person-centred care a pressing issue. The communities of practice, i.e. where providers and recipients are on an equal footing, and communities of everyday living for all citizens is an essential foundation to practice development (PD).

The core of person-centred care approaches can be implemented in any setting, not just the healthcare arena, including an individual's home, school or workplace (Harden 2017), as long as individuals fully understand what the principles are in order to ensure they are effective in every relationship, every setting and organisation. If, however, it is viewed negatively by professionals within the health and care sector as yet another model or imposed way of working (Mahony 2015), it will not be embraced as a culture and therefore will fail to be embedded.

Embedding this approach requires several key actions (Harden 2017). In the sections that follow we describe a story from each of the three authors to provide clear examples of an approach to person-centred care across communities that embodies the principles that McCormack and McCance (2006) describe at three levels – micro, meso and macro.

Case 1 Tobba's story: Developing person-centred relationships – the heart of a person-centred community

The story I want to share is about a couple I met almost weekly for a year, Elliot and Louise (names changed to protect anonymity). Elliot participated in a three-armed randomised control trial (RCT) aimed at studying how brain changes (i.e. neuroplasticity) could affect, amend or ameliorate the symptoms or progression of cognitive decline and dementia. The three arms of the RCT were physical activity (I was project leader), music therapy and one-year delayed intervention (either physical activity or music therapy). The team responsible for the physical activity intervention (physical therapist, sports teachers and students on the BA programme in public health) undertook physical tests on all participants in the project and were responsible for a weekly physical activity session indoors or outdoors depending on weather and season. Activities were organised to be fun and playful, and to facilitate physical, cognitive and social engagement in the group, e.g. as circuit training and physical education stations. Whenever possible, we tried to utilise the participants' experiences or knowledge in physical education or sports.

Elliot and Louise came together to the sessions, often hand in hand. Louise was obviously very fond of her husband and he of her, so it was quite moving to see them together. I also observed how much fun and support both got from the group of participants.

During springtime, Elliot once came to the session wearing a Lakers basketball t-shirt, and by asking Louise we learned he used to be a keen player and a big fan of several basketball teams. Right from the start of the project he had moved slowly, struggling to understand and follow the group's activities, and he struggled even if he had two students guiding and helping him. When we gave him a proper American basketball, he started moving with grace in just a few minutes, bouncing the ball to the perfect position to be able to jump and put the ball right into the basket. We were all so happy, and the smile on his face, and on his wife's face, was unforgettable. Alas, we did not capture this magic moment on video.

Elliot became increasingly affected by his dementia and his problems with following the group's activities were bothering him as time went by. The dementia progressed and it was hard to motivate him to take part in activities as he found it difficult to master and follow. Not too many months later they had to withdraw from the project due to a rapid deterioration of his health.

Losing function and health is part of living, but losing health and days to incurable diseases is very hard for everyone involved, whether due to cancer or dementia. My encounter with this couple is narrated here as an example of 'love and sadness beyond intervention' which I have met several times in my professional and private life. For me, this magical moment was one of a few select epoch-making clinical experiences in my professional life, where I discovered generosity and hospitality or their obvious absence. I learned a lesson about how to meet, greet and create ephemeral communities with people in grief and distress (Thille et al. 2020). The t-shirt prompted me to find the basketball, which subsequently gave Elliot and Louise an unforgettable experience. After Elliot's death, Louise told me that our ability to pick up and act on subtle and insignificant cues in Elliot (e.g. clothes, mood, movements, glances, utterances, sounds) made them look forward to the sessions and take joy in the activities and the embodied experiences derived.

Case 2 Mayur's story: Developing systems leaders who are collective and person-centred

The National Health Service (NHS) in England is strategically led by NHS England. In 2014 it published the 'Five Year Forward View' (NHS England, 2014) and 'The NHS Long Term Plan' (2019) to provide a more integrated, collaborative service model for the NHS over the next 10 years. Primary care in England has always focused on a person-centred care ethos; however, over the years care has become more fragmented, not only between organisations such as community care, social care and even medical practices but also between professionals within practices delivering care to the same population of patients as one team. These professionals include practice managers, general practitioners, practice-based nurses and, more recently, newer roles, such as practice-based pharmacists and physician associates. It is generally agreed by all their respective professional bodies that all have key leadership roles to play in creating safe, high-quality person-centred care.

As a general practitioner, in a multidisciplinary general practice serving over 5000 registered patients, I found I was continually challenged with 1) adapting our service to changes in our population, 2) facilitating the learning of skills required of our clinical and administrative team and 3) meeting new contractual demands of NHS England, such as shifting primary care to a more preventative health service, in addition to everything we were already doing. I realised we were all operating in our professional silos on a day-to-day basis and were losing our shared purpose and the values that brought us together as one team on one mission to help patients. As a medical educator interested in leadership, this started a journey to launch a community-based multiprofessional programme where different healthcare and managerial professionals could learn leadership skills together in a safe space, away from the frontline demands of service provision.

This culminated in an eight-day multiprofessional programme which ran monthly over eight months. It was open to all types of practice-based clinicians and practice managers. Key sessions included self-awareness development with standardised personality testing, team role assessments, change theory, digital advances in primary care, networking and presentation skills.

A key learning component of each day were 'peer consulting' action learning sets, which allowed a safe space for individuals to be vulnerable and describe a work-related issue that they were facing at that time. Having non-judgemental thoughts and opinions from different clinical and non-clinical viewpoints, as well as different personality types in their group, helped the problem holder take a more rounded view of their issue with practical next steps to take forward. Each participant took it in turns to facilitate a peer consulting session so they could utilise this tool back in their practice.

Prior to joining the programme, I found that participants at the meso level felt they had very few opportunities to discuss openly work-related organisational problems and stress, which were part of their own organisational cultures. When given an opportunity on the programme to air these issues during the peer consulting sessions, they were almost universally shared by all participants. These open discussions empowered collaborative problem solving and peer support. Building relationships across professionals and between general practices, based on their willingness to show vulnerability, provided a solid, sustainable basis for longer-term change across the healthcare system.

The formal evaluation of our programme (Manley and Jackson 2019) showed significant impact on:

- collaboration;
- multidisciplinary teamworking and learning;
- developing a more explicit and specific sense of purpose.

Underpinning this impact were three key successful strategies of the programme:

- creating a safe environment for learning;
- a daily peer consulting session creating a reflective space for collaborative problem-solving;
- learning about practical tools and skills through facilitated workshops.

I personally reflect from facilitating this programme that the values desired by all of the participants were remarkably similar and they all shared a wish to empower their teams to join them in their mission to provide excellent person-centred care. Simply providing permission, time and a safe space within a reflective framework increased their listening, empathy and relationship-building skills, all key leadership skills for healthcare teams. As time passed on the programme, they were able to apply tools and working practices which improved their service with the support of their newly found local peer network. As participant feedback noted:

'The Leadership Masterclass has made me realise that change starts with me.'

'By attending this course, I feel that I have grown in confidence and feel that I have the tools to inspire and motivate staff to continue to grow as a team and to effect the changes we would like to bring to the surgery.'

Case 3 Sharon's story: Commissioning and supporting systems-wide person-centred approaches to health and social care – the Esther Model

An example of the principles of person-centred care is clearly articulated in the 'Esther model' which originated in Sweden over a decade ago (Esseling et al. 2018; Gardner 2020; Gray et al. 2016). It followed the case of an individual (named Esther to protect identity) whose poor experience of the care system was like that of many patients and service users. The care staff involved in Esther's care recognised that there was a different way of doing things that would lead to better outcomes for both the individual and the system. The model focused on 'what is best for Esther' from Esther's own perspective, to ensure person-centred care. User involvement is integral to the model, building a network around the individual including family, friends and key staff from health and social care. The key enabler of this example was collaboration between health and social care. In adopting this approach, Gardner (2020) reported that the evidence suggested that the Esther project had contributed to a decline in hospital admissions, from 9,300 in 1998 to 6,500 in 2013. In addition, closer integration between health and social care led to a reduction in the length of hospital stay between 2009 and 2014 (from 3.6 to 3.0 days) and rehabilitation (from 19.2 to 9.2 days), with hospital readmissions within 30 days for patients aged 65 and older reduced from 17.4 per cent in 2012 to 15.9 per cent in 2014.

As a result of this success, the model was a clear demonstration of promoting a positive culture that is person-centred, collaborative and enabling. Currently, the Esther model is being implemented across Kent and Medway as part of integrated care in response to the national Long Term Plan (NHS England 2019) supported by Kent's Design and Learning Centre. One of the unique factors about the model centred on the fact that it embraced a multisystem approach and not just the health domain. The fundamental principles of the model in Kent and Medway are based on four areas of quality improvement to drive person-centred care. These are:

- listening and learning from Esther's experience of care to drive future improvement projects;
- providing training and support programmes to the health and social care workforce, including the care sector, to support the implementation of the Esther culture;
- ensuring all members of the teams above feel empowered to ask the question 'What matters to Esther?';
- introducing and holding Esther cafes, which are owned by local communities and provide a platform for Esthers to share their experiences of care and their ideas about how these could be improved, while health and social care professionals listen, develop and feed back conclusions to their organisations and commissioners.

To date, there has been no formal evaluation in Kent. However, anecdotal feedback to the Kent team from health and social care professionals has included the following comments:

'It gave me my mojo back.'
'I realised that small things matter.'
'It has given me a better understanding that every individual has unique needs.'
'Esther means what the individual wants, not what professionals think they should have.'
'I have gained a better understanding of my partner organisations.'

Consideration is now being given to adopting the Esther ethos in the new Kent and Medway Medical School to embed the philosophy with undergraduate medical students.

The litmus test – what are sustainable person-centred communities?

Delivery of health and social care was previously based on the model of citizens being supported by customs and procedures that the health and social care professionals felt were most relevant to their needs (Ham et al. 2012). However, to transform the way in which care and support are provided, in order to be person-centred services need to change and be more flexible to meet people's needs in a manner that is right for them. The benefits are well documented (Kim and Park 2017; Rubashkin et al. 2018) and highlight improvements in quality-of-life measures for individuals as well as job satisfaction for health and care professionals.

The shift from 'What's the matter with you?' towards 'What matters to you?' is presently gaining a foothold (Kebede 2016).

The stories presented are designed to demonstrate the essence of person-centred care. At the heart of healthcare is the ability to develop person-centred relationships, as clearly demonstrated in the first case about Elliot, which is a key enabler of the process. By positively engaging with what matters, we can enable individuals to be active participants in the support provided, creating a sense of happiness for everyone involved. The relationship between the clinician, Elliott and Louise clearly demonstrated co-production and this enhanced the experience and outcome for Elliott. When we are unable to create and sustain these relationships, drop-out rates of people accessing services tend to increase and satisfaction with services is poorer.

Development towards person-centred approaches needs not only the right skills and capabilities but leadership at all levels to ensure it is truly sustainable (see Chapters 12, 13 and 14). The second case about developing leaders demonstrates that organisations need systems in place to support learning, development and improvement to build on what works, and to embrace and support innovation and solutions towards transformation. System leaders can enable person-centred approaches and collective leadership across the system and are therefore enablers of person-centred care. As important, however, is commitment to developing the wider workforce. System leaders, in story two, enabled the workforce to develop and own the values and principles collaboratively with coaches and ambassadors so that the values and principles became a tool to facilitate the change they wanted to happen. Being a skilled professional who has developed advanced leadership skills focused on achieving the key values of being person-centred, and the ways of working that are collaborative, inclusive and participative, is therefore identified as another enabler. Enabling a 'bottom-up' approach to teams to enable sustainable system change that is people-centred doesn't happen in isolation. Effective teams in one organisation can influence others through sharing best practice initiatives, as demonstrated through publication of the Esther model.

The final piece of the jigsaw, exemplified in the third story about Esther, are commissioners who understand the impact of the model from Sweden and are willing to adopt the ways of working and the learning and development required to enable system leaders to implement this approach. Transformation of a workforce with the values, skills and capabilities to support a person-centred approach, such as the Esther model, is a key driver for person-centred approaches to education and training applicable to all stakeholders (Harden 2017). Whilst valuable skills frameworks can be easily applied across a variety of organisations, without the right leadership to embed this ethos, person-centred values and systems may not be sustained.

Currie et al. (2015) experienced this finding when exploring how nursing students understand the concept of person-centred care during the first year of their programme. Helping students to understand the concept of person-centred care during their training could enable students to build connections in their knowledge and skills progression, which could permeate throughout their career. However, their findings suggested that whilst students were aware of the concepts, principles and professional values of person-centred care, many appeared to be preoccupied by learning about what nurses 'do' rather than 'how patients experience care'. In order to sustain the ethos, the authors argue that there is a need for targeted support from mentors to help students gain confidence in reflecting on how patients experience care. In the multi-professional leadership programme described in story two, facilitation expertise was required to train the delegates in peer consulting so they could then support open conversations in their own workplaces to enable their staff to consider different perspectives about how care could be delivered. The Esther model adopted in Kent, UK, is congruent with this suggestion as it uses an Esther ambassador or coach to promote and develop the workforce. The Esther ambassador applies the ethos of 'Esther' in their day-to-day activities to promote and raise awareness of the model. An 'Esther coach' identifies areas or opportunities that would benefit from the model as well as supporting teams or colleagues to implement improvements that may be of benefit to their local population. Essentially, they become the targeted support that Currie et al. (2015) suggest is needed. Development towards person-centred approaches needs not only the right skills and competence but leadership at all levels to ensure it is truly sustainable. The second case clearly articulated the need for support to individuals to feel empowered to be the leaders of that change. Moore et al. (2017) showed that one of the key challenges, as well as the enabling factors, in the delivery of person-centred care in different settings and scenarios was time allocated to care delivery. Since time constraints are a particularly pressing issue, we need leaders and healthcare workers who are considerate with their time use and who prioritise engagement in person-centred care.

Facilitating creative and brave practitioners – critical appreciation of sustainable person-centred communities' design and practice

Three key enablers have been evidenced in the cases for building and designing sustainable person-centred communities, namely the ability to develop person-centred relationships, leadership that enables person-centred systems, and models of care based on person-centred values and ways of working (see Chapter 8). Current health systems, through commissioning, therefore need to actively support staff to 1) implement change based on person-centred approaches, and 2) develop collective leadership with service users to embed sustainable change.

Stories one and two demonstrated this was necessary if progress is to be made with person-centred approaches. Progress was evident within the Kent model, when commissioners embraced this new ethos and provided the support required. Notwithstanding this progress, however, the current health and social care delivery system needs system leaders who can co-create shared values with stakeholders, have the skills to give people and organisations the space to implement these approaches, whilst keeping pace with the changing needs of society as people live longer and new medicines and technologies are identified.

Keeping pace with a changing society necessitates all professionals updating knowledge and skills to meet the changing needs, with the subsequent implications for educators. Learning and development for person-centred practice will become an integral part of the ongoing learner journey for sustainable person-centred care work. This point is illustrated in a review of professional development for psychiatrists undertaken by the Person-Centred Training and Curriculum (PCTC) Scoping Group, comprising members and non-members of the Royal College of Psychiatrists in the UK (2018). The review set out to examine the implications of person-centred care for learning and practice of core trainee psychiatrists. A survey of accredited courses showed patchy availability of person-centred learning and development across the country, notwithstanding an aspiration for it to be an integral part of psychiatric training by both trainers and trainees. So, whilst the review used a collaborative approach and worked with a shared purpose – prerequisites for success (Manley et al. 2018) – a particular gap was identified in learning objectives relating to building therapeutic relationships, one of the three key components identified for building person-centred communities.

Achieving positive engagement with those who use the services is an essential component of person-centred care. Understanding what it feels like to experience person-centred care so that we know we are achieving the desired outcomes can only help to enhance this approach with individuals. However, for this to be effective also requires organisations and teams with shared values and purpose (Manley et al. 2018). This includes the system leaders who enable person-centred approaches and collective leadership across the system as well as the commissioners who understand the ways of working and the learning and development required.

Concluding remarks

To transform how care is delivered at both a system and an individual level to reflect the essence of person-centred care and ensure sustainability will require change. This change will become a reality if the following are enabled:

- person-centred relationships developed with communities and people;
- system leaders who can enable person-centred approaches and collective leadership across the system;
- commissioners who understand and actively support the ways of working and the learning and development required to enable the system leaders to implement this approach.

Sustaining person-centred care will require brave and creative health and care workers at every level of the system and a foundation of trust and relationships to ensure change is sustained. Leadership is seen as the most influential factor in shaping organisational culture (Beckett et al. 2013; Greenfield and Marshall 2013; Lynch et al. 2018; West et al. 2015) and so ensuring the necessary leadership behaviours, strategies and qualities are developed is fundamental to sustaining a person-centred culture across communities.

References

Barnes, M. (1999). *Public Expectations: From Paternalism to Partnership: Changing Relationships in Health and Health Services*. London: Nuffield Trust.

Barry, M.J. and Edgman-Levitan, S. (2012). Shared decision making – the pinnacle of patient-centered care. *New England Journal of Medicine* 366 (9): 780–781.

Beckett, P., Field, J., Molloy, L. et al. (2013). Practice what you preach: developing person-centred culture in inpatient mental health settings through strengths-based, transformational leadership. *Issues in Mental Health Nursing* 34 (8): 595–601.

Cooke, B. and Kothari, U. (2001). *Participation – the New Tyranny?* London: Zed Books.

Currie, K., Bannerman, S., Howatson, V. et al. (2015). 'Stepping in' or 'stepping back': how first year nursing students begin to learn about person-centred care. *Nurse Education Today* 35 (1): 239–244.

Esseling, P., Ford, A. and Trigonoplos, P. (2018). The Esther model: how one patient redefined en entire system vision in Sweden. Retrieved from https://www.advisory.com/research/care-transformation-center/care-transformation-center-blog/2018/06/esther-model (accessed 16 April 2020).

Fix, G.M., VanDeusen L.C., Bolton, R.E. et al. (2018). Patient-centred care is a way of doing things: how healthcare employees conceptualize patient-centred care. *Health Expectations* 21 (1): 300–307.

Gardner, S. (2020). A Swedish approach to intergration: connecting the dots. https://www.caremanagementmatters.co.uk/feature/esther-project-an-integrated-approach/ (accessed 5 May 2020).

Gheaus, A. (2018). Personal relationship goods. *The Stanford Encylopedia of Philosophy*. https://plato.stanford.edu/entries/personal-relationship-goods/ (accessed 5 May 2020).

Gilburt, H. (2016). Supporting integration through new roles and working across boundaries. https://www.kingsfund.org.uk/sites/default/files/field/field_publication_file/Supporting_integration_web.pdf (accessed 16 April 2020).

Gluyas, H. (2015). Patient-centred care: improving healthcare outcomes. *Nursing Standard (2014+)* 30 (4): 50.

Gray, B.H., Winblad, U. and Sarnak, D.O. (2016). Sweden's Esther model: improving care for elderly patients with complex needs. *The Commonwealth Fund*. https://www.commonwealthfund.org/publications/case-study/2016/sep/swedens-esther-model-improving-care-elderly-patients-complex-needs

Greenfield, M. and Marshall, C. (2013). Developing a patient-centred culture through strong leadership. *HSJ*. https://www.hsj.co.uk/leadership/developing-a-patient-centred-culture-through-strong-leadership/5055981.article (accessed 16 April 2020).

Ham, C., Dixon, A. and Brooke, B. (2012). *Transforming the delivery of health and social care. The case for fundamental change*. London: The King's Fund.

Harden, B. (2017). Person-centred approaches: empowering people in their lives and communities to enable an upgrade in prevention, wellbeing, health, care and support. A core skills education and training framework. http://tvscn.nhs.uk/wp-content/uploads/2017/06/40-Beverley-Harden.pdf (accessed 16 April 2020).

Kebede, S. (2016). Ask patients 'What matters to you?' rather than 'What's the matter?' *BMJ* 354: i4045. https://doi.org/10.1136/bmj.i4045

Kim, S.K. and Park, M. (2017). Effectiveness of person-centered care on people with dementia: a systematic review and meta-analysis. *Clinical Interventions in Aging* 12: 381.

Kittay, E.F. (1999). *Love's Labor: Essays on Women, Equality and Dependency*. London: Routledge.

Lynch, B.M., McCance, T., McCormack, B. et al. (2018). The development of the Person-Centred Situational Leadership Framework: revealing the being of person-centredness in nursing homes. *Journal of Clinical Nursing* 27 (1–2): 427–440.

Mahony, C. (2015). The NHS must consider the negative impacts of new care models. *HSJ*. https://www.hsj.co.uk/commissioning/the-nhs-must-consider-the-negative-impacts-of-new-care-models/5084450.article (accessed 16 April 2020).

Manley, K. and Jackson, C. (2019). *Multi-Professional Leadership Masterclass Series Evaluation Report*. Unpublished Evaluation Report. London: England Centre for Practice Development, Canterbury Christ Church University.

Manley, K., Martin, A., Jackson, C. et al. (2018). A realist synthesis of effective continuing professional development (CPD): a case study of healthcare practitioners' CPD. *Nurse Education Today* 69: 134–141.

McCormack, B. and McCance, T.V. (2006). Development of a framework for person-centred nursing. *Journal of Advanced Nursing* 56 (5): 472–479.

Moore, L., Britten, N., Lydahl, D. et al. (2017). Barriers and facilitators to the implementation of person-centred care in different healthcare contexts. *Scandinavian Journal of Caring Sciences* 31(4): 662–673.

Munthe, C., Sandman, L. and Cutas, D. (2012). Person-centred care and shared decision making: implications for ethics, public health and research. *Health Care Analysis* 20 (3): 231–249.

NHS England. (2014). *Five Year Forward View*. London: NHS England.

NHS England. (2016). *Implementing the Cancer Taskforce Recommendations: commissioning person-centred care for people affected by cancer*. London: NHS England.

NHS England. (2019). *The NHS Long Term Plan*. London: NHS England.

Paparella, G. (2016). Person-centred care in Europe: a cross-country comparison of health system performance, strategies and structures. *Policy Briefing*. Oxford: Picker Institute Europe. https://www.picker.org/wp-content/uploads/2016/02/12-02-16-Policy-briefing-on-patient-centred-care-in-Europe.pdf (accessed 16 April 2020).

Penderis, S. (2012). Theorizing participation: from tyranny to emancipation. *The Journal of African & Asian Local Government Studies* 3 (1). https://pdfs.semanticscholar.org/585a/cbc101d963cdb6e65338de878875d2643a65.pdf?_ga=2.249552709.319214579.1595823099-2017242506.1583120697

Person-Centred Training and Curriculum (PCTC) Scoping Group: Special committee on professional practice and ethics. (2018). *Person-centred care: implications for training in psychiatry Person-Centred Training and Curriculum (PCTC) Scoping Group (CR 215)*. London: The Royal College of Psychiatrists.

Rubashkin, N., Warnock, R. and Diamond-Smith, N. (2018). A systematic review of person-centered care interventions to improve quality of facility-based delivery. *Reproductive Health* 15 (1): 169.

The Health Foundation (2016). Person-centred Care Made Simple. What Everyone Should Know About Person-centred Care. London: The Health Foundation.

Thille, P., Frank, A.W. and Sudmann, T.T. (2020). Finding the right track: embodied reflecting teams for generous physiotherapy. In: *Mobilizing Knowledge in Physiotherapy* (eds. D.A. Nicholls et al.), 256–282. Abingdon, Oxon: Routledge.

West, M., Armit, K., Loewenthal, L. et al. (2015). *Leadership and Leadership Development in Health Care: The Evidence Base*. London: Faculty of Medical Leadership and Management, Center for Creative Leadership, The King's Fund.

5. *Promoting Person-Centred Care for Older People*

Victoria Traynor, Hui Chen (Rita) Chang, Andreas Büscher, and Duncan McKellar

Introduction

Older people, across the spectrum of life, experience socio-demographic changes (United Nations (UN) 2019) that easily hinder the capacity of health and social care practitioners to promote person-centred care within this group. The changes associated with ageing are compounded by the ageism that pervades the everyday life of older people (World Health Organization (WHO) 2020). The authors of this chapter are passionate advocates of practice development (PD) as a strategy to enable older people to experience person-centred health and social care. The purpose of this chapter is to share three case studies demonstrating the promotion of person-centred care for people with dementia in Taiwan, Germany and Australia. The case studies demonstrate interdisciplinary implementation of PD projects by practitioners in medicine, nursing and occupational therapy in community and nursing home care settings.

Due to their complex needs, older people are the highest users of health and social care services and effective interdisciplinary teamworking is therefore more crucial than it is in any other population group (Kirst et al. 2017). Only by understanding the complex needs of older people, from an interdisciplinary perspective, can practitioners provide person-centred health and social care services. In addition, genuine understanding can be achieved only by working in partnership with older people and their family carers. PD is ideally placed to provide a strategy for health and social care practitioners to achieve these goals. This is never

International Practice Development in Health and Social Care, Second Edition.
Edited by Kim Manley, Valerie Wilson, and Christine Øye.

truer than it is for people with dementia, who so often experience discrimination and are excluded from decisions about their care (Alzheimer's Disease International (ADI) 2019). Our case studies demonstrate how the care of people with dementia can be improved through the implementation of PD strategies.

In the UK, there are many examples of effectively implementing PD to improve the care of older people. This might not be surprising given that PD grew in the UK in the 1990s (Bradd et al. 2017) from roots wholly grounded in gerontological nursing. In other countries there are fewer examples of using PD with older people, so the aim of this chapter is to demonstrate how PD can be successfully implemented to promote person-centred care practices for older people, in particular people with dementia, in three contrasting healthcare systems. The contribution of PD in the care of older people has never been so important for providing support and guidance to practitioners and policymakers tackling what is no longer a 'future' ageing population trend (United Nations (UN) 2019).

Illustrating the application of claims, concerns and issues

Claims, concerns and issues (CCIs) are used by facilitators to negotiate a shared interpretation among a wide range of stakeholder groups (Guba and Lincoln 1989) or to reach a consensus on constructions about workplace experiences (McCance et al. 2015). The appeal of fourth-generation evaluation is that it argues for all stakeholders to have a right to place their claims, concerns and issues on the negotiating table. The 'evaluator' acts as a facilitator of the evaluation process. 'Stakeholders' refers to all groups in the setting who are affected by the evaluation, including managers, evaluators, medical and nursing staff, and participation of patients/clients is central in the negotiation process (Koch 1994). Demonstrations of how to use CCIs activities are available in written (Foundation of Nursing Studies 2016) and filmed role-play scenarios (NSW Health Essentials of Care (EOC) 2012).

The claims, concerns and issues activity is a commonly used technique to start a PD project to negotiate positive statements about a current way of working (claims), negative statements about a chosen focus topic about care practices (concerns), and to ask reasonable questions about the claims and concerns (issues). A successful claims, concerns and issues activity helps teams undertaking a PD project negotiate an action plan to achieve shared goals.

Case studies

The three case studies presented in this chapter illustrate how authors from three countries implemented CCIs as part of their PD projects to promote person-centred dementia care. Demonstrating our case studies through a CCIs activity gives the reader real-life work-based examples of how to engage colleagues to actively participate in a PD project. Each author presents their case study using this framework to help the reader imagine how person-centred dementia care was promoted using PD. Each case study is illustrated using a vignette of a person with dementia that inspired the change to policy and practice using the CCIs activity described in this chapter. When you read the case studies we invite you to ask these questions: 'How can I use these case studies in my work to promote person-centred care?' and 'How could my team learn from what the practitioners in these case studies achieved?'

Case study 1 Dementia and driving in Taiwan

The University of Wollongong (UOW) in Australia is collaborating with the Taiwanese Alzheimer's Disease Association (TADA) to implement and evaluate a person-centred strategy to help people with dementia make decisions about driving retirement. At the start of the collaboration a CCIs activity was undertaken to better understand the topic of dementia and driving in Taiwan and to develop an authentic partnership between UOW and TADA, creating mutual respect and making use of complementary skills. Vignette 5.1 illustrates a common challenge, in Australia and Taiwan, for people with dementia and family carers and an insight into why this topic was an appropriate international collaboration.

Vignette 5.1 Driving and dementia scenario from Taiwan

Mr Liu is an 80-year-old gentleman. He lives with his son in a Taiwan city suburb. Mr Liu has a diagnosis of dementia. Mr Liu has no difficulties communicating his needs but limited reading skills. Recently, Mr Liu had a fight with his family and, filled with anger, he rode on his motorcycle to see his friend. On the way, Mr Liu crashed and suffered minor injuries that required treatment in hospital. When he recovered, Mr Liu's family wanted to discuss with him how he could prevent something like this from happening again. Mr Liu refused to consider giving up riding his motorcycle. The family were at a loss about how to help Mr Liu keep safe. The family sought help from their doctor but the doctor naively suggested they simply tell Mr Liu to stop riding. Mr Liu and his family met with the occupational therapist (OT), Miss Wang, who took time to share the 'Dementia and Driving Decision Aid' booklet with them and demonstrated how to use the booklet. At the next meeting Mr Liu had decided to make a plan for giving up his motocycle and his family were helping him find other ways to get out and about.

One claim is that in Taiwan, recent policy developments include clear guidelines on driving licences which support driving retirement for people living with dementia. TADA takes an active role in implementing these guidelines using a person-centred approach, enabling people with dementia to participate in decision-making. In addition, Taiwan has a national network of expert practitioners in its memory clinics (Taiwan Ministry of Health and Welfare 2018) to support people with dementia to make driving retirement decisions. Concerns are that it is common for decisions about driving retirement for people with dementia to cause much distress because driving retirement can result in an immediate loss of independence. Conversations about driving retirement are therefore avoided until an accident occurs (as with Mr Liu) and when this happens, people with dementia are disempowered by their driving being taken away from them. The issue of not having a positive strategy to address driving retirement in Taiwan from a person-centred approach could then be addressed by adapting and implementing the Australian initiative.

UOW developed an evidence-based 'Dementia and Driving Decision Aid' (DDDA) booklet to support people with dementia, their family carers and healthcare practitioners to enable person-centred decisions about driving retirement (Carmody et al. 2014). The DDDA Australian booklet is translated into Chinese, Greek, Italian and Vietnamese (Ageing and Dementia Health Education and Research (ADHERe) 2020). TADA was committed to finding a person-centred solution to driving and dementia problems in Taiwan. UOW and TADA collaborated to engage practitioners, experts in dementia care and transport policymakers to create a Taiwanese DDDA booklet (TADA 2020). UOW and TADA are now evaluating the implementation of the DDDA Taiwanese booklet nationally through their memory clinics.

The CCIs framework was used to create a successful collaboration between UOW and TADA. TADA has the best interests of its target client group at the centre of its work and an excellent network of clinicians and service providers committed to improving the health and wellbeing of people with dementia, and UOW had research evidence that using the DDDA booklets promotes person-centred decisions about driving retirement (claims). UOW and TADA had not worked together previously. They needed to develop a strategy to replicate the Australian work in Taiwan and had the long-distance and time differences to overcome to create a successful collaboration (concerns). They set up an excellent project management system, and successfully applied for funding to enable annual face-to-face meetings to create an evidence-based resource and a strategy for troubleshooting bumps along the way, with clear lines of communication between group members (issues).

Now the evidence-based DDDA Taiwanese booklet is available for people like Mr Liu, his family and healthcare practitioners to help achieve person-centred driving retirement decisions by people with dementia (TADA 2020). The collaboration grew every year as their work together expanded and now includes a national network of clinical practitioners working in the memory clinics and Taipei Medical University (TMU) to develop, implement and evaluate the impact of using the DDDA Taiwanese booklet.

Action plan: education project

In addition to the DDDA booklet, UOW created a face-to-face workshop and online module which was translated into Chinese for practitioners to demonstrate how to use the DDDA booklet with people with dementia and family carers (TADA 2020). In Australia, the module is accredited by the Royal Australian College of General Practitioners (RACGP) for continuing professional development points. The content focuses on enabling practitioners learn how to use the DDDA booklet and includes videos of people with dementia and family carers explaining the difficulties of driving decisions, role-playing scenarios and action planning to implement the DDDA booklet. In 2017, 2018 and 2020, the UOW team delivered face-to-face workshops in Taipei to large groups of practitioners from across disciplines to test the reliability and validity of the workshop.

The UOW team administered a pre-post test survey asking participants to rate themselves in the areas of dementia and driving knowledge, and confidence and competence in using the DDDA booklet. Post-test results demonstrated overwhelmingly statistically significant improvements among the participants across all categories of knowledge about driving and dementia, and confidence and competence in addressing driving retirement with people with dementia and their family carers (Veerhuis and Traynor 2019). TADA was satisfied that the UOW dementia and driving workshop would work in Taiwan. A team from UOW visited Taiwan regularly and on one occasion ran a 'train the trainer' workshop to enable a select group of practitioners to become independent trainers as part of the strategy to implement the DDDA booklets across Taiwan. In 2020, due to COVID-19 and social distancing, the workshop was run virtually, including the pre–post surveys to monitor the effects of the education. PD principles are once again shown to be applicable across cultures.

Case study 2 Relationship care in nursing homes for people with dementia

The German Network for Quality Development in Nursing (DNQP) has developed evidence-based expert standards to improve quality of nursing care in core areas of nursing practice (Büscher 2013). After various standards on clinical areas such as pressure injury prevention and pain management, a standard on 'Forming relationships in the care of people with dementia' was developed (Deutsches Netzwerk für Qualitätsentwicklung in der Pflege – DNQPed 2019b) that addresses ways in which nurses can form relationships with people with dementia. Vignette 5.2 demonstrates the need for a different approach to care for people with dementia living in nursing homes and focuses on development of a new standard providing guidance in the way relationships are formed with people with dementia.

Vignette 5.2 Moving to a nursing home

Maria has been cared for in her house by her son and daughter-in-law for the last two years. The care process began because Maria was no longer able to take care of her daily activities as usual. Her son offered support with grocery shopping, cleaning, laundry and preparing meals. It soon became obvious that Maria's needs had rapidly moved beyond what her son could offer. After seeing her GP and having further diagnostic procedures she was diagnosed with dementia. Due to the rapid progress of her memory loss and ability to live independently, her son found a nursing home. After moving into the nursing home, Maria showed indications of 'challenging behaviour'. Her son was stunned as Maria was always a very friendly character.

Claims: description of relationships and stakeholders

By moving into a nursing home Maria lost her familiar surroundings and had to face new circumstances, including a range of people formerly unknown to her.

She did not talk much to anybody. She refused any kind of personal care. Maria lost her familiar relationships and has not had a chance to form new ones. Nurses are willing to support her as best they can, but they lack ideas of how to overcome these challenges and meet Maria's needs. They try to form a relationship with Maria, but would appreciate further support about how to do that.

Concerns: factors that enable the relationship to work

The aim of the expert standard 'Forming relationships in the care of people with dementia' is that all people with dementia receive an offer of support for the formation of relationships, which keeps and supports the feeling of being heard, understood and accepted as well as being connected to other people. The rationale for this is that relationships are rated among the essential factors which constitute and influence quality of life (O'Rourke et al. 2015). Person-centred interaction and communication enable relationships between people with dementia, professional caregivers and other persons in the social environment to be maintained and supported. Staff failed to get to know Maria or develop a relationship with her, and her expressed needs were attributed as symptoms of dementia. According to the steps in the nursing process, the standard addresses five principles aimed at helping to support and form relationships:

- At the beginning the need of support is recorded based on criteria. In order to do this, nurses need a person-centred attitude in the care of people with dementia.
- The care plan is based on a formulation-led hypothesis to which people with dementia, their relatives and the professionals involved have contributed. This is the explicit formulation of staff's understanding, reflection and empathy for the care recipients' behaviour (Jackman et al. 2014).
- People with dementia and their relatives receive information and advice about options for forming relationships.
- The interventions are coordinated by the primary nurse.
- The interventions are constantly monitored and, if necessary, modified by the nurses in coordination with a person with dementia and their relatives.

Issues: challenges

Explicating criteria in an expert standard does not automatically result in their implementation into practice. An individual as well as an organisational approach is needed to actualise the recommendations of the standard. Practicability and acceptance of the standard was piloted in 29 health and long-term care institutions (hospitals, home care providers, homes, day care and shared housing facilities for people with dementia) across Germany and evaluated (Deutsches Netzwerk für Qualitätsentwicklung in der Pflege – DNQPed 2019a). The pilot project followed a four-phase model to implement expert standards into practice settings that is used for all implementation projects of the DNQP: 1) it starts with educational activities for nurses to make them familiar with the intentions and principles of the standard; 2) there are adaptations of the standard to reflect the institutional context – the overall principles described on a national level need to be adapted to the local context, e.g. regarding assessment of the need for support in forming relationships. The standard describes the overall principles. Every organisation is asked to specify these principles without falling below the recommendation; (3) the implementation is guided by supervision; and (4) there is an evaluation using a standardised audit instrument evaluating organisational and personal prerequisites, the process of implementation and its results. The pilot findings revealed general practicability of the standard, but also indicated that the extent of implementation depended on attitudes, professional understanding, institutional frameworks and competencies of the nurses.

Action plan: overview of the benefits for the client group and their evaluation

The implementation of the standard provided promising results in all settings. However, context and purpose differed between settings. They have in common that a professional attitude of nurses and other professionals is a prerequisite to forming relationships with people with dementia. The development of this attitude can be promoted by organisational efforts that depend on organisational cultures and approaches to dementia care. The sustained utilisation of the standard for supporting organisational and individual readiness and attitude to person-centred care should go along with regular audits using the standardised audit instrument. It evaluates the degree of goal attainment across the principles of the standard. These should be used as indicators for areas that need more (or less) attention in team meetings, organisational value clarifications and other approaches to quality development. Having nurses confident in their abilities of forming relationships would help people like Maria to transition to living in a nursing home.

Case study 3 Trauma, complexity and person-centred dementia care

In April 2017, the Oakden Report documented failures at a state-run residential older persons' mental health service in Adelaide, South Australia, for people with complex needs resulting from dementia or mental illness (Groves et al. 2017). The Report precipitated further identification of failures in aged care, triggering the Australian Royal Commission into Aged Care Quality and Safety (Australian Government Department of Health (DoH) 2018).

Vignette 5.3 Considering trauma in dementia care

Maisie was a 70-year-old woman living with dementia. She was rejected by multiple nursing homes because of behaviours including swearing, spitting, hitting and biting. She was admitted to Oakden, having 'nowhere else to go'. At Oakden, Maisie communicated using repetitive syllables, punctuated by swear words. Anxiety during personal care was interpreted by staff as hostility. Up to five staff held Maisie firmly to wash and dress her.

After the Oakden Report, Maisie moved to Northgate House, a service adopting a person-centred and trauma-informed care approach. A rich biography of Maisie was gathered. Staff discovered Maisie was a migrant, lived in multiple places, experienced domestic abuse and had had a motor vehicle accident followed by post-traumatic stress disorder. She experienced depression, anxiety and harmful substance use. Maisie had memory difficulties and was diagnosed with younger onset dementia. Maisie's life story also revealed a woman who was dedicated to personal grooming, had faith, loved gardening, had a passion for 1970s' music and whose family was important to her.

Through understanding Maisie's trauma, staff recognised that her behaviours expressed distress. Realising how they caused re-traumatisation, staff changed their approach. During personal care Maisie was never fully unclothed. Fewer staff provided care, washing her through soft towels, while talking to her about the process. Maisie was transformed. She accepted personal care, was no longer defensive, put on weight and was always well-groomed. Her family were deeply relieved.

Maisie's story demonstrates the vulnerability of people with dementia living in nursing homes. Fortunately for Maisie, she received person-centred care when she re-located to a different service where staff understood trauma-informed care (TIC).

Claims: TIC is part of person-centred care and benefits everyone

TIC acknowledges the possibility that anyone engaging within a service, whether user or provider, may have experienced trauma which impacts on their interactions (Fallot and Harris 2008). Trauma includes physical, emotional or sexual abuse, neglect, serious illness, forced displacement, traumatic grief, and experiencing or witnessing violence (Substance Abuse and Mental Health Services Administration (SAMHSA) 2016). Between 50 per cent and 90 per cent of people have experienced trauma (Key 2008). Being sensitive to the impact of trauma when interacting with people makes sense.

TIC is inherently person-centred, taking a holistic view rather than seeing people as a list of problems (National Association of State Mental Health Program Directors (NASMHPD) 2017). When encountering 'challenging' behaviours, staff will shift from asking 'What's wrong with you' to the more curious and non-judgemental 'What happened to you?' (Key 2008).

TIC aims to protect people from re-traumatisation (Kusmaul and Anderson 2018). Interdependence between service users and staff, the care environment and organisational culture are important elements (Key 2008). People with dementia who have experienced trauma will encounter safer care when TIC is adopted. Maisie's story highlights how trauma-informed, person-centred care can promote wellbeing.

Concerns: nursing home providers and staff are not aware of trauma-informed care

Maisie's story illustrates the relationship between how dementia is experienced and previous trauma. Without TIC, there is a risk of misunderstanding behaviours and re-traumatising people with dementia. All aged care staff encounter people with trauma histories, but staff are generally not aware of or equipped to provide TIC as a component of person-centred care. Systemic ageist assumptions limit understanding of trauma in older people, with the loss of a partner, forced relocation and acquired disability being minimised as 'normal' parts of ageing (Kusmaul and Anderson 2018). Specific populations with high prevalence rates of trauma need more sensitive approaches, including for example people who identify from Aboriginal and Torres Strait Islander communities. Awareness and skills in TIC will be essential in delivering person-centred care to people from all backgrounds in aged care.

Issues: integrating TIC into person-centred aged care

What might we expect the Australian Royal Commission into Aged Care Quality and Safety (Australian Government Department of Health (DoH) 2018) to recommend regarding TIC in aged care? Mapping organisational policies and practices against TIC could enable aged care providers to identify gaps in their capability to deliver TIC. Values-based recruitment will engage empathic, emotionally intelligent staff open to TIC. Education and training are essential. Translation to enculturated practice is a challenge (Bateman et al. 2014). National policy changes are required. The Centers for Medicare & Medicaid Services, in the US, introduced aged care regulations incorporating trauma-informed principles to recognise people who lived through the holocaust and childhood sexual abuse. Changes to aged care standards are indicated. Existing knowledge from programmes such as the US Substance Abuse and Mental Health Services Administration (SAMHSA 2014) and the Sanctuary (Bloom and Farragher 2013; SAMHSA 2016) can inform change but should be embedded at a policy level.

Action plan: what are the benefits of trauma-informed care and how will we know?

There is increasing evidence about the benefits of TIC (Hanson and Lang 2016), including reducing vulnerability, boosting resilience, improving access to healthcare services, decreasing demand for crisis services and reducing cost (Hopper et al. 2010; Wiggall 2017). Further research, including co-design, is needed to explore integrating TIC within person-centred aged care. As Maisie's story illustrates, TIC can transform care to be more compassionate. As this book goes to press, Australia awaits the findings and recommendations from the Royal Commission into Aged Care Quality and Safety, triggered by events at Oakden. It is hoped that awareness of trauma and its impact on people with dementia and those who care for them is an outcome.

International, cross-setting and interdisciplinary learning

The ways in which the stakeholders were engaged in each case study demonstrated the application of the principles of PD (see Chapter 8) to achieve person-centred dementia care. The focus of these case studies was the use of Guba and Lincoln's (1989) fourth-generation evaluation using CCIs as a cornerstone of rigorous PD projects. Skilled facilitation was key to enable the changes and human flourishing to occur.

The outcomes from the case studies demonstrated the application of different aspects of the person-centred framework (McCormack and McCance 2016). At the heart of each case study were strategies to deliver person-centred dementia care. In case study 2, the focus was creating a positive macro context with a policy framework that creates structures that enable people with dementia to receive person-centred care. In case study 3, the prequisite for a person-centred organisation was created with 'competent practitioners' delivering TIC as one way of achieving person-centred dementia care. In case study 1, a person-centred practice environment was achieved through the DDDA booklet implementation, with 'power sharing' empowering people with dementia to make decisions about driving retirement and plan for alternatives to driving rather being forced to give up driving immediately following a crisis such as a car accident.

One area where these case studies could be enhanced is greater involvement of the service users. In dementia care, we still have a long way to go in ensuring the service user voice is commonplace in projects like the ones presented (an example of how this was done in maternity care is outlined in Chapter 3). One positive spin-off of COVID-19 lockdown has been seeing dementia care PD projects adopt more creative approaches to engaging people with dementia. These changes could be sustained with a cultural shift about the minimum expectations to involve service users. The lockdown has made access to information technology a priority strategy to enable people with dementia to maintain their community engagement. Practitioners, researchers and service providers are now using more information technology in their everyday practice. Policy changes will also ensure people with dementia are authentically engaged in research. In Australia, the National Health and Medical Research Council (NHMRC) eligibility criteria for dementia grants is actively including people with dementia in decisions about the topic, design and management of a study. The CCIs guidelines explain that a wide range of stakeholders is essential to negotiating an understanding about healthcare services. This chapter provides a reminder to re-visit the original texts to ensure fourth-generation evaluations are authentically followed and services users are included.

Across the three case studies there was the focus on achieving a 'healthful culture' (McCormack and McCance 2019). In case study 1, developing a successful partnership required the collaborators to understand and respect each other's 'values and beliefs', and crucial to the implementation of the DDDA booklet was practitioners 'sharing decision-making'. In case study 2, the DNQP group was successful in adding a new domain of care focused on relationships for people with dementia to the national nursing care standards. This ensures the attention to physical health is complemented with social and psychological care to guarantee dementia care practitioners in Germany work in a person-centred way. In case study 3, it was clear that TIC enabled practitioners to 'be sympathetically present' to people with dementia. In different ways these three case studies demonstrate the importance of reflecting on relationships through their CCIs activities, which contribute to achieving a person-centred care experience for people with dementia.

Conclusion and implications for undertaken practice development in aged care services

The purpose of this chapter was to illustrate how PD projects aimed at promoting person-centred care for older people are boundaryless, in different care settings and across countries. We presented case studies from different countries, care settings and disciplines. We demonstrated the implementation of a 'tried and tested' PD method of a 'claims, concerns and issues' activity, including developing an action plan to demonstrate how to successfully undertake a PD project in health and social care services for older people. The focus on dementia demonstrated that even when working with a vulnerable population group, practitioners, service providers, non-governmental organisations (NGOs) and policymakers can work towards empowering service users and their family carers to achieve person-centred care experiences. We hope readers from different countries, disciplines and care settings are inspired by our case studies to start a PD project which promotes person-centred healthcare and social care services for older people.

References

Ageing and Dementia Health Education and Research (ADHERe). (2020). Dementia and Driving Decision Aid (DDDA). http://www.adhere.org.au/drivingdementia.html (accessed 30 July 2020).

Alzheimer's Disease International (ADI). (2019). World Alzheimer Report 2019: Attitudes to Dementia. https://www.alz.co.uk/research/WorldAlzheimerReport2019.pdf (accessed 21 July 2020).

Australian Government Department of Health (DoH). (2018). Royal Commission into Aged Care Quality and Safety. https://www.health.gov.au/health-topics/aged-care/aged-care-reforms-and-reviews/royal-commission-into-aged-care-quality-and-safety (accessed 22 July 2020).

Bateman, J., Henderson, C. and Kezelman, C. (2014). Trauma-informed care and practice: towards a cultural shift in policy reform across mental health and human services in Australia: a national strategic direction. https://www.mhcc.org.au/wp-content/uploads/2018/05/nticp_strategic_direction_journal_article__vf4_-_jan_2014_.pdf (accessed 30 July 2020).

Bloom, S. and Farragher, B. (2013). *Restoring Sanctuary – A New Operating System for Trauma-Informed Systems of Care*. New York;: Oxford University Press.

Bradd, P., Travaglia, J. and Hayen, A. (2017). Practice development and allied health – a review of the literature. *International Practice Development Journal* 7 (2): 1–25.

Büscher, A. (2013). 20 Jahre Deutsches Netzwerk für Qualitätsentwicklung in der Pflege: Die Entwicklung in der Pflege vorantreiben [20 years German network for quality development in nursing: promoting the development in nursing]. *Pflege Zeitschrift* 66 (2): 68–70.

Carmody, J., Carey, M., Potter, J. et al. (2014). Driving with dementia: equity, obligation, and insurance. *Australasian Medical Journal* 7 (9): 384–387.

Deutsches Netzwerk für Qualitätsentwicklung in der Pflege – DNQPed. (2019a). *Die modellhafte Implementierung des Expertenstandards Beziehungsgestaltung in der Pflege von Menschen mit Demenz. Projektbericht und Ergebnisse.*

Deutsches Netzwerk für Qualitätsentwicklung in der Pflege – DNQPed. (2019b). *Expertenstandard Beziehungsgestaltung in der Pflege von Menschen mit Demenz, einschließlich Kommentierung und Literaturstudie.*

Fallot, R. and Harris, M. (2008). Trauma-informed approaches to systems of care. *Trauma Psychology Newsletter* 3: 6–7.

Foundation of Nursing Studies. (2016). Develop action plans through shared decision making: claims, concerns and issues. https://www.fons.org/resources/documents/Creating-Caring-Cultures/CCIs.pdf (accessed 23 July 2020).

Groves, A., Thomson, D., McKellar, D. et al. (2017). The Oakden Report. https://www.sahealth.sa.gov.au/wps/wcm/connect/4ae57e8040d7d0d58d52af3ee9bece4b/Oakden+Report+Final+Email+Version.pdf?MOD=AJPERES&CACHEID=ROOTWORKSPACE-4ae57e8040d7d0d58d52af3ee9bece4b-n5hvsmI (accessed 29 July 2020).

Guba, E.G. and Lincoln, Y.S. (1989). *Fourth Generation Evaluation*. Newbury Park, CA: Sage Publications.

Hanson, R.F. and Lang, J. (2016). A critical look at trauma-informed care among agencies and systems serving maltreated youth and their families. *Child Maltreatment* 21 (2): 95–100.

Hopper, E., Bassuk, E. and Olivet, J. (2010). Shelter from the storm: trauma-informed care in homelessness services settings. *The Open Health Services and Policy Journal* 3: 80–100.

Jackman, L.J., Wood-Mitchell, A. and James, I.A. (2014). Micro-skills of group formulations in care settings. *Dementia* 13 (1): 23–32.

Key, K. (2008). Foundations of trauma-informed care: an introductory primer. LeadingAge. https://www.leadingage.org/sites/default/files/RFA%20Primer%20_%20RGB.pdf (accessed 21 July 2020).

Kirst, M., Im, J., Burns, T. et al. (2017). What works in implementation of integrated care programs for older adults with complex needs? A realist review. *International Journal for Quality in Health Care* 29 (5): 612–624.

Koch, T. (1994). Beyond measurement: fourth-generation evaluation in nursing. *Journal of Advanced Nursing* 20 (6): 1148–1155.

Kusmaul, N. and Anderson, K. (2018). Applying a trauma-informed perspective to loss and change in the lives of older adults. *Social Work in Health Care* 57 (5): 355–375.

McCance, T., Hastings, J. and Dowler, H. (2015). Evaluating the use of key performance indicators to evidence the patient experience. *Journal of Clinical Nursing* 24 (21–22): 3084–3094.

McCormack, B. and McCance, T. (2016). A considered reflection and re-presenting the Person-centred Practice Framework. In: *Person-centred Practice in Nursing and Health 2nd Edition* (eds. B. McCormack and T. McCance), 259–264. London: Wiley-Blackwell.

McCormack, B. and McCance, T. (2019). Person-centred Practice Framework. https://www.cpcpr.org/resources (accessed 23 July 2020).

National Association of State Mental Health Program Directors (NASMHPD). (2017). Quantitative Benefits of Trauma-Informed Care. https://www.nasmhpd.org/

sites/default/files/TAC.Paper_.5.Quantitative_Benefits_TraumaInformedCare_Final.pdf (accessed 30 July 2020).

NSW Health Essentials of Care (EOC). (2012). Take the lead: claims concerns and issues meeting essentials of care. NSW Health. https://www.youtube.com/watch?v=6FZFQX-GTjE (accessed 21 July 2020).

O'Rourke, H.M., Duggleby, W., Fraser, K. D. et al. (2015). Factors that affect quality of life from the perspective of people with dementia: a metasynthesis. *Journal of the American Geriatrics Society* 63 (1): 24–38.

Substance Abuse and Mental Health Services Administration (SAMHSA). (2014). SAMHSA's concept of trauma and guidance for a trauma-informed approach. HHS Publication No. (SMA) 14-4884. Rockville, MD: Substance Abuse and Mental Health Services Administration. http://store.samhsa.gov/shin/content//SMA14-4884/SMA14-4884.pdf (accessed 20 July 2020).

Substance Abuse and Mental Health Services Administration (SAMHSA). (2016). Types of trauma and violence. https://www.samhsa.gov/trauma-violence/types (accessed 28 July 2020).

Taiwan Ministry of Health and Welfare. (2018). Dementia Prevention and Care Policy and Action Plan 2.0 2018–2025. https://www.mohw.gov.tw/cp-139-541-2.html (accessed 27 October 2020).

Taiwanese Alzheimer's Disease Association (TADA). (2020). Dementia and driving. http://www.tada2002.org.tw/Download/BookVideo/1?page=2 (accessed 27 October 2020).

United Nations (UN). (2019). World Population Ageing 2019. In Department of Economic and Social Affairs, Population Division. https://www.un.org/en/development/desa/population/publications/pdf/ageing/WorldPopulationAgeing2019-Report.pdf (accessed 23 July 2020).

Veerhuis, N. and Traynor, V. (2019). *Evaluation of a 'Dementia and Driving' education workshop for primary healthcare practitioners*. Unpublished report. Wollongong: University of Wollongong.

Wiggall, S. (2017). The UC San Francisco Trauma Recovery Center Manual: a model for removing barriers to care and transforming services for survivors of violent crime. http://traumarecoverycenter.org/trc-manual/ (accessed 23 July 2020).

World Health Organization (WHO). (2020). Ageing and life-course: ageism. https://www.who.int/ageing/ageism/en/ (accessed 30 July 2020).

6. *Education Models Embedding PD Philosophy, Values and Impact – Using the Workplace as the Main Resource for Learning, Developing and Improving*

Rebekkah Middleton, Tracey Moroney, Carolyn Jackson, and Ruth Germaine

Introduction

A key purpose of practice development (PD) is to create an effective workplace culture that enables everyone to flourish, or put more simply, to create good places to work. PD is underpinned by a commitment to using the workplace as the main resource for continuing professional learning and development through enhancing knowledge, skill and practice wisdom, improvement and innovation (Manley et al. 2013). This chapter focuses on work undertaken in Australia and the UK using the workplace for learning, development and innovation. We will present two case studies: (1) implementing a person-centred undergraduate nursing curriculum, and (2) place-based learning (PBL) in a general practice context. We will follow these with findings from a research study measuring the impact of interprofessional learning in the workplace, which highlights indicators used to demonstrate change in practice for individuals and teams.

International Practice Development in Health and Social Care, Second Edition.
Edited by Kim Manley, Valerie Wilson, and Christine Øye.

Case study 1: The value of integrating a person-centred curriculum

Background

Education providers are faced with preparing a workforce that can contribute to better health outcomes for people. The role of education is to develop personal and professional growth, facilitate and equip graduates with the skills to think critically challenging established processes in the pursuit of excellence. These are all elements aligned to the purpose of PD.

Person-centred pre-registration programmes supported by academic excellence, facilitation of professional and personal growth, and development of student-led, facilitator-assisted communities of practice are key to building the transformative workforce of the future. Embedding person-centred practice by placing values at the heart of the curriculum and the learning environment is essential to transforming workplace culture by preparing registered nurses for future leadership and practice.

Implementation of a person-centred curriculum

Person-centred theory, practices and principles have emerged as a framework for undergraduate nursing curricula and are increasingly adopted in higher education as an underpinning philosophy for education curricula (Cook et al. 2018). A key element of this approach is use of the Person-Centred Practice Framework (PCPF) (McCormack and McCance 2017). While the PCPF has previously been used to structure learning and teaching activities, rather than in the curriculum development or design stages, the benefits of using the PCPF as a core conceptual framework (Middleton and Moroney 2019) facilitate an environment where students can flourish, are respected, appreciated, celebrated and heard (McCormack and McCance 2017).

In order to develop graduates who use person-centred approaches, it is essential that nurse education places the PCPF at the core of all nursing curricula decisions. Throughout their experience, students are presented with pedagogical processes that use PD principles and processes, thereby being transformative and inclusive of activities that use co-facilitation and foster collaboration, shared decision-making and the core principles of person-centredness (Niessen and Jacobs 2014).

Aspects of a person-centred curriculum

Person-centred curricula value the voice of all those involved – academics, students, industry, clinical facilitators, people receiving care. They are supported by a clear structure that demonstrates how decisions are made and how the curriculum is operationalised. An example of a person-centred curriculum that was developed and implemented in a school of nursing in Australia is outlined below, including the conceptual framework and principles of preparation and action.

Conceptual framework

Conceptual frameworks should be an extension of the values espoused by the school or faculty, reflecting beliefs about education and nursing practice. The conceptual framework developed is outlined in Figure 6.1. This framework demonstrates how components fit together, being developed from an in-depth analysis of the schools' values and commitment to person-centred practice.

Co-design

Experience-based co-design, a participatory approach, draws together multiple experiences and ways of thinking to bring about shared ways of working (Bowen et al. 2013; Donetto et al. 2015). This enables positive working relationships to be fostered and inclusive processes representative of all stakeholders needs (Voorberg et al. 2015). Co-design principles were used to review components of the curriculum and engage stakeholders in designing and developing learning, teaching and assessment strategies, ensuring connections were consistently applied to the overarching philosophy of person-centred practice. PD principles (e.g. collaboration, inclusion, participation (CIP), shared values) prompted respect for ideas and diversity, inclusivity, use of appropriate language, facilitation, collaboration and creativity. The process is outlined in Figure 6.2.

Our way of working: **Person-centred practice** (Overarching philosophy)
Our theoretical approach to learning and teaching: **Constructivist learning theory**
How we will achieve this: **Active and collaborative learning, student led, facilitator guided**

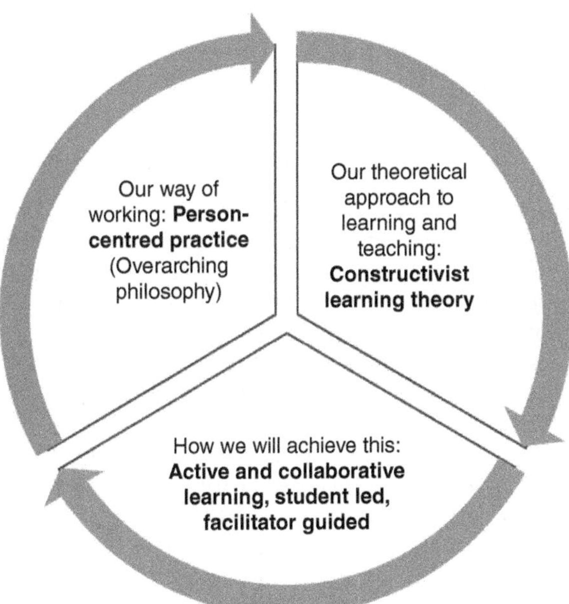

Figure 6.1 Conceptual framework

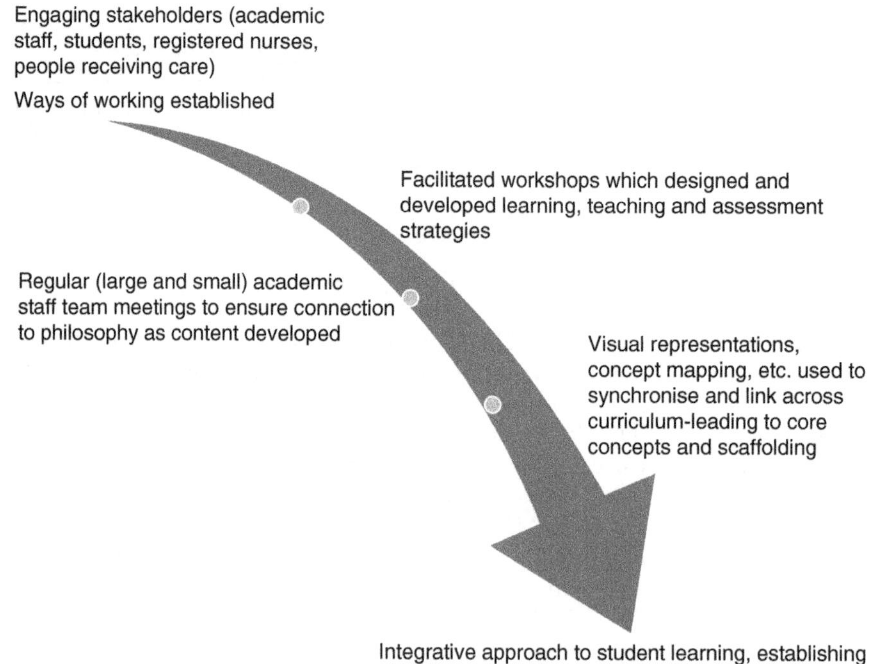

Figure 6.2 Co-design process

Active learning

All teaching and learning activities within the Bachelor of Nursing, including the online space, were designed and developed using principles of active learning. The traditional lecture was reimagined to include facilitated discussions to guide student-led learning, and the tenets of the flipped classroom were applied to ensure students were well prepared with foundational knowledge prior to coming to class.

Key to learning is using active engagement to entice students to use their prior experiences. Active learning is an approach for in-depth learning that draws on creativity and synthesizes and integrates numerous learning methods, such as critical reflection, engagement with the senses, using multiple intelligences and interacting with other people (Dewing 2010). It embeds critical thinking in the learner and encourages life-long learning, retention of knowledge and skills, supporting whole person learning, thereby making learning deeper and more meaningful (Middleton 2013).

Creativity was frequently adopted as a way to generate ideas (PD principle 3). This is an important aspect of person-centred curriculum implementation as it allows participants to cultivate 'independent feeling and thought for themselves as part of their own transformation' (Dewing 2010, p. 24). Creativity helps readiness and responsiveness to change and challenging processes, bringing a more critical approach to decisions (Middleton et al. 2018), which in turn increases personal commitment to learning and taking action as needed (Dewing 2010). This stimulates movement towards transforming practice and looking for creative approaches to develop professional growth and provide person-centred care (Middleton et al. 2018).

For students, this approach provides a learning environment that is safe yet challenging, and creates a critical dialogue with self and content. These techniques provide strong synergy with the PCPF (McCormack and McCance 2017) and with PD principles.

Critical thinking and reflection

Central to learning experiences is enabling space to reflect. Critical reflection increases the student's capacity for learning and to identify their own strengths and areas for improvement. Critical reflection is key to connecting theory and practice (Boud et al. 1985). Students are asked to reflect on practice to assist them in identifying skills and knowledge underpinning person-centred care. To develop critical thinking and reflective skills, activities and assessments that encourage collaboration, investigation, questioning, analysis and drawing together of rational conclusions are essential for transformative practice. These are scaffolded throughout the degree to assist students to learn and practise using the concepts.

Case study 2: Place-based learning

The impact of learning in case study 1 sets the scene for this next section, where learning in action is demonstrated in a living example in a primary care setting or *place*. There is limited reference to place-based learning in relation to health and social care. However, Reid (2011, p. 1) discusses how a 'pedagogy of place' is relevant to healthcare as it 'recognizes the importance of the context of learning and allows the uniqueness of a local community to integrate learning at all levels'. Eggleton et al (2020) considered PBL as an important factor in learning outcomes in general practice, stating it increases understanding through experience of the local population as well as increasing clinical roles as advocates, communicators and leaders. This approach builds upon the concept of PD, using the workplace as a key resource for learning (PD principle 4). Considering the wider context of community and the roles clinicians play highlights the person-centred nature of learning.

Primary care demands/population needs

General practice in the United Kingdom is in crisis due to increased demand, compounded by an aging workforce, difficulties with recruitment and retention, and increasingly complex patient needs (Baird et al. 2016). Furthermore, consultations in general practice are not always person-centred, focusing upon the presenting complaint rather than need (Bodegård et al. 2019). Clay and Stern (2015) consider that burnout due to increased demands leads to depersonalisation of care, compromising outcomes for clinicians and patients. In the UK, primary care networks (PCNs) have been considered as a vehicle that will address these issues through improved partnership across health and social care (NHS 2019). This includes a drive for new ways of working, increased skill mix and a focus upon population health. These changes require leadership that cultivates the culture and capabilities, maximises team potential and supports new ways of working (NHS 2019).

The East Kent Training Hub (south-east England) considered that in order to ensure a workforce able to make the transformation required for this large-scale change, a learning culture through PBL needed to be imbedded within the PCNs. This would allow for the change required, improve recruitment and retention whilst developing a future workforce that shifts focus from demand to need.

To ensure involvement and stakeholder engagement across the system,[1] workshops were developed to co-create a shared vision/purpose and an implementation and impact framework for PBL across PCNs. To underpin the framework, workshops focused first upon co-creating a shared purpose of PBL, allowing participants to share their knowledge, skills and expertise, with everyone considered an asset (see Box 6.1).

Participants were then asked to consider what matters to them, clarifying core values considered necessary to underpin an effective learning culture. These included compassion, care, happy people,[2] respect, positive culture and a willingness to learn, grow, value, support and work together. All values expressed were embraced and synthesized into a mnemonic by PCNs (Box 6.2) and shared to underpin the framework.

Box 6.1 Co-created purpose of PBL across PCNs

Grow, develop and sustain an effective health and social care workforce equipped with the skills, knowledge and expertise to deliver effective safe, compassionate, consistent holistic care. The aim is to improve patient pathways, outcomes and the wellbeing of the local population and evolve with changing needs.

Box 6.2 PCN mnemonic

Person-centred learning, that recognises everyone is an asset, invests in all people and sees the educative potential of all
Cultures of learning at the heart of everyday work in teams
Networks that enable learning together across the PCN, and the sharing of best practice and what works well.

[1] Those invited to the workshops included citizens, primary, secondary and community care providers, third sector and voluntary providers, the local clinical commissioning group and sustainability and transformation partnership and educators, education providers and learners.

[2] For the purpose of this chapter, people refers to all people including citizens and all staff across the system.

Box 6.3 PBL definition and benefits

All learning that takes place in the environment and/or context of where the learning will be used, allowing for the use of a variety of learning methods across health and social care settings. The focus is upon experiential learning where meaning is constructed through interaction, allowing development of knowledge. The benefit of developing knowledge in this way is that it can be applied in practice and evaluated to ensure that broad understanding has been achieved rather than focusing upon individual skills and one aspect of care delivery.

As initially PBL was not defined, instead described loosely as immersive learning that occurs where the learning is used, it allowed understanding of the local context. This enabled participants to consider a range of collaborative interprofessional approaches in real settings that are evolutionary and improve patient care, through development of a learning culture where everyone can flourish and develop (PD principles 1, 4, 6). Following the workshops, the inputs from participants were used to co-create a deeper understanding of PBL and its benefits (Box 6.3).

The core values continued to shape the implementation and impact framework, embedding them within the facilitation strategies, enablers, attributes and consequences of effective PBL across the PCNs.

Facilitation strategies

The facilitation strategies identified many aspects usually associated with facilitation, including expected attributes, ways of teaching, learning new skills and knowledge, taking responsibility for personal learning and developing others. It was also identified that facilitators should embrace the vision, invest in all people, identify and review individual, personal, team and organisational learning needs based upon the requirements of the local population and what matters to people. To achieve this, facilitators needed to network across the system, using resources effectively to create opportunities that help learners understand patient pathways, the wider system and the implications of individual actions, focusing upon need.

Enabling a good learning environment

The enablers required for a good learning environment start with a shared vision and values that can flex and evolve. Additional enablers expressed were divided into two groups. The first was team learning cultures. To underpin this each PCN requires a PBL champion, designated facilitators of learning, and all staff committed to, supporting and/or delivering PBL. Learning opportunities need to be based upon feedback, care priorities and local population data, ensuring citizen, learner and staff engagement supported by systems that allow, recognise, record and value all learning.

The second group of enablers was those needing to happen at PCN and system level. This included having multidisciplinary developmental frameworks giving consistency of career development and continuity of learning that provide equal opportunity across the system. Furthermore, there is a need to have systems in place and appropriate governance to allow the ultimate purpose to be achieved. These include listening to what matters to people, seeing everyone's education as having equal value, and widening participation to health and social care carers. The system also needs to build integrated care partnerships, enabling networking to share learning and good practice as well as access to skills, knowledge, expertise and resources.

Recognising a good learning environment

The attributes that would be seen in a good PBL culture are based upon the values mnemonic PCN (Box 6.2) being observed in action, where everyone feels respected, is recognised as an asset and is invested in, in order to reach their potential. Being supported, teams, staff and learners feel able to seek understanding and ask for help, and all are committed to engaging in and with learning. Through development of trust and shared responsibility, a positive team culture develops that enables people to reflect, respond and be creative, thereby challenging traditional ways of learning. Teams have systems to celebrate and share success they identify, analyse and review learning, give feedback, reflecting and acting constructively to inform improvement and innovation with freedom to try, and a process to learn from mistakes. They use all options to develop learning through innovative, flexible, proactive, pragmatic and adaptable ways of working to utilise, manage and organise resources effectively and efficiently. As a result of this way of working and learning, networks collaborate, share resources and enable learning together across the PCNs.

Outcomes of a good learning environment

The outcomes of effective PBL were considered to be the following.

Staff and learners:

- experiencing an inviting, positive, creative, supportive, happy, learning environment enabling them to feel respected, cared for, recognised and empowered, with a sense of belonging;
- having courage and confidence to ask, speak up and challenge without blame, thereby building resilience and emotional intelligence;
- enjoying being at work, wanting to learn, being current, and having equitable access to learning and career development opportunities;
- having less sickness, improved staff wellbeing and morale, and increased capability and capacity in facilitation of learning;
- having increased input to identifying needs, learning and service design across the PCN with increased indicators of high-quality, safe, effective care.

PCNs and systems:

- seeing increased capability and capacity in interprofessional facilitation of learning and development across the system;

- having positive feedback from all people with improved standards and key performance indicators;
- developing and enjoying a good reputation;
- having better reporting of incidents and learning from mistakes, allowing the system to demonstrate the value and impact of PBL;
- having positive impact upon the local people as health inequalities are addressed, resulting in improved population health with a reduction in over-medicalisation;
- attracting research funding and team investment, and the workforce increasing its effectiveness and productivity;
- having improved retention and recruitment with appropriate multiprofessional skill mix and new roles to meet identified needs and what matters to people.

The full framework is shown in Table 6.1.

In this final section we explore the concept of interprofessional continuing professional development (CPD) in the workplace and how to measure its impact on individuals (micro-), teams (meso-) and organisations (macro-level) using contemporary evidence-based theories about learning.

Measuring the impact of CPD in the workplace

There is no universally agreed definition of CPD, although Box 6.4 provides a comprehensive summary.

Jackson et al. (2015) and Manley et al. (2018) identify CPD's main purpose as being to enhance the delivery of person-centred, safe and effective evidence-informed care in the workplace, which echoes Principles 1 and 6 of PD. CPD that maximises the opportunity to learn at work, through work and for work (Tynjälä 2013) using the workplace as the main resource for learning, development, innovation and improvement helps to shape practice in real time and enables practitioners to make a meaningful contribution to their team, service and organisation (Manley et al. 2019; Manley and Jackson 2020).

An international realist evaluation study undertaken by Jackson et al. (2015) developed a theoretical framework for effective CPD encompassing impact indicators for a range of different stakeholder groups, at micro-, meso- and macro-levels of an organisation. Taking a whole-systems approach to interprofessional learning, the study developed four new transformational theories to describe and explain the relationships between what works (contexts=C) and why it works (mechanisms=M) to achieve specific outcomes (O) of CPD learning in practice, linking these in turn to impact and potential indicators of effectiveness and the principles of PD (for further details relating to this study see Table 6.2). This approach enables identification of the potential impact of CPD on individual practitioners, multidisciplinary teams, and the wider organisation and systems of healthcare delivery across all professions in any context (Manley et al. 2018;

Table 6.1 Place-based learning across the East Kent PCNs – implementation and impact framework

ENABLERS: **required for place-based learning**	*ATTRIBUTES:* **describe what would be happening in good place-based learning cultures**	*CONSEQUENCES*: **including impact, outcomes and outputs**
SHARED VISION, VALUES, PURPOSE, DIRECTION • A shared vision, values, purpose and direction that can evolve flexibly across the PCN. **TEAM-LEARNING CULTURES have:** • a PBL champion in every PCN • designated facilitators of learning to support staff • all staff committed to, supporting and/or delivering PBL • a menu of learning and development activities available to all staff • systems to: o allow, recognise, record and value all learning o ensure citizen, learner and staff engagement from across the PCN and collect and use feedback to inform learning and care priorities • access to data regarding local population/people needs to inform learning needs • opportunities to: o participate in and be supported by learning networks across the PCN o contribute to research and evaluation that informs learning, development and improvement.	**VALUES OBSERVED IN ACTION** • **Person-centred learning:** o everyone is recognised as an asset and invested in to develop their individual potential o respectful relationships and peer support o staff and learners seek understanding and can ask for help and support. • **Cultures of learning** Staff in teams: • understand, engage with and are committed to learning and support • involve and include all people in learning • take ownership for and prioritise learning • are responsive and reflective, positive and creative • challenge traditional ways of learning • develop trust, team bonding and share responsibly.	**STAFF/WORKFORCE/LEARNERS** • **Experience an inviting positive, creative supportive, happy, learning environment that enables them to:** o feel respected, cared for, recognised, empowered and a sense of belonging o have the courage and confidence to ask, speak up and challenge without blame o want to learn, exceed expectations and be ambitious, o build resilience and emotional intelligence o enjoy being at work and have job satisfaction o become skilled, up to date and have equitable access to learning and career development opportunities. **TEAM** • Increased capability and capacity in facilitation of learning and development across the team. • Increased input to identifying needs, learning and service design across the PCN. • Improved staff wellbeing and morale, less sickness and stress. • Improved indicators of high-quality (patient experience), safe and effective care.

PRIMARY CARE NETWORK AND SYSTEM:

- **Multidisciplinary developmental frameworks** for consistent career development and continuity of learning across the system that are inclusive and provide equal opportunity:
  - consistency of roles related to learning and development, including terms and conditions
  - curricula and competencies
  - facilitators of learning and development
  - leadership for developing learning cultures.
- **Systems in place,** i.e. organisational structures, managerial support and governance with clear and transparent processes to:
  - listen to and acknowledge what matters to people
  - review learning and development provision relevant to changes in roles, practice and population needs
  - recognise, value and evaluate learning and development outcomes
  - See everyone's education as having an equal value
  - grow and retain workforce, widening participation, promoting health and social care careers, working with schools, colleges and higher education institutes, increasing capacity and capability and succession planning

Team systems in place to:

- celebrate and share success
- identify, analyse and review learning, feedback and all outcomes, reflecting and acting constructively to inform improvement and innovation
- allow the freedom to try and the right to fail, and a process to learn from mistakes
- use all options to develop learning through innovative, flexible, proactive, pragmatic and adaptable ways of working to utilise, manage and organise resources effectively and efficiently.
- **Networks that enable learning together across the PCN** and the sharing of best practice and 'what works':
- teams work together, network, collaborate and share resources
- teams participate across systems to share learning, best practice, improvement and innovation.

PRIMARY CARE NETWORKS AND SYSTEM:

Learning system

- Increased capability and capacity in interprofessional facilitation of learning and development across the system.
- Improved outcomes:
  - positive feedback from all learners and people
  - improved standards and key performance indicators
  - good reputation
  - outstanding CQC results/
- Increased reporting of incidents and adverse incidents and learning from mistakes and significant events.
- Demonstrable value and impact of PBL across the system.

System outcomes

- Citizens are signposted correctly to see the right people at the right time.
- Positive impact on local people, addressed health inequalities and improved population health.
- Reduced over-medicalisation.
- Attract research funding and investment.

Workforce outcomes

- Increased effectiveness and productivity of organisations/teams across system.
- Improved retention and recruitment of workforce.
- Appropriate multiprofessional skill mix and new roles to meet identified needs and what matters to people.

(Conti.)

Table 6.1 *(conti.)*

ENABLERS: **required for place-based learning**	*ATTRIBUTES:* **describe what would be happening in good place-based learning cultures**	*CONSEQUENCES:* **including impact, outcomes and outputs**
○ review attrition and how to reduce this where needed ○ build integrated care partnerships across health and social care including all stakeholders to ensure seamless working across boundaries ○ allow rotational placements across the PCN ○ identify people's needs with consideration of geography (access/location), sustainability and environmental footprint. • **Networks to enable**: ○ shared learning and good practice across the health and social care system ○ access to skills development, knowledge and expertise. • **Access to resources to support learning, including**: ○ technology and all being digitally informed ○ learning opportunities, information and resources.		

Box 6.4 Definition of CPD

> *'The systematic maintenance, improvement and continuous acquisition and/or reinforcement of the life-long knowledge, skills and competences of health professionals. It is pivotal to meeting patient, health service delivery and individual professional learning needs. The term acknowledges not only the wide-ranging competences needed to practise high quality care delivery but also the multi-disciplinary context of patient care' (EAHC, EU report 2013: 6).*

Table 6.2 CPD transformation theories illustrating contexts (C), mechanisms (M) and outcomes (O) relationships for effective CPD (Jackson et al. 2015; Manley et al. 2018)

Context (C)	Mechanism (M)	Outcome (O)
Theory 1: Transformation of individual's professional practice **Hypothesis:** CPD that is work-based, driven by the learner, provides facilitated support and reflection and includes 360-degree feedback will increase self-confidence, self-awareness, role clarity, a positive attitude to change and opportunities for career development.		
Workplace context: **C1.** Opportunities for CPD that are work-based **C2.** Culture of inquiry, learning and implementation **Organisational context:** **C3.** Supportive organisations that value work-based learning and development	**M1.** Facilitated support and reflection **M2.** Developing skill in reflection and self-awareness **M3.** Self-assessment **M4.** Learning that is self-driven	**For the individual:** **O1.** Increased self-awareness **O2.** Increased self-confidence and perceived self-efficacy **O3.** Transformational learning, new knowledge and continuing motivation to learn **O4.** Empowerment, self-sufficiency and self-directing **For the individual's role:** **O5.** Person-centred, safe and compassionate practice **O6.** Role clarity and opportunities for role innovation and development **O7.** Career progression **O8.** Meaningful positive engagement with change
Theory 2: Transformation of skills to meet society's changing healthcare needs **Hypothesis:** CPD that focuses on self-assessment expanding skills to meet a changing service will be reflected in outcomes around better integration and continuity of service provision, greater employability and opportunities for career progression.		

(Conti.)

Table 6.2 *(conti.)*

Context (C)	Mechanism (M)	Outcome (O)
Workplace context: **C4.** A focus on team competences and effectiveness rather than just the individual **Organisational context:** **C5.** Value for money in the use of human resources and investment **Healthcare context:** **C6.** The need for staff in contemporary healthcare to be adaptable and flexible in responding to changing healthcare needs	**M5.** Assessment of systems and team skills and competences **M6.** Identifying gaps in systems and service needs **M7.** Expanding and maintaining skills and competences through a range of different ways **M8.** Developing team effectiveness	**For service users:** **O9.** Improved continuity and consistency experienced by service users **For individual/team:** **O10.** Better and sustained employability **O11.** Career progression **O12.** An effective, cohesive team **For the organisation/system:** **O13.** Better integration of services **O14.** Better partnerships with services and agencies **O15.** Better value for money through effective use of human resources, e.g. substitution and reduced duplication
Theory 3: Transformation that enables knowledge translation **Hypothesis:** CPD that focuses on providing up-to-date knowledge about effective, safe practice will achieve knowledge transition if participants are supported to develop their skills in facilitation of others' learning and the blending of different knowledges, leadership and workplace contexts and cultures.		
Workplace context: **C7.** Engaging with and using different types of knowledge in everyday practice **C8.** Active sharing of knowledge in the workplace	**M9.** Helping people to reflect on the quality and range of knowledge they use in practice **M10.** Blending different types of knowledge to guide practice **M11.** Facilitating dialogue about using knowledge in practice **M12.** Facilitating active inquiry and evaluation of own and collective practice and learning **M13.** Developing practical and theoretical knowledge of leadership, facilitation, evaluation and cultural aspects influencing knowledge translation in practice	**Workplace/team:** **O16.** Knowledge used in and developed from practice **O17.** A knowledge-rich culture **Team and organisational:** **O18.** Active contribution to practice development **O19.** Innovation and creativity
Theory 4: Transformation of workplace culture to implement workplace and organisational values and purpose relating to person-centred, safe and effective care **Hypothesis:** CPD that focuses on living shared organisational values across different boundaries will increase team effectiveness and organisational effectiveness that makes a positive difference to the experience of service users.		

Table 6.2 *(conti.)*

Context (C)	Mechanism (M)	Outcome (O)
C9. Context has explicit shared values and purposes **C10** Organisational readiness to change	**M14.** Developing shared values and a shared purpose **M15.** Facilitating the implementation of shared values through feedback, critical reflection, peer support and challenge **M16.** Evaluating experiences of shared values relating to person-centred, safe and effective care from both service users and staff **M17.** Creating a culture that enables individual personal growth, effective relationships and teamwork **M18.** Developing leadership behaviours	**Service users:** **O20.** Improved service user and provider experiences, outcomes and impact **Staff/team:** **O21.** Sustained person-centred, safe and effective workplace culture **O22.** An effective, cohesive team **Organisational:** **O23.** Increased employee commitment to work and learning **O24.** Organisational leadership and human behaviours **O25.** Increased organisational effectiveness

Theory 1 transformation of an individual's professional practice through CPD

CPD that is work-based within a context that is enabling, inquiring and supportive and learner-driven, and centred on the provision of facilitated support and reflection and includes self-assessment and a focus on self-awareness, will increase self-confidence, self-awareness, self-efficacy, role clarity, as well as create a positive attitude to change with opportunities for role and career development.

Manley and Jackson 2020). The theories and practical examples of how these can be measured in practice are presented below mapped to the PD principles outlined in Chapter 8.

This theory focuses on contextual opportunities for CPD that are work-based, fostering a culture of inquiry, active and reflective learning, application and implementation of theory and evidence in and from practice (principles 3–6). At an organisational level there must be real investment in the value of workplace learning and development for organisational transformation (PD principles 4, 6, 7). Both the workplace and the organisation are key influencers on whether the outcomes of CPD are achieved for the individual practitioner because both the workplace and the organisation can negatively or positively impact on i) what content is considered important to focus on in terms of learning and development, ii) whether the workplace is valued and used as a resource for learning and development, and iii) how the workplace is used to enable learning and development (principles 1, 2, 4, 7). Key mechanisms for supporting individual professional practice are:

- enabling facilitated support and reflection;
- developing skills in reflection and self-awareness;
- undertaking self-assessment;
- learning that is self-driven by the individual and their interests.

The transformation outcomes for individual professional practice fall into two areas: (1) the individual person, such as confidence and self-efficacy, which encompasses aspects such as how people feel, think, motivate themselves and behave, and (2) their role, for example the provision of person-centred, safe and effective care to their own patients/clients, role clarity, career progression.

A number of different tools and strategies can evidence the impact of CPD learning on the individual practitioner, including personal profiles and portfolios, reflective journaling and critical incident analysis, self-assessment against competence frameworks, 360-degree feedback and personal development action planning, personal stories and narratives about professional transformation, presentations and articles for publication. These enable the practitioner to demonstrate impact at both individual and team level, through increased self-awareness and growth of self-confidence and self-efficacy, critical reflection, role clarity, person-centred practice, using evidence systematically in practice to make a positive impact on patient experience, and using creative problem-solving skills to help themselves and their team to learn from patient feedback.

Theory 2 transformation of skills to meet society's changing healthcare needs through CPD

CPD that focuses on the transformation of skills to meet society's changing healthcare needs, embracing team and system assessment to identify gaps and expand skills to meet a changing healthcare context, will be reflected in better service user experiences of continuity and consistency of service provision, better employability and opportunities for career progression for individuals, more effective teams, better organisational/systems outcomes around integration, partnerships and more effective use of human resources.

This theory focuses on team competences and effectiveness, ensuring that healthcare is adaptable and flexible to ever-changing healthcare needs (principles 3, 4, 7). It is underpinned by concern for social justice that is focused on the provision of equality of opportunity for all learners, irrespective of their personal characteristics or social background, as well as the concept of moral agency, i.e. we all have a responsibility to provide health and social care services that are inclusive and fit for purpose, meeting the needs of everyone in society (principles 1, 2, 4). Four mechanisms for achieving the predicted outcomes are identified as (1) the assessment of systems, team skills and competences, (2) identifying systems and service needs/gaps, (3) expanding and maintaining skills and competences through a range of different strategies, and (4) developing team effectiveness. The outcomes impact on:

- service users and clients – a continuity of service experience;
- the team and its members – opportunities for career progression, better and sustained employability and an effective cohesive team with increased team effectiveness;
- the organisation and system – better integration of services, better partnerships with services and agencies, and better value for money from human resources through substitution and reduced duplication.

Strategies to demonstrate impact include service user feedback, standards reached as part of a registration or revalidation process, and assessment of competence in practice. Measurement of impact indicators include shared purpose and values, patient safety metrics and compliance with national standards. Given that this theory posits the impact of CPD on the whole workforce, other impact indicators that could be evidenced include effective staffing levels, patient experience, improved patient flow and discharge, systematic ways of capturing best practice, and reviewing and improving standards.

Theory 3 transformation of knowledge enabling knowledge translation through CPD

CPD in workplace contexts that both support and encourage engagement with and use of different types of knowledge in everyday practice and active sharing through CPD strategies that focus on using and blending multiple knowledge[3] *to inform professional decision-making; skills in facilitating dialogue, active inquiry and evaluation; and developing practical and theoretical knowledge fostering leadership, evaluation and culture will achieve knowledge-rich cultures recognised by knowledge use and development, active inquiry, innovation and creativity.*

This theory focuses on the immediate workplace in which people work. There is an expectation that staff value and recognise the different types of knowledge required to enable person-centred, safe and effective care to be achieved, e.g. knowledge of the person being cared for; research evidence; expertise that has been rigorously deconstructed through reflection and peer review; local knowledge; policy and so on. Contextual factors include an explicit engagement with and use of different types of knowledge in everyday practice and a workplace culture that enables active sharing of knowledge (principles 1-8). Outcomes identify that knowledge is used in the workplace and the potential to impact on developing knowledge-rich cultures where there is active contribution by staff to

[3] Knowledges encompasses theoretical and practical knowledge, knowledge of the person being cared for/worked with, experience, expertise, artistry, creativity and local knowledge.

development, inquiry creativity and innovation. The mechanisms through which these outcomes arise relate to three levels of activity:

- focus on the everyday decisions that inform professional practice with clients, such as reflecting on the quality and range of knowledge used in practice, and blending and melding different types of knowledge to guide practice;
- focus on a facilitation skillset required across workplace teams to enable others through dialogue to learn about how to use knowledge in practice and through facilitating active inquiry and evaluation of own and collective practice and learning;
- involve developing practical and theoretical knowledge about contextual factors that influence knowledge translation in practice, specifically: leadership, facilitation, evaluation and cultural aspects.

Methods of assessment and evaluation focus on the impact of learning on the practitioner, team and wider service or organisation. Impact indicators to measure include shared vision for the service, KPIs for person-centred practice, patient safety metrics, integrated working, patient at the heart of decision-making, systematic ways of capturing best practice, patient experience, and reviewing and improving standards.

Theory 4 transformation of workplace culture/context to implement workplace and organisational values and purpose relating to person-centred, safe and effective care through CPD

CPD that takes place within contexts where there are shared values and purposes and organisational readiness that draws on CPD strategies which focus on developing and implementing shared values; evaluating the experiences of service users and staff in relation to these values; and developing skills in creating effective workplace cultures through leadership will achieve improved service user and provider experiences, outcomes and impact, sustained person-centred, safe and effective workplace cultures and team effectiveness, increased employee commitment, organisational leadership and effectiveness.

The fourth theory addresses the immediate workplace culture and the implementation of shared values within the workplace, across the organisation and in the wider health economy. Contextually this is dependent on organisational readiness. Six key mechanisms are clustered around three areas (principles 1, 2, 3, 4, 6):

1. *Developing and implementing shared values and beliefs*, specifically:
   - developing shared values and purpose;
   - facilitating the implementation of shared values through feedback, critical reflection, peer support and challenge.
2. *Evaluating experiences of shared values for staff and patients*, specifically:

- evaluating experiences of shared values relating to person-centred, safe and effective care from both service users and staff.

3. *Cultural and leadership skills required to achieve effective workplaces*, specifically:
   - creating a culture that enables individual personal growth, effective relationships and teamwork;
   - developing leadership behaviours.

These four theories help PD practitioners to link ongoing learning in and to their practice at all levels within organisations. Learning with other disciplines facilitates transformational workplace culture change and development.

Summary and conclusion

Undergraduate students who learn person-centred principles and can translate knowledge into person-centred practice help to create flourishing workplaces. This helps to establish a future workforce of person-centred practitioners. Since workplaces bring a wealth of opportunity to learn, develop and improve, applied and ongoing professional development is essential for enabling healthcare practitioners to gain deeper understanding and greater appreciation of what it means to be a professional.

This chapter has demonstrated the value of foundational learning for healthcare practitioners to recognise the importance of developing their person-centred philosophy to underpin their values so that impact is authentic and models person-centred practices. This leads to a workforce that uses person-centred theories and PD methodologies, that strives to continually grow knowledge and skills throughout their career, within their context, with their colleagues. Such learning can lead to transfer of person-centred values in the workplace, enabling practitioners to learn and develop knowledge together in their *place* (PBL) so application is contextualised and impacts more broadly. To continue to develop lifelong knowledge, skills and competences of health professionals, CPD can be used strategically to maximise learning, development, innovation and improvement. These outcomes are possible only when education provided to and with practitioners enables shared exploration of values and uses PD principles to enhance the implementation and impact of the education model.

References

Baird, B., Charles, A., Honeyman, M. et al. (2016). *Understanding pressures in general practice*. The Kings Fund. https://www.kingsfund.org.uk/publications/pressures-in-general-practice

Bodegård, H., Helgesson, G., Juth, N. et al. (2019). Challenges to patient centredness – a comparison of patient and doctor experiences from primary care. *BMC Family Practice* 20 (1): 83.

Boud, D., Keogh, R. and Walker, D. ed. (1985). *Reflection: Turning Experience into Learning*. London: Kogan Page.

Bowen, S., McSeveny, K., Lockley, E. et al. (2013). How was it for you? Experiences of participatory design in the UK health service. *CoDesign* 9 (4): 230–246.

Clay, H. and Stern, R. (2015). *Making time in general practice*. Primary Care Foundation and NHS Alliance. http://www.primarycarefoundation.co.uk/images/PrimaryCare Foundation

Cook, N.F., McCance, T., McCormack, B. et al. (2018). Perceived caring attributes and priorities of preregistration nursing students throughout a nursing curriculum underpinned by person-centredness. *Journal of Clinical Nursing* 27: 2847–2858.

Dewing, J. (2010). Moments of movement: active learning and practice development. *Nurse Education in Practice* 10 (1): 22–26.

Donetto, S., Pierri, P., Tsianakas, V. et al. (2015). Experience-based co-design and healthcare improvement: realizing participatory design in the public sector. *The Design Journal* 18 (2): 227–248.

Eggleton, K., Wearn, A. and Goodyear-Smith, F. (2020). Determining rural learning outcomes for medical student placements using a consensus process with rural clinical teachers. *Education for Primary Care* 31 (1): 24–31.

Executive Agency for Health and Consumers (EAHC) (2013). Study concerning the review and mapping of continuous professional development and lifelong learning for health professionals in the EU. https://ec.europa.eu/health/workforce/key_documents/continuous_professional_development_en

Jackson, C., Manley, K., Wright, T. et al. (2015). Continuing professional development for quality care: context, mechanisms, outcomes and impact. Final Report ECPD ISBN 978-1-909067-39-4

Manley, K. and Jackson, C. (2020). The Venus model for integrating practitioner-led workforce transformation and complex change across the health care system. *Journal of Evaluation in Clinical Practice* 26 (2): 622–634.

Manley, K., Jackson, C. and McKenzie, C. (2019). Microsystems culture change: a refined theory for developing person-centred, safe and effective workplaces based on strategies that embed a safety culture. *International Practice Development Journal* 9 (2) [4].

Manley, K., Martin, A., Jackson, C. et al. (2018). A realist synthesis of effective continuing professional development (CPD): a case study of healthcare practitioners' CPD. *Nurse Education Today* 69: 134–141.

Manley, K., Titchen, A. and McCormack, B. (2013). What is Practice Development and what are the starting points? In: *Practice Development in Nursing and Healthcare* (eds. B. McCormack, K. Manley and A. Titchen), 45–65. Chichester: Wiley-Blackwell.

McCormack, B. and McCance, T. (2017). *Person-centred Practice in Nursing and Health Care: Theory and Practice*. Oxford: John Wiley & Sons Ltd.

Middleton, R. (2013). Active learning and leadership in an undergraduate curriculum: How effective is it for student learning and transition to practice? *Nurse Education in Practice* 13 (2): 83–88.

Middleton, R., Mackay, M., Riley, K. et al. (2018). A creation story of leadership development. *International Practice Development Journal* 8 (1) [9]. https://doi.org/10.19043/ipdj81.009

Middleton, R. and Moroney, T. (2019). Using person-centred principles to inform curriculum. *International Practice Development Journal* 9 (1) [10]: 10-1-10-9.

NHS (2019). NHS England and NHS Improvement funding and resource 2019/20: Supporting 'The NHS long term plan'. https://www.england.nhs.uk/wp-content/uploads/2019/03/nhse-mhsi-funding-and-resource-2019-20-supporting-nhs-ltp.pdf (accessed 2 July 2020).

Niessen, T. and Jacobs, G. (2014). Curriculum design for person-centredness: mindfulness training within a bachelor course in nursing. *International Practice Development Journal* 5 (Special Issue on Person-centredness) [2].

Reid, S.J. (2011). Pedagogy for rural health. *Education for Health* 24 (1): 1–10.

Tynjälä, P. (2013). Toward a 3-P model of workplace learning: a literature review. *Vocational Learning* 6: 11–36.

Voorberg, W.H., Bekkers, V.J.J.M. and Tummers, L.G. (2015). A systematic review of co-creation and co-production. *Public Management Review* 17 (9): 1333–1357.

7. *Critical Ethnography: A Method for Improving Healthcare Cultures in Practice Development and Embedded Research*

Christine Øye, Claudia Green, Katherine Kirk, Cecilia Vindrola-Padros, and Greg Fairbrother

Introduction

Person-centred improvement rests on resolving tensions which may exist between individual knowledge and attitude and collective or work culture-related norms. When resolution occurs, common visions can be targeted and then approached both individually and collectively (Wilson et al. 2020; Collier 2016). Critical ethnography is one of many research approaches which seek to depict and improve workplace care cultures by engaging in collaboration by stakeholders, and where the critical ethnographer works as a facilitator of practice development (PD). Typically, this involves exploring the experiences, cognitions, behaviours and practices of participants within the frames that influence the care work. Critical ethnography can be used to improve healthcare quality, especially when it is used in close collaboration with stakeholders in the co-production of knowledge (Greenhalgh and Swinglehurst 2011). It can be utilised to inform and drive PD in specific unit or workplace cultures and also at the broader organisational culture level in healthcare. Two case studies, one from Australia and one from the UK, are presented and discussed in the chapter. They show how embeddedness and 'internality/externality' can be brought to bear differently, depending on the context. Foundational questions to be asked by a critical ethnographer are: 'What happens here?' and 'What can we learn from this to improve the care culture?'

International Practice Development in Health and Social Care, Second Edition.
Edited by Kim Manley, Valerie Wilson, and Christine Øye.

The critical ethnographer seeks to immerse themselves in the everyday life of differently positioned stakeholders in study sites (Pensoneau-Conway and Toyosaki 2011). This means that critical ethnographers work directly with and for the people they are studying, in natural workplace settings. In this sense, there is a fundamental 'embeddedness' entailed in critical ethnography. It seeks to combine critical perspectives with practical knowledge in order to promote or drive emancipatory change (Madison 2012; Foley and Valenzuela 2005). Critical ethnography extends conventional ethnography's concern with describing 'what is' and tries to speak up on the stakeholders' behalf, and in addition to describing 'what is', asks 'why is this, and what can be done about it?' (Cook 2005, p. 132). Accordingly, the critical ethnographic investigation focuses on what can be improved, not only on what the empirical field looks like (Batch and Windsor 2015). In the workplace context, critical ethnography can be powerfully used, as it allows for investigation, analysis, co-facilitation and learning, to bring about improvement-oriented action and practice transformation (Foley and Valenzuela 2005). The critical ethnographer can challenge stakeholders' points of view and engage participants in analysis and reflection on their experiences and practices. That is, a critical ethnographer can facilitate persons in a workplace to begin to change unsafe, unsatisfactory or poor practices. The ethnographer can become an external co-facilitator who seeks to help participants to reflect on the roots of the problem in order to choose appropriate action in favour of developing and elevating care practices (Cook 2005). The roots of problems are often anchored in structure and culture; therefore, a critical ethnographer will try to discover and unravel these historical, cultural and social frameworks influencing poor or non-person-centred practices observed (Madison 2012). Accordingly, a critical ethnographer will not only seek to grasp the native points of views and their practices but will also try to embed an analysis of macro-theoretical factors by describing, for instance, hierarchy and inequality (Marcus 1998). Considering the 'macro picture' positions the critical ethnographer to shed light on 'unacknowledged biases' that may result from implicit values, in order to provide new avenues for reflexive inquiry and dialogue around transformation and improvement (Foley and Valenzuela 2005). The knowledge produced by critical ethnography is partial and situated in a critical reflexive dialogue within the context of collaboration with stakeholders to resolve the roots of problems. As such, the critical ethnographer will engage in a meaning-making process around what has been seen, heard and interpreted in close collaboration with participants (Shih 2018). Therefore, the 'what is' or cultural traits is a 'co-product' between the researcher and the stakeholders throughout the whole collaborative research process.

Critical ethnographer as an embedded researcher

In PD it is not uncommon that researchers function as embedded co-facilitators (Dahl et al. 2018; Øye et al. 2019; Wilson et al. 2020). This is also the case in the tradition of critical ethnography where knowledge is co-produced (Shih 2018). Accordingly, the researcher is not the representative who presents the social reality as a 'true' reality on behalf of the stakeholders. Rather, the immersed critical ethnographer will be concerned with 'how we come to know what culture means' (Shih 2018, p. 3) in this particular setting, then critically engaging with stakeholders to transform collective experiences and expertise in care improvement work. Instead of being a researcher from the outside looking in as an expert, a critical ethnographer will engage in reflexive inquiry, questioning her/his role as an 'expert' based on how he/she has positioned him/herself (Tedlock 2000; Atkinson and Hammersley 1994). Therefore, a critical ethnographer will often consciously diminish their power by playing the role of a democratic facilitator and consciousness-raiser working with differently positioned stakeholders (Foley and Valenzuela 2005). The facilitator will then function as a cultural broker, challenging implicit values in the workplace culture, as well as pinpointing awareness of powerful structures which frame the care culture. Being a cultural broker in a workplace might be ethically challenging, due to professional pride and reputation (Øye et al. 2019; Mosse 2011). This is because firstly, ethnographic descriptions of the care culture can be perceived as threatening and irrelevant to staff communities, since ethnographic descriptions often examine and reveal the back-stage care practices. In a healthcare setting, for example, back-stage spaces and associated practices may include the rest room or linen cupboard, where staff may behave in ways that are not reflective of their usual behaviour, perhaps using language perceived as unprofessional or offensive or showing intense emotion outwardly. As such, ethnographic descriptions draw attention to the hidden or unnoticed values and effects which staff might not recognise or otherwise agree about (Mosse 2011). Therefore, when presenting their data, a critical ethnographer must pay attention to the overall values, views and vulnerabilities of staff groups they work with (Oeye et al. 2007). In addition, they should be open to how knowledge was produced, based on what has been seen, heard and perceived as a participant observer. Thereafter, the critical ethnographer can engage in reflective dialogue with staff over how to interpret the data (Wilson et al. 2020) in order to avoid a form of negative judgement on care practices that the staff might be proud of (Oeye et al. 2007). The data-sourced feedback, reflective dialogues and collective analysis will all inform the action plan for care improvement (Wilson et al. 2020), and as such the critical ethnographic work can be integral to an action cycle by facilitatively informing the reflection and observation phases, and as a facilitator of improvement targeting action (see Figure 7.1).

Introducing two case studies

Two cases which illustrate the utility of critical ethnography as a PD tool are presented. First, a case from Australia, where critical ethnography using an internal/external facilitator approach was used to drive communication practice improvement in an aged care setting. Second, a case from the UK, which illustrates how an external researcher can be embedded within a care culture to improve practice. The chapter draws from both cases to examine the notion of the positionality of the ethnographer when working on improving care cultures.

The project aimed to employ critical ethnography to raise staff awareness about everyday communication practices between healthcare providers and patients and

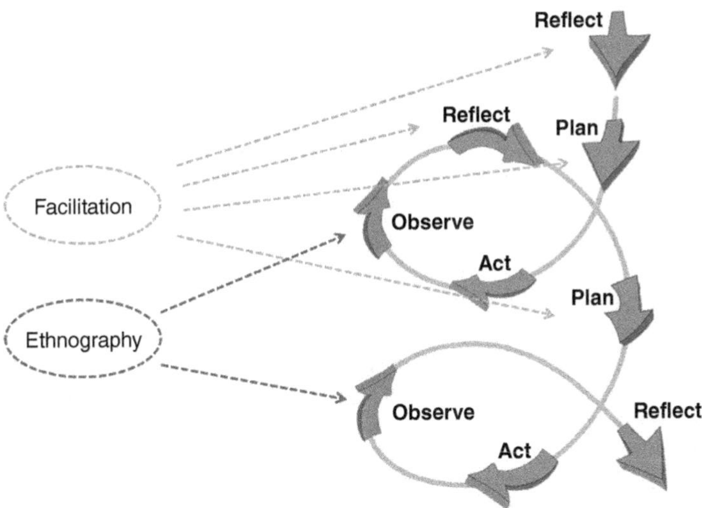

Figure 7.1 Locating critical ethnography in the action cycle (*Source:* Greg Fairbrother and Claudia Green)

Case study 1 Communication practice change in a metropolitan Australian inpatient aged care setting

This work was conducted in two inpatient aged care units in a metropolitan teaching hospital, as part of a state-wide practice development programme (Essentials of Care programme) (NSW Health 2009) whose aim was to improve professional practice using participatory methods such as critical ethnography and facilitation (see Figure 7.1). The Essentials of Care programme targets nine domains for improvement. The three domains relevant to the reported case study were clinical practice (model of care), communication, and staff learning and development.

to investigate the impact of this on person-centred care delivery. A further aim which developed as the project proceeded was to introduce a peer review process to the clinical units. This was achieved by pairing external and internal practice developers to undertake ethnographic activities in order to develop and facilitate ethnographic, facilitation and leadership skillsets. Critical ethnography was considered to be a potentially useful methodological approach to the 'problem' of communication on the units, as it was felt that its observation-based character ought to shed light on the characteristics of everyday communication practices. Two situational contexts for observation were chosen: the clinical shift handover and the patient bedside (four-bed room bays). Three key domains of observational focus were chosen by the project group: i) patient-related communication (e.g. discussing patients at handover and direct patient–staff member communication, ii) process-related communication (e.g. when undertaking procedures, work-related plans), and iii) learning and development related (bedside clinical teaching, clinical questioning, etc.).

An ethnographer (practice developer and external facilitator) with nursing leaders (facilitators) internal to the units being studied observed the quality and depth of clinical and interpersonal communication (1) between nurses at shift handover and (2) between nurses, allied health professionals, medical officers, patients and carers at the bedside throughout the shift. The ethnographer worked with internal facilitators over a 12-month period to feed back observational findings, create space for reflective practice, support staff to make sense of the information arising, challenge perceptions where necessary, and help to identify actions that could result in the team's desired changes and outcomes.

Three processes were employed to build a consistent model of ethnographic and facilitation practice: i) the expert ethnographer/facilitator conducted ethnography and facilitated sessions alongside a unit-based novice (i.e. a staff member who was internal to the work culture); ii) following this, the novice's ethnographic and facilitation practice was observed and feedback provided; iii) the novice independently conducted ethnographic and facilitated sessions independent of the expert, but participated in periodic supervision around their practice.

As a result of conducting this work, it was noted that using ethnography (under an external–internal partnership model) afforded significant benefits to culture change-oriented work. There were two broad benefit areas: i) staff engagement with practice and workplace change; ii) development of local ethnography and facilitation expertise and leadership capability.

The project enabled the creation of a shared unit-based space where:

- staff could have access to real-time, rich, specific and contextual information that they could use to inform change;
- an external ethnographic observer could capture information previously taken for granted (i.e. implicit communication practices which were not ideal) by those immersed in the culture;
- facilitated discussions surrounding the observed staff culture could focus change activities on aspects over which the internal players had influence;
- critical reflection could be activated in real time and imminent to the actual observations – this provided opportunities for learning in practice.

The ethnographic work surfaced three held beliefs that appeared to impact on the progress and outcomes of the staff's communication practices: i) diffusion of responsibility ('it's not my responsibility to fix things, "they" should fix this'), ii) helplessness ('things will never change and we need to just make do'), and iii) a tendency to support rhetoric that change was outside of the staff's influence ('we have no control over what happens, "they" will never let us change this'). The staff regularly expressed that others were responsible for the quality of clinical and relational communication and that it was outside of their control to change anything, despite their feeling that practices were less than optimal. Staff regularly expressed that aspects such as time, lack of staff and busyness were barriers to optimal communication and that these conditions were outside of their control and would never change.

These beliefs were discussed and challenged through the facilitative processes which ensued in unit-based discussion sessions. These discussions yielded meaning-making, a drive for action and finally a locus of control shift whereby collective agreement was reached that actions could proceed positively. A range of emotions and reactions was voiced in the sessions. These included anger, disbelief, suspicion, shock, validation and urgency to fix and change. There was also a group experience of 'crisis' (Fay 1987). The energy generated by this discomfort was directed to planned and systematic change. As a result of the information sharing based on the ethnography findings, the staff were able to evaluate and compare and contrast between actual versus perceived communication practices, cultural enablers and barriers, and from there to shift focus to what could be influenced. This focus shift powered some quick changes and directed long-term plans regarding communication with patients and staff.

The outcomes achieved were encouraging. One unit commenced with implementing a person-centred multidisciplinary team (MDT) communication strategy. MDT meetings were moved to the bedside in order to involve the patient and family/significant people. This shift also allowed for the MDT to have access to contextually relevant clinical, social and psychological information regarding the patient. This team used the Essentials of Care Framework (NSW Health 2009), which prescribes an action research approach as an ongoing structural guide/ informant to the change management process.

The second unit focused their work on the model of care. This involved shifting their approach from a loosely structured individual patient allocation (IPA) model to a team-based model which incorporated some aspects of the IPA approach to account for variations in skills and experience. Research around the clinical impacts of the new model of care is ongoing. The methodologically strong and ongoing nature of the critical ethnography-sparked improvement work (and how such work can 'spin off' into further research) is illustrated in Figure 7.2, the 'PD

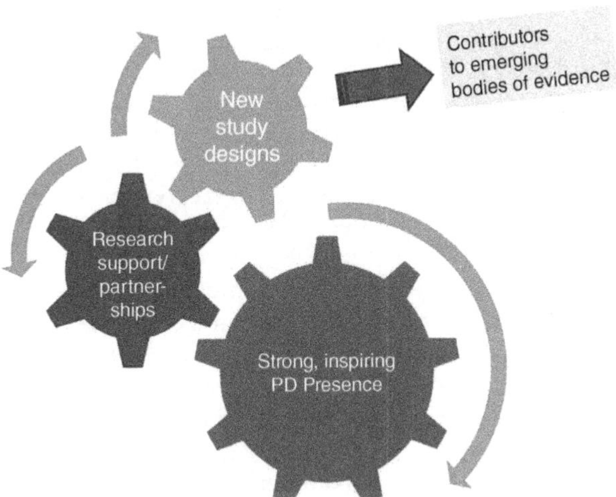

Figure 7.2 The 'PD wheel' – using PD as a starting point to drive research-based change (*Source:* Greg Fairbrother and Claudia Green)

wheel', which seeks to illustrate how a strong unit-based (or organisation-based) PD presence can partner with methodologically strong collaborators (in this case ethnographers) to drive research-based change and ongoing research output.

Case 1 Some summary characteristics of the case study

Project aim	To drive workplace improvement on communication practices and care model through facilitated discussions
Collaboration	Internal–external collaboration was the founding frame for the approach taken
Facilitation	Facilitation by both internal and external partners among clinical staff. Key material for facilitated discussion: findings from the ethnography
Critical ethnography (design)	Internal–external (shared) ethnography. Immersion in the unit culture via participant observation throughout work shifts. Values, attitudes, beliefs and practices were observed
Methods	Participant observation, patient interviews, reflection notes
Feedback	Reflexive inquiry and dialogue among clinical staff
Observed changes	Material changes in approach to staff–patient communication and care model were observed over time

Case study 2 Changes in service delivery in a UK hospital

The case study in the UK was based on the experiences of an embedded researcher with a background in medical anthropology working in a children's hospital. The embedded research role was based on the researcher having dual affiliation (to the hospital and to an academic institution) and being introduced to hospital staff as a member of the team. The researcher's use of anthropological perspectives and her familiarity with ethnographic research were considered assets in the hospital's attempt to explore and change some aspects of organisational culture, particularly in relation to clinicians' willingness to engage with technological innovations to improve care delivery. These fundamental cultural issues within organisations, such as facilitation, competing stakeholder perspectives/expectations and concerns, are intrinsic to PD theory more broadly.

Some hospital managers were trying to implement a new system for scheduling doctor consultations that used a fixed template for assigning appointments. At that time, waiting times for certain outpatient services were long, causing patient dissatisfaction and delays in the delivery of care. Each service organised its own appointments using simple tools such as spreadsheets and, in some cases, paper-based recording. This meant errors were frequent and information was sometimes lost. The new system would ensure all services used the same online template with fixed time slots, with some flexibility for overbooking. Managers anticipated that the hospital would need a 'deep cultural shift' to incorporate this new online system into routine practice. The new system was implemented using a top-down approach and led by senior managers, established as a potentially problematic approach in PD because change is imposed and organisational cultures are characterised by 'command and control' approaches rather than enabling and including frontline staff.

A partnership with a medical anthropologist who could work with staff to understand old and new booking systems, including perceptions and experiences with the new system, seemed like a good approach to help inform and facilitate implementation. The aim of the study was to:

1. use an ethnographic lens to capture and share everyday practices in relation to organisational and cultural aspect
2. document barriers and facilitators in the implementation of the new system and how these varied by context and professionals involved
3. co-produce (with hospital staff) a process for designing and implementing similar future interventions.

The researcher documented processes of design and implementation using participant observation, informal conversations and semi-structured interviews with a purposive sample of staff. The study was carried out over a six-month period. Initial work on the project highlighted the fact that staff views had not been taken into consideration when designing the new system. When the new system was officially introduced to staff, it was not well received, as concerns were voiced regarding its suitability for some services. Most doctors continued to use their own spreadsheets and paper-based booking systems.

Some of the managers who designed the new system indicated that the reason the system was not working was because 'the doctors' culture makes them resistant to change'. Management viewed the new system as part of a 'culture change' where doctors needed to align to a new standard way of working. Their 'culture' was seen as homogeneous, easily identifiable and static.

The study carried out by the embedded researcher pointed to a different, more complex, picture. First, not all doctors thought the new system was a bad idea; some liked it and felt it would help them organise their services better. However, they did not engage with the new system because they felt the hospital would eventually discontinue its use. Other doctors who liked the system were not able to voice their approval because they were in junior positions or had recently transferred from another hospital, and since several senior doctors in the service opposed the new system, they felt they also needed to be seen to be against it. For doctors who did not like the new system, the main reason was that it was not designed in relation to the requirements of their service. Doctors wanted to be able to shape the appointments in relation to their patients' needs and combine outpatient consultations with private practice, inpatient rounds or academic commitments. Some also felt that the fixed timeslot booking method did not reflect the amount of time some patients required during consultation.

This understanding of doctors' daily practices was used to engage with a new way of working with staff, one that was based on open participation as well as the recognition of power relations and hierarchies acting across the organisation, and the wider context of healthcare delivery (for instance, financial pressures that resulted in the cutting of resources for clinicians, staffing reductions and an increase in patient demand). The embedded researcher, a group of hospital managers and a group of clinicians created a working group to redesign the outpatient booking system. The embedded researcher played a facilitator role, translating desires and issues across the group to ensure different points of views were heard and taken into consideration. She also tried to maintain more bottom-up, collaborative practices, by making sure the needs and desires of those who would ultimately be using the system (i.e. clinicians) were at the centre of the redesign of the system. These 'bottom-up' practices, which encourage and empower shared decision-making, again relate back to core PD concepts. Through this approach, the embedded researcher aimed to achieve a sense of shared purpose among the managers and frontline clinicians. The new system was rolled out and was incorporated into routine practice with greater ease. These meetings were also used as a blueprint for future intervention design processes, where relevant stakeholders were brought together during early stages of design to review plans and provide input.

Case 2 Some summary characteristics of the case study

Project aim	To facilitate the implementation of interventions aimed at service improvement
Collaboration	Researcher–hospital manager–clinician collaboration
Facilitation	Ethnographic research on staff perceptions and experiences with a new intervention facilitated conversations about the need to develop a new approach for intervention co-design
Critical ethnography	Immersion in the hospital through an embedded research role
Methods	Participant observation, informal conversations and semi-structured interviews
Feedback	Reflexive inquiry and dialogue with clinical staff and hospital managers
Observed changes	Changes in approaches to design and implement interventions aimed at improving service delivery were observed by the researcher

Critical ethnography: a method for discovering 'hidden' practices and an avenue for practice development

Case Study 1 shows that by using critical ethnography in a sophisticated manner it is possible to improve care cultures in a person-centred way. The case especially highlights the need to improve staff's communication practices based on a baseline perception by staff that 'poor' communication practices were at play. The project highlighted the importance of diffusion of responsibility, helplessness and a view that change was outside the staff's control and influence as key barriers to overcome, using good facilitation practices. These challenges were also highlighted in case study 2. Here, the embedded researcher called on skills of translation and facilitation to mitigate professional boundaries and achieve a shared sense of purpose. Both case studies highlighted challenging staff cultures or even crisis to varying degrees (see Chapter 9) and at first staff were not motivated to engage in improvement work. However, the ethnographic work showed that there was a contrast between communication practice perceived as 'poor' and communication practice that staff understood to be 'better' or ideal. The ethnographic work revealed information unseen as well as taken for granted, and as such revealed habitualised values and beliefs (e.g. Foley and Valenzuela 2005; Atkinson and Hammersley 1994). Barriers outside the control of staff, such as time, staff shortness and busyness, were also revealed. These barriers can be understood as 'roots of problems' anchored in historical structures not easy to reveal or change (Marcus 1998; Madison 2012). Nevertheless, the 'roots of problems' were identified (Cook 2005) and with the help of ethnographic facilitators, new avenues for improvement were pinpointed. The facilitators 'opened up' appropriate person-centred action alternatives. The ethnographic work lay closely alongside the facilitated discussion work in temporal terms. This was an advantage, as observations could be wielded to prompt reflection and action planning in a 'real-time' way.

In case study 2, the ethnographer revealed other kinds of 'roots of problems' such as power relations and hierarchies implementing a new booking system. The ethnographic work shed light on the fact that the view held by management staff that 'the doctors' culture makes them resistant to change' did not account for the complex factors shaping the doctors' attitude towards the new system. Typically, the complex factors were a mixture of structural factors such as financial pressure and cultural stereotypes in relation to the doctors' culture. Moreover, the ethnographic investigation revealed that the management, when first implementing the new system, did not recognise that doctors are a heterogeneous group with different needs, patient types, interests and capacity to influence other doctors. An ethnographic lens discovered this heterogeneity and found avenues for management to work with doctors who actually liked the new system. Furthermore, it was discovered that several doctors had already recognised that waiting time was a problem and had started to make changes in their own booking systems. Accordingly, the critical ethnographic investigation in both cases discovered a complexity of factors either hindering or promoting care, which provide opportunities for building on these factors to find new avenues for PD.

Internal–external partnership in practice development

In case study 1, the work was done using an external–internal partnership model by connecting an external ethnographer with an internal novice PD facilitator, where both were doing ethnographic work. This model proved to be invaluable, as the PD facilitator had insider or situational knowledge and longstanding and important inside relationships. In this way she was able to become a research-informed and positive influencer, not a subjectively informed (and potentially ineffective) influencer. The ethnographic partnership and teamwork also revealed that the work improved leadership skill sets. Action plans for change needed to be led and leadership skills needed to be tested and workshopped as the project moved forward. The external facilitator proved to be invaluable here, as she could 'coach' local leaders over time, once action goals were agreed upon by all. The paired model provided support to the internal facilitator of change, in a role that is often described as isolated and challenging in PD (Dahl et al. 2018), and opportunities for learning for both occurred 'on the run'. Case study 1 demonstrated similarly that initial use of facilitated ethnographic methods can enable change-oriented action plans based on evidence, not subjective opinion, to have a good chance of success, and also prompts skill development on multiple fronts (e.g. leadership, ethnography, research literacy/capacity and facilitation). In case study 2, the embedded ethnographer worked as a cultural broker sharing and translating knowledge across different positioned stakeholders in order to improve the organisational culture. However, being a cultural broker by sharing uncomfortable findings such as preconceived notions of clinical culture might be ethically demanding due to inherent power relations and professional reputation and pride (Øye et al. 2019; Mosse 2011). Nevertheless, in PD a facilitator works continuously with teams and individuals using personal and cultural wisdom in order to preserve pride, reputation and dignity.

Positionality of the embedded ethnographer in practice development

In case study 2, focusing on the positionality of the embedded researcher has highlighted the challenges of being in a dual role in critical ethnographic research. The embedded researcher must maintain a critical distance and at the same time strive for trust by being close to the participants, sharing information with them, described as 'the ambivalence of distance and familiarity' (Atkinson and Hammersley 1994, p. 256). The role of keeping a distance from the healthcare organisation in order to retain their ability to share 'uncomfortable' findings with the wider, and often more senior, team and at the same time being close to discover 'backstage' and implicit values and practices is challenging. This is one of the many roles and dilemmas for the researcher as they 'juggle' competing expectations. It is possible, as in all anthropological studies, that the researcher may become 'native' within the setting (Tedlock 2000) – arguably, more likely in health service research as the success of the research depends largely on the strength of individual relationships, access and 'buy-in'. At the same time the researcher must work hard to maintain their critical distance from both subjects and setting, a challenge that can be partly addressed through maintaining strong academic connections. Moreover, an embedded researcher will often be puzzled by the question of representation (Shih 2018; Marcus 1998): how does the ethnographer as a facilitator present the everyday complexity to the stakeholders? And not least, who they represent when presenting what has been seen, heard and learned since different stakeholders may have different views and interests in the project. Despite the allegiances researchers may or may not feel, it is ultimately the role of the embedded researcher to facilitate representation of all stakeholder groups. Again, the emphasis is on working to achieve a shared voice and vision across organisational, professional and broader cultural barriers for successful PD to work (see Chapters 8 and 16).

Conclusion

The chapter highlights how critical ethnography supports PD and its role in embedded research for the purpose of improving care and healthcare cultures in a more person-centred manner. Critical ethnography can reveal inconsistencies between what people say and utter and what they actually do (see Chapter 15). Case study 1 showed that despite staff being in a collective crisis, a critical ethnographic study with a facilitated discussion component involving ethnographers who were both internal and external to the work culture could reveal promising care practices as well as poor ones. This sets the stage for productive values-based discussion regarding action alternatives, action planning, change management and finally new research-based 'spin-offs' from the originating critical ethnography work. Case study 2 showed that critical ethnography can help unpack preconceived and taken-for-granted notions of organisational culture to allow for dynamic and collaborative ways of working among hospital staff.

Critical ethnography is a strong methodological partner to PD. It motivates action when partnered in PD-facilitated relationships and involves working in close partnership with staff and stakeholders. Positionality and ethical awareness are important as an immersed ethnographer lies betwixt and between different roles and tasks. Involving and mentoring insiders to use critical ethnography has much potential to inform PD across different health and social care contexts, from micro to meso and macro levels.

References

Atkinson, P. and Hammersley, M. (1994). Ethnography and participant observation. In: *Handbook of Qualitative Research* (eds. K. Denzin and Y.S. Lincoln), 83–99. Thousand Oaks: Sage Publications.

Batch, M. and Windsor, C. (2015). Nursing casualization and communication: a critical ethnography. *Journal of Advanced Nursing* 71 (4): 870–880.

Collier, A. (2016). Practice development using video-reflexive ethnography: promoting safe space(s) towards the end of life in hospital. *International Practice Development Journal* 6 (1): 1–16.

Cook, K.E. (2005). Using critical ethnography to explore issues in health promotion. *Qualitative Health Research* 15 (1): 129–138. https://www.doi.org/10.1177/1049732304267751.

Dahl, H., Dewing, J., Mekki, T.E. et al. (2018). Facilitation of a workplace learning intervention in a fluctuating context: an ethnographic, participatory research project in a nursing home in Norway. *International Practice Development Journal* 8 (2): 1–17. http://doi.org/10.19043/ipdj.82.004

Fay, B. (1987). *Critical Social Science: Liberation and Its Limits*. New York: Cornell University Press.

Foley, D. and Valenzuela, A. (2005). Critical ethnography: the politics of collaboration. In: *Handbook of Qualitative Research* (eds. N.K. Denzin and Y.S Lincoln), 217–234. Thousand Oaks, CA: Sage Publications.

Greenhalgh, T. and Swinglehurst, D. (2011). Studying technology use as social practice: the untapped potential for ethnography. *BMC Medicine* 9: 45.

Madison, D.S. (2012). *Critical Ethnography: Methods, Ethics and Performance*. Los Angeles: Sage Publications.

Marcus, G.E. (1998). *Ethnography through Thick and Thin*. New Jersey: Princeton University Press.

Mosse, D. (2011). Politics and ethics: ethnographies of expert knowledge and professional identities. In: *Policy Worlds. Anthropology and the Analysis of Contemporary Power* (eds. C. Shore, S. Wright and D. Però), 50–67. New York: Berghahn Books.

NSW Health (2009). *Essentials of Care: Working with Essentials of Care: A Resource Guide for Facilitators*. Sydney: New South Wales Department of Health.

Oeye, C., Bjelland, A.K. and Skorpen, A. (2007). Doing participant observation in a psychiatric hospital – research ethics resumed. *Social Science & Medicine* 65 (11): 2296–2306.

Øye, C., Sørensen, N.Ø., Dahl, H. and Glasdam, S. (2019). Tight ties in collaborative health research puts research ethics on trial? A discussion on autonomy, confidentiality, and integrity in qualitative research. *Qualitative Health Research* 29 (8): 1227 – 1235. http://Doi:10.1177/1049732318822294

Pensoneau-Conway, S.L. and Toyosaki, S. (2011) Automethodology: tracing a home for praxis-oriented ethnography. *International Journal of Qualitative Methods* 10 (4): 378–399.

Shih, P. (2018). Critical ethnography in public health: politicizing culture and politicizing methodology. In: *Handbook of Research Methods in Health Social Sciences* (ed. P. Liamputtong), 1–15. Singapore: Springer.

Tedlock, B. (2000). Ethnography and ethnographic representation. In: *The Handbook of Qualitative Research* (eds. N.K. Denzin and Y.S. Lincoln), 455–486. Thousand Oaks, CA: Sage Publications.

Wilson, V., Dewing, J., Cardiff, S. et al. (2020). A person-centred observational tool: devising the Workplace Culture Critical Analysis Tool. *International Practice Development Journal* 10 (1). http://doi:org/10.19043/ipdj.101.003

8. *A Global Manifesto for Practice Development: Revisiting Core Principles*

Sally Hardy, Simone Clarke, Irena Anna Frei, Claire Morley, Jo Odell, Chris White, and Valerie Wilson

Introduction

This chapter provides a revision of practice development's core principles through undertaking a stakeholder critical review process to co-create a revised set of principle statements suitable for a contemporary global audience.

Nine practice development (PD) principles, published in the first edition of *International Practice Development in Health and Social Care* (Manley et al. 2008), were derived from PD practice and research across a broad range of contexts, countries and stakeholders. The purpose of having such principles is to provide guidance for those undertaking PD activities and to distinguish these from other improvement initiatives.

PD offers a framework to stimulate values-based and practice-driven realisation of change as worthwhile, yet recognising aspects can provoke anxiety. PD provides a supportive framework that enables people to move through change as a process of enlightenment, towards empowerment, moving further to emancipation and beyond, into a renewed existence, as a culture of transformation (Friere 1973; Grundy 1982; Fay 1987; Morrow and Torres 2002). PD is also a process of self-discovery, enhanced through skilled facilitation. PD uses a variety of evidence required for implementing, monitoring and enhancing effective, evidence-based strategies that achieve systems-wide sustainable change.

PD principles inform the International Practice Development Collaborative's (IPDC) shared curriculum for the Foundation PD School (delivered in the UK

International Practice Development in Health and Social Care, Second Edition.
Edited by Kim Manley, Valerie Wilson, and Christine Øye.

since the mid-1990s, extended internationally from 2001 to Canada, South Africa and across Europe, New Zealand and Australia), plus the Advanced PD School (see Chapter 10), established since 2017 in Australia and Europe.

The use of PD principles within the published literature has focused on increased understanding of facilitation (Timlin et al. 2018; Price et al. 2016; Filmalter et al. 2015), using creativity in research and practice (Roberts and Williams 2017; Yalden et al. 2013), using critical reflection to achieve health-full outcomes (Murray and Tuqiri 2020), blending approaches to incorporate evidence-based practice (Fairbrother et al. 2015) and quality improvement (Manley et al. 2017), further extending understanding and application of systematic evaluation (Wilson and McCance 2015; Odell 2018).

Several years have elapsed since their launch in 2008, so a re-examination was considered timely to ensure the PD principles remain fit for contemporary purposes. It was anticipated that analysis of the principles would provide insight into how they are being used and ways they may be modified to enhance their versatility into the future. While some PD principles have been more readily translated into practice, a revision is timely to ensure they remain relevant and translatable across different contemporary workplace contexts across multiple settings (e.g. education, healthcare, social care and research). An international stakeholder critical review has guided the revision process.

Revising the PD principles through a stakeholder review process

Seven contributing authors from six IPDC member organisations comprised the review team: three members from New South Wales (NSW), two members from the UK and single members from Tasmania and Switzerland. These volunteers led the critical review process, gathering stakeholder feedback from their networks. Although there was a need to remain outcome-focused, PD values guided the process. The review team ensured PD methodologies were used throughout, with each facilitated meeting using PD principles of collaboration, inclusion and participation (Manley et al. 2013).

At the first meeting it was agreed that each of the seven IPDC members would devise their own methods for gaining feedback on the utility and applicability of the 2008 PD principles, taking into consideration which feedback strategies would work best in their local contexts. Although there were slight variations in methods used for gathering feedback, the nine PD principles were shared with a set of questions to stimulate discussion and critique, capturing 184 direct respondents, across a variety of stakeholder participants (refer to Table 8.1). Tasmania participants were asked to consider the following questions: Are they meaningful? Do they draw you in and make you want to know more? Is the wording correct? Other groups (i.e. Switzerland and NSW) used the 'Concerns, Claims and Issues' exercise (Guba and Lincoln 1989) for collective critique. In the UK, invitations to participate in a review were sent out via the Foundation of Nursing Studies

Table 8.1 Stakeholder critical review of PD principles

IPDC member organisation	Method used	Persons involved	Key themes from feedback inspiring the revision
Foundation of Nursing Studies, UK	Email call and subsequently personal conversation Principles sent out via email with a set of questions and then feedback sought verbally over phone and in discussion	7 2 people new to PD 3 attended foundation PD school 2 advanced PD Senior Nurse, PHE Community Practice and Professional Development Nurse, Wales Head of Nursing Professional Development, Leeds Practice Educator, Hospice, Scotland Lecturer and practice development facilitator QMU Scotland FoNS team (2)	• Collaboration, inclusion and participation with all stakeholders are key • Enabling learning for people is key in everything we do • The importance of having or developing self-awareness and the role of critical reflection • The three Es of enlightenment, empowerment and emancipation • Transformation of others and ourselves. Life-long learning • Importance of skilled facilitation and development of this, also linked to three Es • Sphere of influence and change, innovation at different levels within an organisation • Values-led
Imagining Potential Across Complex Teams (ImPACT) hosted by University of East Anglia, England	Newsletter to Council of Deans (to all HEIs) and staff emails	5 Council of Deans, occupational therapist, nurse educator, midwife, mental health nurse educator	• Very useful to have principles • Principles work across disciplines • Language use • Improvement-focused

(Conti.)

Table 8.1 *(cont.)*

IPDC member organisation	Method used	Persons involved	Key themes from feedback inspiring the revision
Network of Practice Development Units of the University Hospitals Basel, Berne and Zurich, Switzerland	Face-to-face sessions in the three network organisations: 'Claims, Concerns and Issues' exercise. Co-creating critical questions around relevance to practice and accessibility of PD principles.	29 CNS working as unit-based practice developers Advanced facilitators Heads of PD units	• Principles are an inspiring source for the daily work with patients and staff. They are helpful for reflection with staff members and in PD projects • The language is overpowering and some terms have been difficult to translate into German • Some principles need to be untangled to get a better understanding
Tasmanian Health Organisation – South and University of Tasmania, Australia	Initial brainstorm session with the leaders of PD Tasmania. Email to all staff who had attended a PD school in Tasmania (76) for comment. Face-to-face session (n=12) to work through revised principles – reached agreement on eight new principles. All staff emailed revised principles and given three weeks to seek comments from colleagues.	76 Staff members who have attended a PD school Members of the PD Tas group, very familiar with PD principles Nursing Directors Senior lecturer at UTAS Advisor to state minister for education and mental health Clinical nurse educators with varying levels of exposure to PD	• We need to understand who the principles are for • Current language is overwhelming and does not draw you in • Current language made PD difficult to explain to the uninitiated

University of Wollongong, NSW, Australia	Group discussion: 'Claims, Concerns and Issues' exercise Co-creating critical questions around relevance to practice and accessibility of PD principles	21 Participants from Advanced Facilitation Course and facilitators of the programme (9) University of Wollongong person-centred community of practice (12)	Language • Simplify language including for the micro-system (staff, patients and families) • Principles could be summed up in a couple of words to help recall Sharing • More focus on relationships • Able to share principles with patients, carers and other consumers Leadership • Add leadership principle (distinct from positional authority) Focus on the unique selling point (USP) of PD and how it complements related improvement work and learning approaches
Sydney Children's Hospital Network, NSW, Australia	Group discussion: 'Claims, Concerns and Issues' exercise Co-creating critical questions around relevance to practice and accessibility of PD principles	39 Experienced PD facilitators as well as varied levels of PD knowledge and skills Essentials of Care programme coordinators, a state-wide programme in NSW that uses practice development as a foundation (30) Child and adolescent mental health nurse managers and clinicians who work with PD (9)	• Language: 'overwhelming' and 'too wordy', requires updating to make it more accessible • Leadership: include specific reference to leadership • Sharing: want to share principles with patients and colleagues in simple ways • Principles guide PD work – 'it's a way of being, not doing' in the way we work, supports working with PD alongside other programmes and initiatives • Importance of examples to illustrate each principle

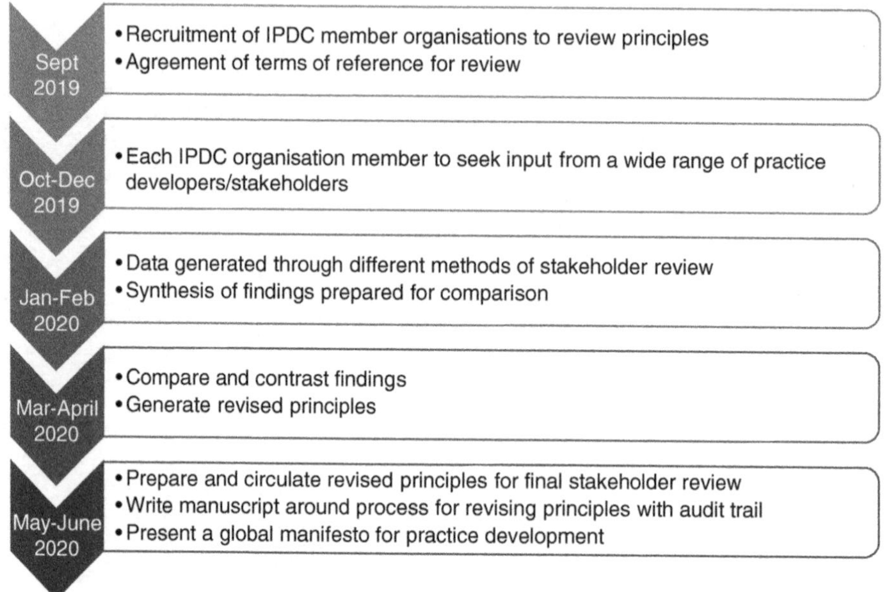

Figure 8.1 Stakeholder critical review timelines

(FoNS) newsletter and all higher education institutes offering health and social care education, via the Council of Deans network.

The revision team themed results from their stakeholders' feedback, identifying findings to be shared at the regular review meetings. Taking on board all feedback and emergent themes, alongside ongoing critique via online discussions, progress was slow (see Figure 8.1). Therefore, as deadlines loomed, each author agreed to take ownership of one or two principles and to propose a new principle statement. An audit trail was maintained, to show how each of the original nine principles have been updated, reshaped and amended to ensure a contemporary re-envisioning. These revised principles were again circulated to a smaller stakeholder group for an external critique. Each team member provided further commentary alongside their suggested revisions, which culminated in the agreed wording for eight revised PD principles, achieved at the review team's online discussion on 27 May 2020 (see Table 8.2).

Emergent themes

Theme 1: Accessible language

Participants recommended the need for short statements that could be more easily recalled and memorised when trying to share PD principles with others. For example, one Australian participant explained:

> *The language is overpowering and just doesn't draw me in, in fact it pushes me away.*

Table 8.2 Audit trail of the process for revising the original practice development principles (Manley et al. 2008) 26 May 2020

PD principles	a. Manley et al. 2008	b. Tasmania, Australia (January 2020)	c. New South Wales, Australia (February 2020)	d. Revision of principles by each person (March 2020)	e. Final revisions May 2020
1	PD aims to achieve person-centred and evidence-based care that is manifested through human flourishing and a workplace culture of effectiveness in all healthcare settings and situations.	PD fosters person-centred care.	Practice development aims to develop effective workplace cultures that have processes, systems and ways of working embedded within them.	The fundamental aspects of practice development are: person-centred practice, positive and effective workplace cultures, flourishing/ growth for all involved.	PD is fundamentally about person-centred practice that promotes safe and effective workplace cultures, where all can flourish.
2	PD directs its attention at the microsystems level - the level at which most healthcare is experienced and provided but requires coherent support from interrelated mezzo and macro levels.	It focuses on the relationships where care is provided and experienced.	It concentrates on all system levels where healthcare is experienced and therefore requires ongoing and interrelated support between the micro, meso and macro levels.	PD requires a systemic view with a focus on where healthcare is experienced (and supported from all levels).	PD focuses on supportive relationships across individuals, teams and systems to stimulate effective change.
3	PD integrates work-based learning with its focus on achieving learning and formal systems for enabling learning in the workplace to transform care.	PD facilitates learning to enable transformation of care.	It is a complex methodology that can be used across healthcare teams and interfaces to involve all internal and external stakeholders.	PD facilitates workplace learning to enable transformation of care.	PD utilises active work-based learning to facilitate individual, practice and cultural transformation.

(Conti.)

Table 8.2 *(cont.)*

PD principles	a. Manley et al. 2008	b. Tasmania, Australia (January 2020)	c. New South Wales, Australia (February 2020)	d. Revision of principles by each person (March 2020)	e. Final revisions May 2020
4	PD integrates and enables both the development of evidence from practice and the use of evidence in practice.	Evidence from practice informs care.	It uses key methods that are utilised according to methodological principles being operationalised and the contextual characteristics of the PD programme of work.	Use of evidence in and evidence from practice informs and transforms (systems wide) notions of practice delivery.	
5	PD integrates creativity with cognition in order to blend mind, heart and soul energies, enabling practitioners to free their thinking and allow opportunities for human flourishing to emerge.	PD blends creativity into learning approaches and supports human flourishing and free thinking.	It integrates work-based learning with its focus on active learning and formal systems for enabling learning in the workplace to transform care.	PD works with people to help them use their creativity (heart, mind and soul), enabling new knowledge, ways of working and being (human flourishing).	PD blends creativity with learning, freeing people's hearts, minds and souls to achieve new ways of thinking, doing and being.

6	PD is a conscious methodology that can be used across healthcare teams and interfaces to involve all internal and external stakeholders.	Practice improvement is enabled by a range of PD approaches: skilled facilitation is a key component; methods are carefully selected to support the purpose; and reflection and critical thinking are essential.	It requires skilled transformational facilitation that can be adopted into a specific skillset required as near to the interface of care as possible.	PD methodology uses a range of carefully selected methods to engage stakeholders in different contexts in learning and developing their practice.	PD is a complex methodology that uses all forms of evidence to inform practice transformation (blend PD 4 and PD 6).
7	PD uses key methods that are utilised according to the methodological principles being operationalised and contextual characteristics of the programme of work.	Evaluation incorporates process and outcomes and takes place throughout.	It integrates and enables both the development of evidence from practice and the use of evidence in practice.		PD uses collaborative, inclusive and participatory approaches.

(Conti.)

Table 8.2 *(cont.)*

PD principles	a. Manley et al. 2008	b. Tasmania, Australia (January 2020)	c. New South Wales, Australia (February 2020)	d. Revision of principles by each person (March 2020)	e. Final revisions May 2020
8	PD is associated with a set of processes, including skills facilitation, that can be translated into a specific skillset as required as near to the interface of care as possible.	PD requires collaborative, participatory and inclusive ways of working.	It integrates critical and creative thinking to blend mind, heart and soul energies, enable practitioners to free their thinking and allow opportunities for human flourishing to emerge.	PD is a facilitated process that creatively seeks to enable critically informed action (praxis) where all can flourish.	PD is a facilitated process that seeks to promote critically informed action.
9	PD integrates evaluation processes that are always inclusive, participative and collaborative.		It integrates evaluation approaches that are always inclusive, participative and collaborative.	PD is an inclusive evaluation approach that integrates all forms of evidence to capture process and outcomes of transformation.	PD uses inclusive evaluation to integrate evidence from process and outcomes of transformation.

PD language can be a barrier to understanding different concepts being described, hindering people's ability to grasp core elements. Even among those familiar with PD, the principles were seen as being presented in stilted language that overpowered any dynamism and energy that PD stimulates. In the UK, feedback about the language reflected this distraction from PD's lived experiences:

> *The language! What do people understand by the words used in the principles? What does person-centred mean? What does human flourishing mean?*

For the Swiss cohort, working with requirements of translation provided some useful insights. When starting to work with PD methodology, the facilitator teams were using the original 2008 version, but it needed to be translated. The translation process and associated discussions led to a reformed understanding. Although the translation process generated insights and discussions, certain challenges remained. For terms like *human flourishing* or *facilitation*, there are no single words in German to express the meaning; therefore, in Switzerland they needed to be paraphrased. Evidence that non-English-speaking countries struggle with the best possible translation to make the principles understood, and other issues of accessibility, underlines the importance of language used in PD.

A revision to increase understanding across different cultures and countries became paramount. The review team therefore attempted to reduce the use of complex terms across the principle statements and keep sentences concise.

Theme 2: Ordering the principles

Stakeholder feedback revealed that the PD principles were not seen as ordered or hierarchical. The Swiss group, for example, discussed PD principles in terms of those seen as more relevant than others because they were more useful in clinical practice. This led to some principles being identified as fundamental, whereas others became more meaningful once working at a deeper, more advanced level of PD.

Several participants questioned why evaluation was identified as principle 9, when considering an evaluation approach is required early on in a project's development. This enables both baseline and ongoing data to be captured throughout the PD intervention, in order to increase potential for improving understanding about where, how and what impact is being achieved. An experienced PD facilitator in the UK gave an insight into how they used and worked with the principles while facilitating PD programmes:

> *Having reflected on how I am working with the PD principles within the PD programme I can see all of the principles being used at one time or another, and certainly some are more pivotal than others. So, for example, principle 2 was very important at the beginning of the programme to engage the fellows, their managers and their organisations in the programme. The use of active learning and creativity was a key theme throughout the workshops and sustained beyond the fellowship. However, there is one key theme throughout the programme and that is working in collaborative, inclusive and participatory ways and using skilled facilitation that enables learning for all.*

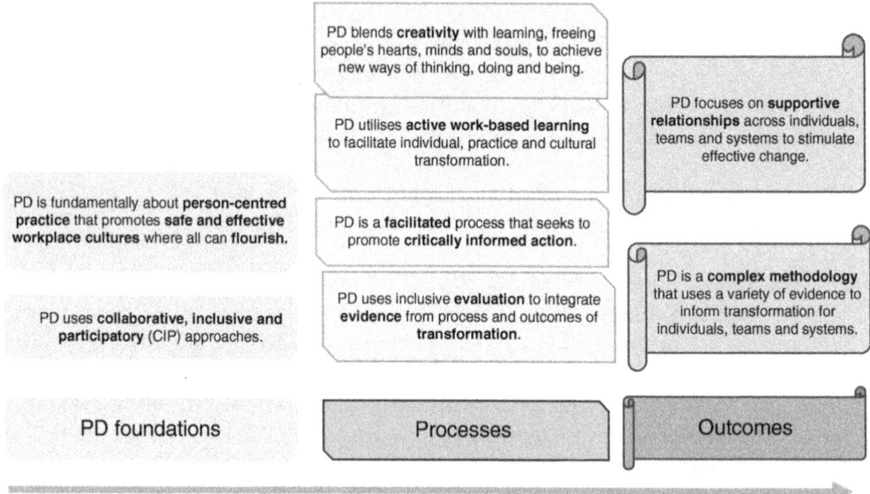

Figure 8.2 A stepped approach to engaging with PD principles – a global manifesto

Using a numbering system to identify the PD principles was seen as a mechanism for helping place some order on a cyclical process, to achieve different goals. The review team found a new way of organising the revised principles, moving from PD foundation level through different approaches towards sustainable transformation (see Figure 8.2). Throughout the review process we aimed to not repeat, or over rely on, certain phrases and terminology. Therefore, our goal to achieve succinct statements that allow a person to move from the foundation of PD through to considering its complexity has underpinned the 2020 PD principles. The order and wording have changed, while retaining the original concepts, to develop the revised principles as a global manifesto for PD.

Comparing the 2008 PD principles with the revised 2020 PD principles

A final step in the critical review process was to send out the revised statements to a smaller group of stakeholders to verify the clarity of the proposed 2020 PD principles. This enabled for some final edits to the revised principles. In keeping with feedback, the revisions provide shorter, simpler sentences (See Boxes 8.1–8.8). The order has also changed. The aim is to contemporise the PD principles, presented here alongside the original version.

Box 8.1 Revised statement

2008: 1. PD aims to achieve person-centred and evidence-based care that is manifested through human flourishing and a workplace culture of effectiveness in all healthcare settings and situations.	2020: PD is fundamentally about person-centred practice that promotes safe and effective workplace cultures, where all can flourish.

The focus of this revision was to specify the fundamental aspect of PD, as person-centred practice, while also acknowledging the importance of effective workplace cultures and how this process impacts on a commitment for all to flourish.

Person-centred practice is often referred to as 'a journey not a destination' (Dewing et al. 2014, p. 7). Being person-centred involves a lifelong commitment to development and refinement, whether that is personal, public, individual and/or group based. It manifests in lived experiences, as a way of influencing and working within the creation of an effective workplace culture. This culture is an environment where the challenges and tensions of practice are part of an open, respectful and inclusive agenda; working from a strengths-based analysis of those involved, resulting in an objectified and supportive strategy to meet challenges posed, regardless of the source. The revision removed *human flourishing* as a concept, instead referring to the outcome of attaining *flourishing* for all as part of a roadmap to excellence, whether that be in service delivery or experience of care/interventions, plus consideration of personal and professional growth.

Box 8.2 Revised statement

2008: 9. PD integrates evaluation processes that are always inclusive, participative and collaborative.	2020: PD uses collaborative, inclusive and participatory (CIP) approaches.

Through the process of revision, collaboration, inclusion and participation (CIP) (Manley et al. 2013) emerged as key concepts. The emergence of CIP as an important concept sees it as a standalone principle in the 2020 version. This contrasted with the 2008 principles, where CIP was associated with the evaluation processes. It is now positioned within the foundation principles, being useful for those starting to work with PD. Identifying foundational principles helps facilitate how these approaches are readily used in practice, as a starting point for PD activity, which underpins other PD approaches.

As one UK PD leader commented on how those new to PD have incorporated CIP into their repertoire of skills: 'they have really embraced the CIP principles and how to enact these in practice.'

Box 8.3 Revised statement

2008: 5. PD integrates creativity with cognition in order to blend mind, heart and soul energies, enabling practitioners to free their thinking and allow opportunities for human flourishing to emerge.	2020: PD blends creativity with learning, freeing people's hearts, minds and souls, to achieve new ways of thinking, doing and being.

This principle emphasises creativity and how PD facilitators work innovatively with people to enable them to expand their repertoire for learning and problem solving. The rewording was primarily aimed at making the language accessible, without losing elements of how people grow/flourish through participation in active learning. Creative expression and critical creativity are an approach or method for PD engagement that incorporates transformation (Titchen and McCormack 2010). A Tasmanian participant commented that this principle gives permission to 'think outside the box and perhaps not feel the need to always be so task orientated when trying to solve issues in the clinical space'.

A UK programme facilitator wrote: 'The participants are encouraged to use creativity (e.g. picture cards, arts and craft, mindfulness exercises and visualisation) to view and reflect on their practice and gain understanding of themselves, their learning and their actions going forward.'

Box 8.4 Revised statement

2008: 3. PD integrates work-based learning with its focus on active learning and formal systems for enabling learning in the workplace to transform care.	2020: PD utilises active work-based learning to facilitate individual, practice and cultural transformation.

The 'active' aspect to work-based learning, both in the moment of practice and when reflecting on work more formally, means that learners and facilitators have equal responsibility for structure, content and processes used for learning. Our refinements reflect developments in other literatures, most notably adult education (Yacek 2020). A co-constructive element to learning aims to increase opportunity for insight, via those 'aha' moments. Transformation results as the fruit of true synthesis, where content blends with application, rather than relying on understanding just the facilitator's viewpoint. When all involved start to shift their thinking, a resultant change in the culture can be seen (e.g. achieving a change in how people talk respectfully towards each other) (Hardy et al. 2013).

Further into the revisions, facilitation is more firmly centred in PD as a process. A realignment of responsibilities gives greater revelation between what is meant by *facilitation* and a more traditional understanding of *teaching* (i.e. formal systems of learning). A dynamic arises in such a paradigm shift, clarifying skills that differentiate teachers from facilitators. In reality, these concepts remain closely connected, but this revision reinforces the argument that they are not synonymous.

Transformation has pride of place in its many dimensions within PD, as an ultimate goal or outcome. The 2020 wording embraces multiplicity of transformation within personal and public domains. These domains are closely connected – a change in one aspect, be it internal to the individual practitioner or through external displays in practice, inevitably leads to a change in the other realms (private/public/practice).

Box 8.5 Revised statement

2008: 8. PD is associated with a set of processes including skilled facilitation that can be translated into a specific skillset required as near to the interface of care as possible.	2020: PD is a facilitated process that seeks to promote critically informed action.

Achieving a process of transformation, whether at individual or team level or across whole systems, requires skilled facilitation. Facilitation as a process of skilled negotiation, movement and charting developments (in self and others) is central to *critically informed action*. Skilled facilitators maintain a clear vision of *from where, to where* and *how* for themselves and those they work with. They foster and generate innovation in both the development process and practices – wrapped in sincerely held values-based tenets of safety, professional responsibility and mutual accountability. Critically informed action is one step of the facilitated process founded in critical social theory. In particular, Fay's idea (1987) that critical reflection enables a process of enlightenment, empowerment and emancipation, through to transformation (Middleton 2017), is employed.

Box 8.6 Revised statement

2008: 9. PD integrates evaluation processes that are always inclusive, participative and collaborative.	2020: PD uses inclusive evaluation to integrate evidence from process and outcomes of transformation.

PD as a complex synthesis of strategies, practices and deftly applied processes marks its uniqueness and comprehensiveness. It encourages qualitative and quantitative measurement of the process of change; it insists that the stories of all involved are heard and included in the assessment summary and therefore is universal and eclectic in its evaluation approach. The seeds of evaluation sown at the inception of the process enable as full a picture as possible of the *then* and *now* situations. The *how* has been mentioned previously as a blend of reflective, critically informed actions, bounded within discreet strategies. These are observed, or collectively agreed, to be deviated from (reflexivity), according to objective and insightful assessment against intended outcomes.

Outcomes are transformative where they represent effective changes in practice, especially where they result from innovative processes. This sets the groundwork for innovation (ergo transformation) to be a feature of an individual's or group's change agenda – rather than a prospect to be approached with apprehension and/or suspicion. The prospect of transformation in a team, relating to both what they do and how they got there, is one of many satisfying rewards within PD.

Box 8.7 Revised statement

2008: 2. PD directs its attention at the micro-systems level – the level at which most healthcare is experienced and provided, but requires coherent support from interrelated mezzo and macro levels.	2020: PD focuses on supportive relationships across individuals, teams and systems to stimulate effective change.

Our review identified confusion as to the meaning of systems levels, as included in the 2008 principle 2. How these levels are distinctively recognised is complex. Each level can depend on many factors, especially pertaining to the individual.

Where, for example, does micro start and end, similarly with meso and macro? All are relative to an almost endless degree (Nelson et al. 2002). This distraction is addressed in the 2020 version; while still referring to system levels (imperative for professions with such significant institutional presence), this emphasis has been balanced by focus upon the relationships. A critical dimension of working with values is that we have a continual restlessness, in that meaning requires constant refining, thereby challenging thinking. The revised principle shows that innovation is an essential part of PD processes, rather than just a random happy accident. This creates space for future innovators to contribute to furthering the ultimate cause of PD transformation in ways not previously imagined (Berwick 2003).

Box 8.8 Revised statement

2008: 4. PD integrates and enables both the development of evidence from practice and the use of evidence in practice. 6. PD is a complex methodology that can be used across healthcare teams and interfaces to involve all internal and external stakeholders.	2020: PD is a complex methodology that uses a variety of evidence to inform transformation for individuals, teams and systems.

The revised principle has combined two 2008 principles (4 and 6) in valuing all forms of evidence and how that can be used in practice, recognising the complexity of working with PD principles, methods and approaches. The importance of working with people and particularly all stakeholders is further endorsed in the new principles.

PD works in the 'swampy lowlands' (Schon 1983, p. 42), where context, practice and people encountered are always changing. PD thereby asks a lot of practitioners, in its invitation to consider practice as a world of endless possibilities. It draws frequently from the relatively unexplored world of broader social and physical sciences for its approach and *ways of knowing* (Carper 1978; Higgs and Titchen 2001; Garrett and Cutting 2015). PD embraces the responsibility of the practitioner to use their intuition and tacit knowledge as an active part of their judgement processes, which connects the spiritual element (the human soul) to the concept of flourishing (Titchen and McCormack 2010).

PD uses complex approaches to understand supportive relationships across teams and systems to stimulate effective, sustainable transformative change. Practice transformation becomes both the end-goal and the jumping-off point for a continuous process, best entered into with full awareness and clear intent. This scope is both freeing and intimidating, which is why we believe that the character and quality of facilitation are vital components in the process of critically informed change.

Practice development principles: a global manifesto

This final version of revised PD principles is presented here as a global manifesto. The goal has always been to ensure the core concepts are included for those new to PD through to those who return to it as a constant renewal of their own and others' transformational development. The outcome of this critically reflective process is a reconsidered, concise and reordered set of eight PD principles.

Conclusion

This chapter has described a critical revision process to achieve a contemporary global perspective on PD principles. Multiple group activities across diverse stakeholders were included in the process. The process was one of co-construction, incorporating feedback received alongside incorporation of our own PD experiences, to realise an updated version of the PD principles that we hope are both engaging and memorable.

Engagement with stakeholders offered precious opportunities to explore current experience of employing the principles and their use in everyday practice. The resounding response was that the principles were valuable as a road map for those engaging with PD, both early on and at various stages of a PD journey. Two areas of critique focused on language and the order of the principles, illustrating that action was needed to enhance their accessibility and usability. A balance of ensuring more simplified language while not losing the nuances and essence of PD, its philosophical underpinnings and consideration of both processes and outcomes was maintained throughout the review process.

Eight principles have evolved from the revisions made to the original nine, supporting a call for simplicity to facilitate early engagement with core PD concepts. Grouping the principles into *foundation, process and transformational outcomes* of PD provided a reordering, as a natural development of the iterative critical review. Elements within the principles relate to the foundations on which transformational change is built, such as collaboration, inclusion and participation. These have become more universal in an individual's or team's approach to PD, rather than relating exclusively to evaluation of PD activity. While the order of the principles does not reflect a ranking as such, the importance of considering evaluation early on in a transformation journey was acknowledged, with this principle placed more prominently in the midst of the revised principles.

To further enhance accessibility, a visual representation of the interrelationships between the 2020 principles and transformational outcomes is provided. This illustrates a stepped approach to engaging with PD (see Figure 8.2), allowing interaction and flow between them, alongside the potential to consider our own relationship to them across a transformation journey or continuum.

The process used for reviewing the PD principles stayed true to PD methodology. The methods align with PD values and philosophies they aim to promote, particularly in relation to collaboration, inclusion and participation. The review sessions with practitioners and cooperation between the review team demonstrate that PD methods are appropriate and relevant for undertaking a critical review. This will provide confidence to others about the relevance and validity of using PD approaches and also the centrality of evaluation in PD work.

The 2020 PD principles are offered for use by all who wish to critically engage in an invigorating journey of transformation. We would love to receive stakeholder feedback on these revised principles, and how you work with them to further inform understanding and provide evidence of PD's effectiveness across different workplace contexts.

References

Berwick, D.M. (2003). Disseminating innovations in health care. *Jama* 289 (15): 1969–1975.

Carper, B. (1978). Fundamental ways of knowing in nursing. *Advances in Nursing Science* 1 (1): 13–23.

Dewing, J., McCormack, B. and Titchen, A. (2014). *Practice Development Workbook for Nursing, Health and Social Care Teams*. Chichester: John Wiley & Sons.

Fairbrother, G., Cashin, A., Mekki, T.E. et al. (2015). Is it possible to bring the emancipatory practice development and evidence-based practice agendas together in nursing and midwifery? *International Practice Development Journal* 5 (1). https://doi.org/10.19043/ipdj.51.004

Fay, B. (1987). *Critical Social Science: Liberation and its Limits*. Cambridge: Polity Press.

Filmalter, C.J., van Eeden, I., de Kock, J. et al. (2015). From fixers to facilitators: the start to our South African journey. *International Practice Development Journal* 5 (1). https://doi.org/10.19043/ipdj.51.008

Friere, P. (1973). *Education for Critical Consciousness*. New York;: Continuum.

Garrett, B.M. and Cutting, R.L. (2015). Ways of knowing: realism, non-realism, nominalism and a typology revisited with a counter perspective for nursing science. *Nursing Inquiry* 22 (2): 95–105.

Grundy, S. (1982). Three modes of action research. *Curriculum Perspectives* 2 (3): 23–34.

Guba, E.G. and Lincoln, Y.S. (1989). *Fourth Generation Evaluation*. Newbury Park, CA: Sage.

Hardy, S., Jackson, C., Webster, J. et al. (2013). Educating advanced level practice within complex health care workplace environments through transformational practice development. *Nurse Education Today* 33 (10): 1099–1103.

Higgs, J. and Titchen, A. (2001). Framing professional practice: knowing and doing in context. In: *Professional Practice in Health, Education and the Creative Arts* (eds. J. Higgs and A. Titchen), 1–15. Oxford: Blackwell Science.

Manley, K., Büscher, A., Jackson, C. et al. (2017). Overcoming synecdoche: why practice development and quality improvement approaches should be better integrated. *International Practice Development Journal* 7 (1). https://doi.org/10.19043/ipdj.71.012

Manley, K., McCormack, B. and Wilson, V. (2008). *International practice development in nursing and healthcare*. Oxford: Blackwell Publishing.

Manley, K., Titchen, A. and McCormack, B. (2013). Introduction. In: *Practice Development in Nursing and Healthcare. 2nd Edition* (eds. B. McCormack, K. Manley and A. Titchen), 50–51. Chichester: Wiley Blackwell.

Middleton, R. (2017). Critical reflection: the struggle of a practice developer. *International Practice Development Journal* 7 (1): 1–6. https://doi.org/10.19043/ipdj.71.004

Morrow, R.A. and Torres, C.A. (2002). *Reading Freire and Habermas: Critical Pedagogy and Transformative Social Change*. New York;: Teachers College Press.

Murray, S.J. and Tuqiri, K.A. (2020). The heart of caring – understanding compassionate care through storytelling. *International Practice Development Journal* 10 (1). https://doi.org/10.19043/ipdj.101.004

Nelson, E.C., Batalden, P.B., Huber, T.P. et al. (2002). Microsystems in health care: part 1. Learning from high-performing front-line clinical units. *The Joint Commission Journal on Quality Improvement* 28 (9): 472–493.

Odell, J. (2018). Reflections on developing a participatory evaluation as part of the Patients First programme. *International Practice Development Journal* 8 (2). https://doi.org/10.19043/ipdj.82.007

Price, A., Hirter, K., Lippiatt, C. et al. (2016). Using creative writing to explore facilitation skills in practice. *International Practice Development Journal* 6 (1). https://doi.org/10.19043/ipdj.61.011

Roberts, D. and Williams, L. (2017). Is it possible to bring the emancipatory practice development and evidence-based practice agendas together in nursing and midwifery? *International Practice Development Journal* 7 (1). https://doi.org/10.19043/ipdj.71.013

Schon, D. (1983). *The Reflective Practitioner: How Professionals Think in Action. 1st edition.* London: Temple Smith.

Timlin, A., Hastings, A. and Hardiman, M. (2018). Workbased facilitators as drivers for the development of person-centred cultures: a shared reflection from novice facilitators of person-centred practice. *International Practice Development Journal* 8 (1). https://doi.org/10.19043/ipdj81.008

Titchen, A. and McCormack, B. (2010). Dancing with stones: critical creativity as methodology for human flourishing. *Educational Action Research* 18 (4): 531–554.

Wilson, V. and McCance, T. (2015). Good enough evaluation. *International Practice Development Journal* 5 (10). https://doi.org/10.19043/ipdj.5SP.012

Yacek, D.W. (2020). Should education be transformative? *Journal of Moral Education* 49 (2): 257–274.

Yalden, J., McCormack, B., O'Connor, M. et al. (2013). Transforming end of life care using practice development: an arts-informed approach in residential aged care. *International Practice Development Journal* 3 (2) [2]. https://www.fons.org/resources/documents/journal/vol3no2/ipdj_0302_02.pdf

9. *Theorising Practice Development*

Emma Radbron, Clint Douglas, and Cheryl Atherfold

Reflections on theory in practice development
Pantoum Poem by Loraine Stephenson

Inspired by webinar on PD and critical theory, 29 November 2019

Theory helps us to connect with practice
Keeps us true to the process
Links knowledge and experience
Keeps us true to the process

Keeps us true to the process
Guides creative ways of thinking
Helps to make meaning of what we experience
Helps us to bring about planned change

Guides creative ways of thinking
Links knowledge and experience
Helps us to bring about planned change
Theory helps us to connect with practice

International Practice Development in Health and Social Care, Second Edition.
Edited by Kim Manley, Valerie Wilson, and Christine Øye.

Introduction

This chapter grew out of our contribution to an International Practice Development Collaborative (IPDc) webinar on theory in practice development (PD). Although working across two countries in different roles across academic, research and health systems, we shared an appreciation of and commitment to PD. We were also interested in understanding, using and critiquing its theoretical base. The webinar created a platform for us not only to engage in discussion but to connect with other like-minded colleagues across the globe (access here: https://eu-lti.bbcollab.com/recording/60e52197428b491e848c09dd149d5b6b). The pantoum poem above was written by one of the webinar participants and reflects their learning in response to the discussion that took place. It also captures a number of themes discussed in this chapter.

This chapter explores the links between PD and critical social science (CSS). We revisit the importance of the critical paradigm in shaping the development of the PD movement. In seeking to make visible these theoretical tools for PD, we share three practical examples from our different roles and contexts: working at the micro and meso levels as PD facilitators and researchers, to a macro level in the development of health workforce strategy. Finally, while practice developers have made remarkable theoretical advances over the past few decades, we argue that a vibrant and flourishing PD scholarship depends on future healthy debate, conceptual critique and theoretical refinement.

Theoretical origins

The political roots of PD reflect its radical and activist origins as practitioner-led enquiry guided by an emancipatory interest. The PD movement emerging in the 1980–1990s crystallised a new wave of critical-emancipatory scholarship in nursing. Nurse-led PD units in hospitals emerged in the UK and Australia during this time of significant reform, as nursing established itself in universities. Unable to pursue doctorates in nursing, many nurses undertook postgraduate study in education and the social sciences, drawing on critical theory (Nelson 2012). Working from a critical perspective, these nursing leaders sought to transform task-focused care and create more democratising, empowering and liberating workplaces (Titchen 2018). One leading PD theorist shared at a recent conference how simple acts of resistance to oppressive and irrational workplace structures — such as physically lying across the ward entrance as a nurse unit manager to prevent an unsafe patient discharge — reflected the critical intent of the early PD movement.

Since the early 2000s, the international PD movement has made major theoretical advances and established emancipatory PD (ePD) as a methodological framework. Early PD colloquiums and later IPDc meetings established international working groups for analysis and development of concepts at the heart of PD: person-centredness, effective workplace cultures, facilitation, active learning — learning in and from practice, and the links with knowledge translation (Manley 2017). Subsequently, a realist synthesis of PD research (McCormack et al. 2006) and Manley et al.'s (2008) nine principles of PD have been widely influential in providing a coherent PD methodology (Chapter 8 revisits these principles). Theoretical critique and development over the last decade have seen further exploration of person-centred workplace cultures (McCormack and McCance 2017; Manley and Jackson 2019) and critical creativity (Titchen 2018). PD has been conceptualised as a social complex intervention (Manley 2017), aiming to develop effective workplace cultures that have embedded within them person-centred processes, systems and ways of working, enabling all to experience person-centredness.

Although key methods are recognised, PD scholars have resisted presenting PD as a set of methods or techniques. In working with methodology (the theory of PD), we are not constrained by methods. Having a deeper appreciation of the theoretical base of PD enables intentionality, critical intent and creativity in application. Theory has a generative function in pushing us to go beyond the surface and opens new possibilities for PD. We hope that in reading this chapter it has a similar impact as you reflect on your own practice. As you move through the following three examples, we encourage you to reflect on and theorise your own PD approaches.

Working with the 'critical' in critical reflection

A facilitator working in the emancipatory worldview explores how workplace culture is shaped by the wider structures of power and dominant ideology. They uncover practices that seem to make their professional lives easier but that actually end up working against their own best long-term interests (Brookfield 2005). They work to facilitate collective action, deconstructing and reconstructing practice structures in accordance with practitioners' values.

My facilitation experience is largely in acute care hospital settings. One focus has been building patient safety cultures – and working with acute care nurses to support their role in recognising and responding to clinical deterioration. Delayed recognition of deterioration on general wards is a complex problem. However, from an acute care nursing standpoint, oppressive ward practices contribute to a troubling example of hegemony: nursing assessment is rendered invisible and unimportant by others – and ultimately by ward nurses themselves (Peet et al. 2019). From this critical lens, patient assessment can be understood as a site of tension between competing professional and organisational interests and priorities. Indeed, who puts the stethoscope on the patient's chest is as much about how the politics of patient assessment are played out on the hospital ward as it is about the individual needs of the patient and rational deployment of nursing skill and knowledge.

I am using the concept of hegemony here as developed by critical theorists like Gramsci et al. (1971). In this tradition, hegemony is about people learning to love their oppression: taking pride in acting on the very assumptions that work against their best interests (Brookfield 2005). Hegemonic assumptions become deeply embedded and invisible to us — part of the cultural air we breathe — and function to stop people challenging the status quo (Brookfield 2017). For example, we see nurses embrace dominant ideologies when organisational imperatives for efficiency drive nursing practice so that assessment becomes task focused. Or when nurses reproduce chain-of-command communication hierarchies that distance the primary registered nurse (RN) from decision-making (Peet et al. 2019).

Working with critical intent then, a goal has been to raise awareness and creatively challenge these assumptions. A simple and powerful example has been the use of story writing. I have facilitated this activity in small group workshops, with hundreds of acute care nurses across Australia. Drawing on the work of Buresh and Gordon (2013), the activity was designed to elicit positive personal experiences and stories, to make visible the significance and consequential nature of nursing assessment in general wards. Each nurse is asked to write a narrative, framed by the statement 'When my assessment made the difference . . .', and reads their story aloud uninterrupted.

Mirroring our workplace observations (Peet et al. 2019), nurses initially write themselves right out of the story, positioning themselves in ways that marginalise or trivialise their contribution to clinical assessment and decision-making. Working with the theoretical tools of CSS (Brookfield 2005), my role as facilitator is to bring hegemonic assumptions to the surface in a generative and often provocative way by pointing out contradictions in language and 'common-sense' understandings of practice. For example, when a nurse goes into great detail about the assessment and actions of everyone else in the team but renders their knowledge and skills invisible, I point out that patients wouldn't be in hospital if they didn't need nursing assessment! When there is nervous laughter as we uncover and challenge irrational assumptions, or tears as nurses re-experience a profound clinical incident, the use of silence and slowing down the process to ask 'what is really going on here?' can bring deeply held assumptions into question. Creating this high-support/high-challenge environment allows for facilitated reflection and at times uncomfortable conversations about power relations and competing interests that subjugate the nursing voice.

Framed by the group's feedback, nurses are invited to revise their story in ways that give voice to their clinical knowledge and skills, highlighting their agency in keeping patients safe. Some prompting questions may help nurses put themselves 'centre stage' in the narrative (Buresh and Gordon 2013, pp. 150–151):

- Start by painting the whole picture – what is this story about and why is it significant to you?
- Paint yourself into the picture – describe your patient assessment, clinical judgements and actions in as much detail as you can remember.
- What was the outcome? And in your opinion, what would have happened without your nursing assessment?

I have found the process generates opportunities for appreciative learning, fostering respect and recognition among the nursing team. For example, with permission we have presented collections of these stories as large posters on the ward.

In reflecting on working with the 'critical' in critical reflection as practice developers in the acute care context over the past few years, my colleague Jacqui Peet offers the metaphor below. I think it captures the complex and messy reality of working in this space – and how with a deepening understanding of critical theory and ePD methodology, facilitation becomes a way of being.

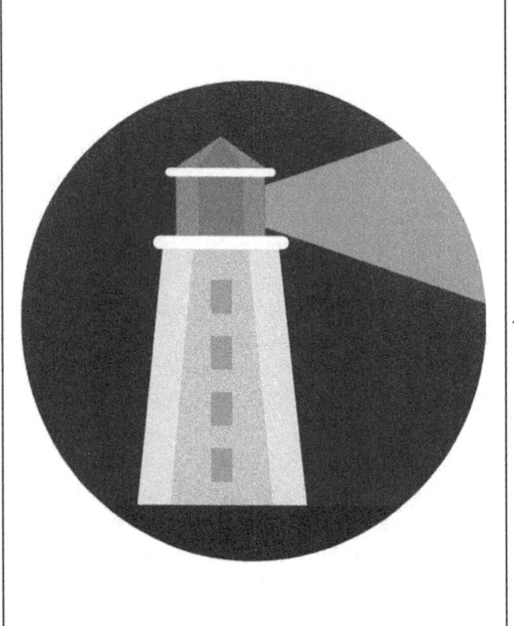

Theory was a guiding light on the turbulent seas of participatory research. It illuminated the direction of how to engage, make decisions and move forward with the ward. It enables researchers to navigate their responses to the reefs and rocks of the status quo and inertia. Abandoning theory would leave emancipatory practice development (ePD) at the mercy of a sea of methods with no lighthouse to guide. My research demonstrates an imperative for ePD to remain true to its emancipatory origins and be explicit about the disruptive nature of emancipation. Disconnection from its political ancestry endangers it to become co-opted to serve the very agendas it seeks liberation. This requires further development of the conceptual framework of PD to bring clarity about facilitation approaches that raise awareness and support social action.

— Jacqueline Peet RN, PhD candidate using emancipatory practice development methodology

Connecting through crisis: critical social science and person-centredness in PD research

This short story helps illustrate the links between theory and PD research through an example from a doctoral study using action research. It describes how CSS informed an aspect of practice within the study and how awareness of theory enabled the researcher to support staff to work through a crisis.

In situations like this where staff are unhappy, CSS sees this 'unhappiness' as an opportunity for enquiry and potential to change. The outcome in this story is consistent with the work of critical social theorist Brian Fay (1975, 1987). His work sees the feelings and experiences of unhappiness and crisis as catalysts for enquiry and change which can be observed in this situation. In this example, rather than trying to bring peace to the crisis, drawing on the work of Fay enabled me as a researcher to identify the potential in the situation to bring transformation. Theory informed my actions in creating a space where the challenging data and surfaced feelings of unhappiness could be explored and then used to improve the current team-nursing practices. Approaches like this example that are guided by CSS in supporting others to critique their feelings and practice in this way can result in transformation of individuals and collective units; however, it is important to note that this process takes time.

While a critical approach enabled reflection on generative potential of the situation, working with the concept of person-centredness enabled the process to be a catalyst for change. At the core of PD there is an explicit focus on person-

> *As a doctoral student I (Emma) was working with staff from a clinical unit as part of a large international study involving three cycles of data collection. Engagement with staff had been challenging due to a number of leadership changes, negative ward culture and transactional past experiences with research and projects. After several efforts (over eight months) to connect as people and understand the context of the unit, traction was slowly building. However, during cycle two of the study, several issues emerged from separate data that was collected relating to the ward leadership team. This data was confronting in both content and the way in which it was delivered. This was very challenging for the team and the distress caused had halted their progress with other intervention studies. This 'crisis' was unpacked in an action research team meeting where the staff expressed that they had never experienced receiving such challenging feedback in this way and were unsure how to respond. The nursing unit manager approached me for assistance, and I worked with the nursing leadership team to develop a plan to work through the data with staff. Through co-facilitation, the nursing unit manager and I unpacked the data with 70 per cent of nursing staff in this unit over several weeks. These sessions provided an opportunity to process the surfaced emotions and review and critique practice using a number of datasets. After reflecting on their feelings and the evidence, staff proposed solutions on how to improve the teamwork model within the unit. These suggestions were themed and prioritised, and changes were implemented before collecting the third and final cycle of data three months later. The process and results of the third cycle of data collection were overwhelmingly positive compared with previous cycles and demonstrated improvements based on the changes staff made. In reflecting on the situation both in the moment and retrospectively, I identified that there was a situational 'crisis' occurring. By engaging with the team over several weeks, supporting them as they unpacked the challenging data, the crisis became a catalyst for entry, engagement and momentum for change.*

centredness and the development of person-centred cultures. However, with numerous definitions and 'interchangeable' terms in healthcare and literature, it is important to define person-centredness within PD. McCormack and McCance (2017, p. 3) define person-centredness as:

> *An approach to practice established through the formation and fostering of healthful relationships between all care providers, service users and others significant to them in their lives. It is underpinned by values of respect for persons, individual right to self-determination, mutual respect and understanding. It is enabled by cultures of empowerment that foster continuous approaches to practice development.*

Within this definition, the values of CSS can be observed. CSS as outlined by Fay (1987) is underpinned by the process of enlightenment, empowerment and emancipation, where understanding leads to motivation to take action, which then results in the transformation of people and cultures (Wilson and McCormack 2006). A key link between PD and person-centredness is that PD (with person-centred cultures at the centre) offers a methodology for healthcare clinicians, researchers and academics to enable flourishing and transformation to take place. This occurs through realising and evaluating person-centredness (or barriers to it) in research and practice in a variety of ways. It occurs as a result of recognising personhood, what matters to individuals and the importance of relationships, as well as context and cultures.

In relation to the story above, person-centredness played a key role in being invited to support the team through their crisis. Connecting as persons and understanding

> *As a research student the person-centred practice framework has been helpful not only in underpinning my research study and evaluating person-centredness but also in informing my approach as a researcher. It has helped me identify gaps in clinical practice as well as areas for improvement in my capacity to be 'professionally competent' in undertaking person-centred research. I appreciate how it depicts not only the person-centred outcomes that as practice developers we all desire (good care experience, involvement in care, feeling of wellbeing, existence of a healthful culture) but clearly outlines the inter-related concepts of the prerequisites, environmental factors and processes required for this to occur. It has been a helpful tool to inform my approach to my research, particularly in challenging situations where I have been reminded of the value of shared decision-making when perhaps it felt 'easier'/more time efficient to be transactional and make decisions for the team. It has also helped me identify when processes such as being sympathetically present or engaging authentically have been key in seeing person-centred outcomes achieved for the research team, nursing staff and patients on the unit I am working with.*

the context and cultures within the clinical unit in the months leading up to this moment had fostered the development of respect and trust between the staff and myself. When the crisis occurred, staff drew on this effective relationship to help them use the data to reflect on practice and inform person-centred practice change. Engaging with the team over several weeks, staff were supported to unpack this data in a safe and respectful way. Connecting as persons at the beginning of each session and the option to provide anonymous feedback provided the environment for staff to take a deeper dive into their practice and participate in shared decision-making. The changes made as a result of this study resulted in improved care experience for patients and staff as well as an enhanced feeling of wellbeing and existence of a healthful culture among the research and broader staff teams.

Action in this situation was also guided by the Person-Centred Practice Framework (McCormack and McCance 2017). This middle-range theory is a practical link between person-centredness and PD. Informed by conceptual frameworks and empirical research, it is able to both explain and predict person-centred practice across a broad range of research and health contexts. Middle-range theories such as the Person-Centred Practice Framework are beneficial as both theoretical underpinnings and guiding frameworks for research studies with person-centred foci. The brief account below from my reflective journal describes how this framework influenced and informed practice in a doctoral research study.

Theory in action: a bicultural perspective

Having explored examples at a micro and meso level, this example provides insight into the links between CSS and PD work at a macro level in health workforce strategy. As a foundation of PD, CSS provides a framework for generating practitioners who understand identity as the basis of who they are and relationship as the connections to others in practice (Hardiman and Dewing 2014; Mooney and Nolan 2006; Titchen 2004). Within the Aotearoa New Zealand context there is a need for healthcare provision to incorporate the governing agreement of the Tiriti o Waitangi 1840

(Treaty of Waitangi). This Treaty assures bicultural application of partnership, protection and participation between Māori as the indigenous people of the land and others who have settled there later. Health outcomes for Māori demonstrate that western systems have not been effective in achieving the health outcomes that would be evident had these elements been honoured (Kidd et al. 2019). This aligns with the CSS concept of false consciousness where healthcare has been delivered in a way that was well intended but not effective or appropriate. Subsequently this has generated a social crisis as Māori are disadvantaged in terms of mortality, with reduced life expectancy, and morbidity, with overrepresentation in long-term conditions which impacts the ability to provide for self and family because of high representation within all long-term conditions and associated disability (New Zealand Ministry of Health 2019). This sense of crisis has prompted a phase of education to enlighten and to bring insight and understanding to identify the conditions that enable transformation to occur as an emancipatory process (Fay 1987).

Growing a Māori workforce forms an active strategy towards addressing inequity. The nature of CSS and PD enables this to be developed in order to achieve justice in terms of equity of health outcomes in person-centred ways that incorporate individuals as part of whānau (family) and community (social systems). This ideal requires a workforce that prepares and employs Māori nurses and facilitates practice environs that enable authentic ways of being, reflecting authentic identity and connections. To generate sufficient Māori nurses for our population demographic a minimum would be 23% of this District Health Board's nursing workforce. Recruitment begins from early secondary school subject choice and support to prepare for student nursing (or other health professional roles). Undergraduate curriculums and practice placements incorporate pursuit of Māori ways of being based in holistic approaches and linked to navigation of health that align with cultural priorities such as whānau rather than individual. On employment, graduates transitioning to the registered nurse role receive in-practice and on-practice support from Māori educators to reflect and continue the development of 'self' as a Māori nurse (or other health professional) rather than a nurse who happens to be Māori (C. Baker, personal communication).

Over four consecutive years the proportion of Māori recruited into this District Health Board's graduate nurse entry to practice programmes fluctuates between 17% and 23%. This is significant given the total number on the programme is 176. The limitation is the number of Māori nurses in the undergraduate programmes, which is why there is such a priority on the early part of the pipeline attracting Māori students to a career in nursing or health. The graduate nurse employment model prioritises a place for Māori nurses in all settings (primary, acute and mental health) across a diverse geographical area with high proportions of rural and deprived populations. Within this approach, Titchen's (2018) metaphor of flowing like a river is used to link the ancient ways of knowing to the origins of knowledge and learning in cultures. As with many indigenous and first nation peoples, Māori historically value relationships and connections, the land and water as part of the journey and their provisions, and holistic approaches that incorporate mind, body, spirit, family and community in its most comprehensive sense. By applying such approaches, it is possible to come away from technical reflection which focuses on problem solving and solutions, to the type of dialogue and knowledge development that is dynamic and achieved via connections aimed at achieving just outcomes (Fay 1987; Mooney and Nolan 2006). At the centre of Figure 9.1 is the imagery of the koru; an unfurling frond of a native New Zealand plant provides a way to consider the links between CSS, PD and bicultural concepts. All components are connected to create movement in action within ideas; the koru connects these and they unfurl to deliver the aspects it relates to. As a visual representation of the development process there are links to a systematic approach while the imagery and creative context of the koru may facilitate creative thinking and depth of insight for others.

The six Pou form strong pillars for each of the bicultural concepts.
'Pou Timata': Establish identity
'Pou Hononga': Establish connection
'Pou Raruraru': Crisis, sense of something needs to be different
'Pou Tikanga': Beliefs, systems, bias
'Pou Ako': Education, insight, learning
'Pou Whakaahu Whakamua': Bring about the change

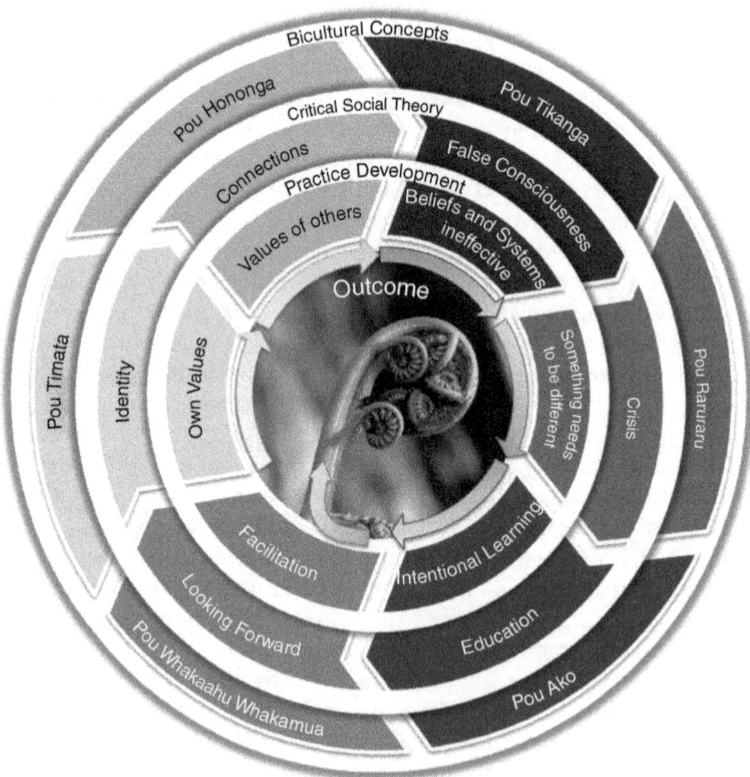

Figure 9.1 Author-developed synthesis of bicultural principles, CSS and PD informed by Fay (1987), McCormack et al. (2013) and Lacey et al. (2011). Acknowledgement and thanks to Chris Baker and Faye Blossom (Cultural Workforce Development Team) regarding application of bicultural concepts, Jean Michel Burgess and Lin Marriott for articulation of the model.

Lacey et al.'s (2011) Hui process has been used as an indigenous process for the recruitment interviews of graduate nurses, including time for greeting and engagement (Mihi); making a connection that links where a person is from, who their significant people are, (whanaungatanga); progressing the purpose of the interview (kaupapa); and concluding (poroporoaki), summarising, clarifying expectations from this point in time, closing and release. These processes facilitate person-centredness for graduates and model ways that affirm their identity and connect with those in their care when in practice. The way the room is set up facilitates this, with open space to include family and support people (whānau) to attend, and often a family member comes to add value (tautoko) to the contribution of the graduate. While the graduate speaks for themselves, this support provides a sense of 'standing' with strength and confidence. Family and support people may speak to affirm the graduate as humility is a valued attribute, and the graduate may underrepresent themselves. Because of this, when interviewing graduates in the same way as all other graduates, Māori scored poorly in the recruitment measures. This was incongruent with how they were achieving academically and performing in practice. Using a culturally appropriate approach enabled the attributes and skills being assessed to be accurately represented. Such person-centredness is the difference between equity and equality, resulting in recruitment outcomes that more closely align with the population demographic as part of an overall strategy to improve health outcomes.

Reflecting on the future of theory and practice development

A fundamental theme in each of the examples in this chapter is the need for critical reflection on the use of theory in PD. Critical reflection has been beneficial as individuals and as a collective when writing this chapter. It has resulted in a number of realisations about the power of theory to generate momentum in practice and research. Progressive growth requires an extension of the boundaries into different theoretical orientations, and the examples provided in this chapter from a micro, meso and macro level aim to do just that. Challenging the way theoretical tools are used creates a tension and the methods of application or 'doing' generate an opportunity to evolve PD approaches. This requires courage. Using PD methods in a formulaic way can reproduce the dynamics of power they are seeking to disrupt. Awareness of this and generative discussions while using PD methods and theoretical concepts mitigates this and enables theory and concepts to be movement oriented and active: they come to life.

Although practice developers have made remarkable theoretical advances over the past few decades, we argue that a vibrant and flourishing PD scholarship depends on future healthy debate, conceptual critique and theoretical refinement. This will require a shift in focus advocated by Kislov et al. (2019) from 'theory' as a relatively isolated, static, reified source guiding PD towards embracing 'theorising' as a set of processes that aim to use evaluation data actively in developing, validating, modifying and advancing conceptual knowledge in the field. There are excellent examples of rigorous PD research contributing to this two-way theory–practice relationship in advancing PD. Manley and Jackson's (2019) refined PD theory of cultural change in frontline teams offers a model for others to go beyond descriptive 'shopping list' conceptual frameworks to develop and test mechanism-based explanations of PD facilitation. Not all projects need to make such large-scale refinements to middle-range theory, but all can make meaningful contributions to PD's theoretical base. An example is Brown and McCormack's (2016) contribution of psychological safety to holistic facilitation models, based on their emancipatory research with an acute care frontline team.

Kislov et al.'s (2019, p. 4) call to shift perspectives from 'theories' as finished products to 'theorising' as an iterative process has significance for the future of PD:

> *Here, theory is a tool which should be improved with each subsequent application, rather than merely having its utility confirmed. Theorising becomes an iterative and recursive process: theory is no longer seen as 'fixed and immutable' — a holy text to be corrupted at one's peril — but as 'a fluid collection of principles and hypotheses'.*

Our collective reflection in writing this chapter is that a deepening appreciation of CSS also demands just that. Continually analysing our assumptions when working with PD principles opens up possibilities for creatively and fluidly working with theoretical tools in different contexts. Sharing our theorising with each other is what builds PD's contribution to healthcare. We have started by sharing our stories with you. We look forward to hearing yours.

Invited commentary – Dr Deborah Baldie

This chapter contains illuminating examples of how theory has supported practice developers and researchers to 'tune in' to their own and others' experiences and connect with theory to help sense-making, decision-making and actions. While such to-ing and fro-ing between realities and theory is crucial, I worry that we often move in two dimensions – between what we initially see in practice into familiar theories that serve the purpose of verifying our initial assumptions and sense-making rather than challenging our assumptions and unpacking the reality of the context.

The authors remind us of Fay's false consciousness and how it stifles further exploration of issues and more appropriate forms of action. I wonder if some of us as PD scholars have false consciousnesses? Do we step off from that two-dimensional to-ing and fro-ing often enough to explore alternative theories that test our worldviews? I am not sure that we all do, or at least, perhaps not often enough.

Complexity and network theories have highlighted many of the concepts represented in Fay's critical social science theory and the Person-Centred Practice Framework (Kitson et al. 2017; Greenhalgh et al. 2004). They do, however, help widen our lens beyond the power imbalances frequently referred to in this chapter to consider the unpredictable and constantly changing nature of the behaviour of individuals and networks; the different worldviews held by disciplines and persons that influence perceived credibility of evidence and the need for and purpose of change. While I agree that we are not curtailed by methods within PD, we also need to increasingly consider alternative theories to help make sense of the realities we work in and thus become more effective.

We, like the practitioners we seek to support, need to challenge our individual and collective false consciousness as we take into account the role of power, networks, our embodied theory and evolving methods to support PD.

References

Brookfield, S.D. (2005). *Power of Critical Theory for Adult Learning and Teaching*. Berkshire: McGraw-Hill Education.

Brookfield, S.D. (2017). *Becoming a Critically Reflective Teacher, 2nd Edition*. Somerset: Jossey-Bass.

Brown, D. and McCormack, B. (2016). Exploring psychological safety as a component of facilitation within the Promoting Action on Research Implementation in Health Services framework. *Journal of Clinical Nursing* 25 (19–20): 2921–2932.

Buresh, B. and Gordon, S. (2013). *From Silence to Voice: What Nurses Know and Must Communicate to the Public, 3rd Edition*. Ithaca, NY: ILR Press.

Fay, B. (1975). *Social Theory and Political Practice*. London: Allen and Unwin.

Fay, B. (1987). *Critical Social Science: Liberation and its Limits*. Oxford, New York;: Polity Press.

Gramsci, A., Hoare, Q. and Nowel-Smith, G. (1971). *Selections from the Prison Notebooks of Antonio Gramsci/. Edited and translated by Quinton Hoare and Geoffrey Nowell-Smith*. London: Lawrence & Wishart.

Greenhalgh, T., Robert, G., Macfarlane, F. et al. (2004). Diffusion of innovations in service organizations: systematic review and recommendations. *The Milbank Quarterly* 82 (4): 581–629.

Hardiman, M. and Dewing, J. (2014). Critical ally and critical friend: stepping stones to facilitating practice development. *International Practice Development Journal* 4 (1): 3-1–3-19.

Kidd, J., Warbrick, I., Hall, A. et al. (2019). *Briefing on: Waitangi Tribunal health kaupapa report WAI-2575*. Auckland New Zealand Taupua Waiora Research Centre. Auckland University of Technology.

Kislov, R., Pope, C., Martin, G.P. et al. (2019). Harnessing the power of theorising in implementation science. *Implementation Science* 14 (1): 103.

Kitson, A., Brook, A., Harvey, G. et al. (2017). Using complexity and network concepts to inform healthcare knowledge translation. *International Journal of Health Policy and Management* 7 (3): 231–243.

Lacey, C., Huria, T., Beckert, L. et al. (2011). The Hui Process: a framework to enhance the doctor–patient relationship with Māori. *New Zealand Medical Journal* 124 (1347): 72–78.

Manley, K. (2017). An overview of practice development. In: *Person-centred Practice in Nursing and Health Care: Theory and Practice* (ed. B. McCormack and T. McCance), 133–149. Oxford: Wiley.

Manley, K. and Jackson, C. (2019). Microsystems culture change: a refined theory for developing person-centred, safe and effective workplaces based on strategies that embed a safety culture. *International Practice Development Journal* 9 (2). http://dx.doi.org/10.19043/ipdj.92.004

Manley, K., McCormack, B. and Wilson, V. (2008). Introduction. In: *International Practice Development in Nursing and Healthcare* (eds. K. Manley, B. McCormack and V. Wilson), 1–16. Oxford: Blackwell Publishing.

McCormack, B., Dewar, B., Wright, J. et al. (2006). *A Realist Synthesis of Evidence Relating to Practice Development: Executive Summary*. NHS Quality Improvement Scotland and NHS Education for Scotland, Edinburgh.

McCormack, B., Manley, K. and Titchen, A. (2013). *International Practice Development in Nursing and Healthcare*. Oxford: Blackwell Publishing.

McCormack, B. and McCance, T. (2017). *Person-centred Practice in Nursing and Healthcare: Theory and Practice*. Oxford: Wiley Blackwell.

Mooney, M. and Nolan, L. (2006). A critique of Freire's perspective on critical social theory in nursing education. *Nurse Education Today* 26 (3): 240–244.

Nelson, S. (2012). The lost path to emancipatory practice: towards a history of reflective practice in nursing. *Nursing Philosophy* 13 (3): 202–213.

New Zealand Ministry of Health (2019). *Health and Disability System Review Report*. Hauora Manaaki ki Aotearoa Whanui – Purongo mo Tenei Wa. Wellington: HDSR.

Peet, J., Theobald, K. and Douglas, C. (2019). Strengthening nursing surveillance in general wards: a practice development approach. *Journal of Clinical Nursing* 28 (15–16): 2924–2933.

Tiriti o Waitangi (1840). (Treaty of Waitangi). https://nzhistory.govt.nz/politics/treaty-of-waitangi

Titchen, A. (2004). Helping relationships for practice development: critical companionship. In: *Practice Development in Nursing* (eds. B. McCormack et al.), 148–174. Oxford: Blackwell Publishing.

Titchen, A. (2018). Flowing like a river: facilitation in practice development and the evolution of a critical-creative companionship. *International Practice Development Journal* 8 (1). http://dx.doi.org/10.19043/ipdj81.004

Wilson, V. and McCormack, B. (2006). Critical realism as emancipatory action: the case for realistic evaluation in practice development. *Nursing Philosophy* 7 (1): 45–57.

10. *Unpacking and Developing Facilitation*

Rebekkah Middleton, Margaret Kelly, Caroline Dickson, Valerie Wilson, Famke van Lieshout, Kathrin Hirter, and Christine Boomer

Introduction

Skilled facilitation is key to the success of practice development (PD) and can be practised by professionals, leaders, educators, consultants, clinicians, at any level. Using a person-centred approach to facilitation is an essential aspect of engaging stakeholders, of working *with* people rather than working *on* people through change processes, and in supporting systematic approaches to enhancing the practice context. The importance of relationality in facilitation cannot be understated, enabling impact at individual, group and system levels. Facilitation centres on co-producing knowledge using critical reflection and critical conversation and supporting (active) learning in and about practice.

This chapter considers the breadth and depth of facilitation, including an overview of what facilitation is, from a doctoral research study, and providing two examples of facilitator development programmes. One programme is aimed at developing novice facilitators, the other designed for those at the stage of developing advanced facilitation.

Unpacking facilitation – an overview

Enacting skilled transformational facilitation is complex as individuals develop requisite skills, knowledge, attitudes and experiences. Key findings are shared from a doctoral study that aimed to uncover the nature of skilled facilitation and

International Practice Development in Health and Social Care, Second Edition.
Edited by Kim Manley, Valerie Wilson, and Christine Øye.

explore facilitators' development (Kelly 2018). This two-stage research used critical reflection and in-depth interviews with 22 facilitators of all levels of experience across four countries, to inform construction of a global picture of transformational facilitation and development.

The research revealed a clear continuum of development from novice facilitators to those with expertise. The continuum reflected increasing sophistication of facilitators' thinking and practice as they became highly skilled. The themes and subthemes interlinked and overlapped, forming three distinct groupings (Figure 10.1). These groupings are examined in more detail in the rest of this section.

Internal to the facilitator

This group of themes uncovered the nature of the inner dialogue, internal feelings and thought processes. These could constrict a novice facilitator's practice but allowed sophisticated decision-making by skilled facilitators.

Inside your own head

A key finding was uncovering the way facilitators navigated between internal dialogue and facilitation process. All facilitators described having an inner dialogue as they engaged in the practice of facilitation. This influenced *what* facilitators were

Internal to the facilitator

Inside your own head
- The inner dialogue
- Strategies to stay in control
- Changing the inner dialogue
- Externalising the inner dialogue

Walking a fine line
- Balancing challenge and support
- Manipulation versus guidance
- Use of power

Being Me
- Developing your facilitation
- Finding your own style
- Gaining insight

External to the facilitator

A lens on facilitation
- Working with others
- Making the art of facilitation explicit

Making sense of theory
- Making sense of theory for yourself
- Using theory in practice

Enacting transformational facilitation

Being fluid
- Growing in confidence
- Incorporating flexibility

Understanding people in context
- Understanding the context
- Working with people in their context

Figure 10.1 Research themes and sub-themes (Kelly 2018)

doing and *how* they did it. However, the nature of the inner dialogue was different for inexperienced facilitators compared with highly skilled individuals. New facilitators experienced the inner dialogue as constant chatter, indicating the unease they often felt. Molly described this as 'my heart was churning, and my brain was actually jelly'. To reduce anxiety, these facilitators employed strategies to stay in control, creating plans they adhered to, regardless of the needs of people they were working with. The nature of the inner dialogue changed as facilitators gained skills, experience and confidence. The stress and chaos faded, while decision-making came to the forefront. Skilled facilitators were able to assess situations rapidly and decide interventions that would enable individuals or groups to progress work. These individuals were able to endure, and help resolve, discomfort or dissonance within a group. Their decisions were linked to the aims of work undertaken, rather than any predetermined plan. Lucy explained how skilled facilitators were able to externalise their inner dialogue, as 'it's more likely that I'll bring people into the space and say "what's happening?"'. This was not an option usually taken by new facilitators, who needed to be seen as experts, not wanting to reveal their internal turmoil.

Walking a fine line

Facilitators' dialogue and thinking were vital in managing different elements of facilitation practice. Achieving balance required facilitators to consider levels of challenge offered, alongside appropriate support. Inexperienced facilitators often found this difficult to gauge and ended up under- or overchallenging. As skill and knowledge levels increased, facilitators fine-tuned ways to challenge, incorporating several elements into their decision-making. While inexperienced facilitators focused on learning how much challenge to offer, more experienced facilitators, like Amanda, highlighted how they could 'help people to stretch themselves by using different strategies that don't require it to be all about the challenge'.

Lack of confidence sometimes led inexperienced facilitators to push people in a direction they themselves felt more comfortable with. This was not considered manipulation; rather, that groups benefited from structure and guidance. As skill increased, facilitators recognised the fine line between guidance and manipulation. They learned to avoid manipulating a group into following their path, focusing instead on group needs and direction. Manipulation, as described by study participants, related to use of power, who holds or should hold power, and different ways of using power. While skilled facilitators identified and worked with multiple levels and layers of power in context, less experienced individuals might not consider power at all. Jennifer summed up a general feeling among experienced facilitators that they should be 'sharing power, delegating, achieving things through supporting others rather than doing them yourself'.

Being me

An integral part of facilitation uncovered in this research was the idea of being authentic, which reflected the movement of individuals as they developed. Finding their own facilitation style incorporated facilitators' personal sense of being, values and beliefs, plus facilitation knowledge, skills and experience.

In early stages of development, facilitators could be quite technical in their thinking, focusing on learning approaches and skills. This evolved as facilitators developed their craft, building confidence, becoming more knowledgeable and skilled, working with everyone's values and beliefs, including their own. New facilitators did not have the confidence to be themselves, so they copied facilitators they admired. They felt they could achieve similar outcomes by reproducing strategies they saw other facilitators use. As facilitators increasingly gained insight, they realised simply copying would not work. Rebecca articulated this as 'I moved from "I want to be just like them!" to "I want to be myself"'.

External to the facilitator

The second group of themes highlighted elements outside the facilitator's own person, incorporating valuable aspects of facilitators' development.

A lens on facilitation

Interacting with other facilitators was identified by participants as adding value to learning and development. Inexperienced facilitators enjoyed working with more experienced colleagues because it helped them gain insight into skilled facilitation. It provided an environment where they felt safe to practise and take risks. Skilled facilitators, like Debra, set up a space for novices to 'take the risks, to use the tools in safe environments where they can make mistakes and practise it'. In general, working with other facilitators resulted in positive experiences that enabled novices to develop skills and gain confidence in supportive environments. As facilitators gained expertise, they became role models and engaged in developing others. An integral part of this process, for Vanessa, was to 'help them surface this hidden, embedded, embodied knowledge'.

Making sense of theory

It was important for facilitators to underpin their practice with a diverse range of theories. People's thinking is influenced by their personal and professional lives, meaning each person is unique regarding theories they know and the approach they take to engaging with theory in their facilitation practice. Facilitators varied in their delving into the theory of PD and facilitation. Some new facilitators found theory hard to understand and tended to avoid it. These individuals focused more on the 'doing' of facilitation, practising and trying things out. Over time, those facilitators, like Molly, realised 'it's much more about how can theory help me, how do I draw on that to make me a better facilitator?'. Immersing in theory helped facilitators make sense of their own practice in addition to helping others understand and use theory to change their thinking and practice. As facilitators became more skilled, connections between new assimilated theory and previously learned theories were made. This allowed embedding of theoretical principles in a way that helped facilitators understand and enact their practice more comprehensively.

Enacting transformational facilitation

The final group of themes conveys how facilitators assimilate learning and experiences to enable them to work effectively.

Being fluid

Central to this theme was facilitators' ability to be agile in practice. Skilled facilitators described the way they responded in the moment to people and the situations they found themselves in as 'being fluid'. Fluidity came as knowledge, skills and experience were gained. It was not possible for inexperienced facilitators to be fluid because they were too busy learning facilitation, trying to make sense of it for themselves and control their anxiety about getting things wrong. Growing confidence with increasing skill allowed facilitators to, as Amanda stated, 'just let it all go and just do it. You know you know it'. This led to flexibility that all facilitators in the study identified as being essential to practice, the ability to change direction and 'go with the flow'.

Understanding people in context

Facilitators worked with many different groups across a wide range of contexts. To be fluid and effective, facilitators needed to understand people and the context in which they practised. Understanding context included considering available supports or challenges present. Inexperienced facilitators recognised context was important but did not necessarily understand it, how it could impact on activity or how to work with it. This changed as facilitators became more skilled and learned how to work with people within their particular context. As they did so, facilitators helped people understand their own context and work towards transformation of culture.

Embodying facilitation

By synthesising everything articulated in this doctoral research, participants embodied facilitation as a 'way of being'. Embodying facilitation stemmed from individuals gaining personal insights and understanding what facilitation meant to them. This was a constant state of becoming, enabled by facilitators focusing on their development as well as that of others (van Lieshout and Cardiff 2015). Embodying reflected how the internal milieu of facilitators changed as they gained skills, knowledge and experience, going from chaos and self-focus for new facilitators to the theoretical juggling of the expert facilitator. Titchen (2018) describes the professional artistry of critical companionship as a dance to meet people's needs. Skilled facilitation, evidenced by this research study, is a complex intervention of embodiment. It reflects the expertise required to 'dance' and integrate, into a way of being, knowledge, skills and experiences with the internal self.

Facilitator development – developing person-centred facilitators

Drawing on the principles of facilitation above, an example of a facilitator development programme aimed at novice facilitators is shared in this section. As part of ongoing commitment to developing person-centred cultures, a new team of PD facilitators (PDFs) was formed within Marie Curie, a UK-based charity supporting people with palliative care needs towards the end of their life. To support their learning and development as facilitators, a 12-month facilitation programme was commissioned from Queen Margaret University, Edinburgh in 2016 (Dickson et al. 2018). Since programme completion in 2017, ongoing support including a three-day workshop in 2019, ad-hoc co-facilitation and mentorship, has occurred. This next section outlines the original programme aim, methods and evaluation (more detailed evaluation can be found in Dickson et al. 2018). Further evaluation data from the 2017 programme and evaluation carried out in 2020, following ongoing support, is used for this evaluative account. Rather than transformational facilitators, the explicit purpose of the programme was to develop person-centred facilitators.

'Developing Person-centred facilitators': initial programme

This programme aimed to develop PDFs to be catalysts in the transformation of person-centred workplace cultures, through development of their facilitation expertise. There was an expectation of a shift from a technical focus of their role to a holistic approach, helping others thrive within the organisation and promote person-centred practices (Dewing and McCormack 2015). The five programme intentions are outlined in Box 10.1.

Evidence of facilitator development

The PDF programme, in three phases, is outlined in Figure 10.2. Theoretical frameworks underpinning programme methodology were the Person-Centred Practice Framework (McCance and McCormack 2017), emancipatory PD, and active learning (Dewing 2010). Evaluation methods for each programme included claims, concerns, issues (Guba and Lincoln 1989), facilitator stories and reflective accounts.

During the programme and since, a high turnover of the team occurred, perhaps accounting for different rates of progression of individuals along the novice to expert continuum, as well as highlighting different rates people learn and develop.

Box 10.1 Programme intentions

1. Enhance facilitation skills to enable transformation of cultures and contexts of care.
2. Increase understanding of emancipatory PD and knowledge of evaluation processes.
3. Develop a community of practice around person-centred practice.
4. Develop a suite of resources available across Marie Curie.
5. Create a communication and engagement strategy to enhance and sustain person-centred culture of care.

2016–2017	2018–2019	2020
Developing Person-centred PD Facilitators	Ongoing support/mentorship	Three-day workshop: 'Developing person-centred facilitators to enhance a culture of person-centredness'
Four monthly workshops: 1. Key concepts of facilitation, person-centredness and PD 2. Developing facilitation skills and tools 3. Ways of intentionally developing person-centred cultures 4. Different participatory evaluation methods Monthly active learning sessions over 6-months	External facilitation (Caroline) through ad-hoc workshops, co-facilitation in workplaces; Being a critical friend (Hardiman and Dewing 2019).	Learning outcomes: 1. Participants will feel re-connected as a PDF team and feel prepared for the ongoing facilitation of person-centred cultures in their workplaces 2. A shared understanding of person-centred culture for learning will be created collaboratively to be the anchor for person-centred practice 3. Participants will understand patterns and routines in practice and be able to draw on PD to create person-centred patterns 4. Individual and co-designed team objectives and action plans will be created to be embedded in systems and processes

Figure 10.2 Theoretical underpinnings

During the initial programme, there was general aspiration for facilitation to become a 'way of being', but some reticence in believing in personal ability to achieve this. For most, at the start of their journey, they wanted direction and were focused on the 'doing' aspects of facilitation. As novice facilitators, there was a sense that to be person-centred facilitators, the organisational context would have to change. However, during the programme PDFs realised they needed to look inside themselves to be the facilitator, indicating the inner dialogue going on *inside their head*. Through time they understood their potential role in facilitating culture change, but needed to find opportunities to make that happen. *Being me*, one aspect of internal facilitation, was evident in their reflections about treading carefully initially, gauging when to reveal themselves as people and contribute to articulating shared values. One PDF highlighted the need for open trust in the team and to progress at her own pace:

> *'The openness to challenging was at my pace as a new PDF and at their pace as a team.'*

PDF's articulated challenges experienced in raising consciousness and walking the fine line between support and challenge. Growing expertise in this regard was revealed in the 2020 evaluation data from a clinical nurse specialist:

> *'The session was really powerful and has made me think about a lot of things including the relationship I have with [others]. It's really helped me put a few things into perspective'*

In their reflective accounts in 2017, the PDFs were developing skills in creating conditions for themselves and others to be authentic, helping in *being me* and enabling engagement at an increasingly deep level, to be courageous and develop resilience. The safe spaces created within their team environments, where they felt able to share more of themselves, were viewed as liberating as they felt no fear of failure. According to Martin and Manley (2018), motivated, engaged, self-directing teams are a strong indicator of the outcome and impact of facilitation.

Participants were intentional about external factors needed in learning and development to transition to being person-centred facilitators. In the beginning, supported by the PD Leaders, they sought opportunities to practise their developing skills. They used existing opportunities within their role (e.g. induction, clinical supervision, clinical skills training). As the theme *inside your own head* suggests, for novice facilitators there was comfort in organising these workshops and setting up meetings and groups, with scripted plans to support them. Over time, there was evidence that generally they relied less on structure. Rather, they could introduce more flexibility comfortably, as the theme *being fluid* suggests. In 2019, one PDF realised this:

'I came away understanding various PD tools and an understanding that I don't need to have a structured "action plan" leading to a pre-planned destination. I don't need to have as much control. I can let go and trust in the process, see where the sessions we plan lead us.'

As the theme *lens of facilitation* suggests is important in facilitator development, the team set up ways to learn from others. There is ongoing commitment to continue personal development and support others. To move along the continuum from novice to expert, they actively seek opportunities to practise facilitation skills. They use technology and have established triads, mentorships sessions, weekly teleconferences and team 'time-outs' (critical dialogue, giving and receiving support and challenge). In the early days of development, focus on scripted frameworks meant less intentionality of *making sense of theory*. Involving more experienced facilitators as co-facilitators/mentors, however, helped PDFs try different facilitation tools and generate their own theory. Using critical creativity was viewed at the beginning as risky, but over time, the 2020 data revealed they began to value and integrate critical creativity into their role as a method for achieving in-depth understanding of topics, skills and scenarios.

There is also evidence in the 2020 evaluation data that some PDFs were enacting transformational facilitation. As the PDF team have become more confident in facilitation, they perceive the culture has simultaneously become more open to their role. This confirms their role as a catalyst for culture change, moving them far from the concerns they had as novices. One quote from a regional manager in the 2020 evaluation data demonstrates how she viewed the PDF's facilitation leadership and its significance in culture change:

'Initially we were all a bit sceptical about being creative and using that to explore person-centred care, our vision and culture, but you have won us over by allowing us to take it at our own pace and in a non-threatening way.'

This embodiment of facilitation is also evident as the PDFs reflected on the embeddedness of using CIP principles. This is a shift from the original, top-down approach to facilitation they adopted as novice facilitators. They report how they are now able to use a range of tools to encourage involvement in critically creative methods for learning. The variety of tools is being used to promote participation in different scenarios, such as shown in Box 10.2.

Participants' skills in articulating shared values, asking critical questions, guiding critical reflection, using scenarios from practice as positive learning opportunities, developing a shared vision, giving and receiving feedback, and using feedback to develop practice demonstrate their growing ability to embed theoretical principles. For some, the transition reflects flexibility and movement from being facilitator to co-facilitator, in response to the group dynamic and feedback advocated by Heron (2001). One PDF gave an example of where team managers in a leadership group made this transition into co-facilitators, identifying differences they wanted to make to session structure and the control they wanted within that. On page XXX this is referred to as *holding the power*.

Evaluation of the PDF facilitator development at Marie Curie demonstrates how, over time, they are beginning to *embody facilitation*. The data gives examples of their changing internal milieu and how the intentionality of seeking external opportunities is enabling more fluidity and responsiveness in facilitation.

Box 10.2 Examples of tools to promote participation

- Reframing learning contracts as 'ways of working' – helping groups promote feelings of safety, creating conditions for courageousness.
- Checking in and out, gauging the 'mood' of the group or the learning achieved.
- Using observational tools, focusing on moments of person-centredness and person-centred language.
- Using poetry to gauge feelings/morale

Facilitator development – moving to advanced facilitation

It is clear from the previous sections that those who facilitate PD are enabling themselves and others to grow. But how do facilitators themselves further develop skills, strengthen theoretical knowledge, find unique ways/strengths, evaluate, and advance the art and science of their facilitation practice?

Facilitation at a foundational level is supported through various programmes (e.g. the International Practice Development Collaborative (IPDC) five-day PD foundation programme). Developing beyond foundational level has been an individual activity (for most) with no formal opportunities to spend time focussed on advancing facilitation within PD. In a complex and ever-changing healthcare environment, advanced facilitation is required to help people, at all levels and in all roles, navigate the challenges of applying PD principles, theories and implementation models to healthcare environments.

To bridge this gap, IPDC members worked together using CIP principles (see Chapter 8 for details) to create a principle-based programme focusing on advancing facilitation skills within the context of person-centred practice. The development of the course was co-constructed using principles of facilitation, person-centredness, PD, reflexivity, leadership, and critical social science theory. An example of the advanced course is provided to demonstrate aspects of extending and enhancing facilitation knowledge and skills, broadening facilitation scope, and challenging participants to adapt to local societal and organisational developments and changes, moving towards being a propositional facilitator (Crisp and Wilson 2011), where person-centred facilitation becomes embodied.

Advanced facilitation course

To actively engage participants in growing their facilitation, co-production of knowledge needs to occur using critical reflection and critical conversation, and by enabling (active) learning in and about practice. This occurs only when facilitators become aware of their skills, strengthen their theoretical knowledge, evaluate their facilitation, and advance the art and science of facilitation practice. In challenging facilitators to extend their seeing, doing, ways of knowing, and being as a facilitator, using the Person-Centred Practice Framework (PCPF) (McCance and McCormack 2017) is critical. This framework helps facilitators consider context and self (van Lieshout 2013), preparation, reflection and reflexivity. Considering the constructs of the PCPF, learning outcomes were developed by the IPDC and are listed in Box 10.3.

Theory is required for growth as a facilitator, and the advanced facilitation course focuses on person-centredness, critical social theory, leadership and facilitation and their links to PD. Theories of person-centredness centre on facilitating an individual's authenticity so their full potential can be realised (McCance and McCormack 2017). Theories of critical social theory reveal how knowledge is structured by existing sets of social relations (Fay 1987) (see Chapter 9 by past participants for more detailed information). Theories of facilitation manifest

Box 10.3 Learning outcomes

- Develop deeper awareness of self and others in person-centred ways of working.
- Demonstrate and apply advanced knowledge of theoretical principles underpinning person-centredness, critical social science and facilitation practice.
- Use theoretical principles to underpin holistic facilitation practice across a range of different practice contexts reflexively.
- Evaluate effectiveness and impact of facilitation practice across a spectrum of contexts and complexity.
- Contribute to advancing the PD paradigm.
- Become critical companions for the IPDC.

facilitation as an art and knowing intuitively when to use specific strategies and theoretical underpinnings in practice (Manley et al. 2015).

Participants are allocated a theory to explore prior to day 1. Participants share learning and application of theory in the safety of active learning groups. Critical reflection is fostered using multiple creative means, engaging reflection at a deeper level, and through insights into self, remembering the work of John Dewey: 'We do not learn from experience. . . we learn from reflecting on experience' (Dewey 1910, p. 78). Participants use a personal portfolio with the purpose of encouraging them to document their learning and 'moments' to timeline growth and highlight aspects for follow-up. Creativity is encouraged to stimulate thoughts, help creative imagination and reflection (Titchen et al. 2011).

A pilot of the programme was delivered in Australia, commencing in October 2017 and ending in February 2018. Since this time, three more programmes have been completed in Australia and one in Europe. Various delivery methods are used to suit the context, with Australia using a 2/1/1-day (face-to-face) model and Europe using a 3/1/1-day (face-to-face and virtual) model. Participant numbers ranged from 6 to 16 for each course held, with people from a broad and diverse range of health roles and facilitation experience.

The intent of the programme was to focus on what matters to individuals and teams in the context of their work and the workplace, in order to achieve person-centred cultures and improved health outcomes (Manley et al. 2015). A key factor of the advanced facilitation course was person-centred co-design, which included participants setting their own collective learning objectives for the course on day 1. Some examples are given in Box 10.4.

> *'The first two days were great as it allowed submersion in the concepts and allowed a concentrated time to get to know and trust each other. The following separate days were spread out enough to allow time to try out and practise the concepts and "do homework" that we could then reflect on and bring back to the group the next time we met. It was also an environment that challenged and extended me (us) and that is rare to find in my workplace, and many others I imagine.' (Australia)*

Facilitation critique lists were developed and used in conjunction with Manley et al.'s (2015) facilitation standards. Various means of reflecting on facilitation were adapted. These reflections and critical conversations enabled participants,

Box 10.4 Learning outcome examples

- Develop my understanding of theory and how it links to practice, using it in a creative, flexible and meaningful way.
- Explore myself as an authentic facilitator who has the courage and vulnerability to enhance my facilitation practice, especially when challenged.
- Enhance my skills and confidence in how to articulate PD to multiple stakeholders.
- Develop strategically around PD and my role as an influencer.

as facilitators, to revisit and revise principles of facilitation as core aspects of engaging and promoting effective PD (e.g. Figure 10.3). Facilitation strategies are mapped to Manley et al.'s (2015) standards and compared and plotted to the PCPF (McCance and McCormack 2017).

A minimum of two days are co-designed and offer participants space to practise in a safe environment, enabling challenge to be provided in a supportive milieu. See Box 10.5 for examples of programme topics.

Participants reported co-design as challenging but a point of real growth and trust in self and others:

> *'I loved that we lived what was espoused. We should be co-designing with others, bringing to the group our version of things, opening it up to discuss and explore. It also meant that we were required to think about the topic we had and pre-read, which in turn increased our development on each subject. There was a good balance of support and challenge offered by [lead facilitators] and each other.' (Australia)*

The European course held two virtual days, working in sub-groups per country on case studies highlighting the possibilities and challenges of doing PD with

Critical Friends
Support
Inquiry
Co-creation
Listening
Focus on leaders first
Having the same vision
multiple-purpose framework
Socratic questions
Starting
Need for change
Leadership
Share ideas together
VISIONING
look for allies in the organisation
clarity about purposes
Relationship
celebrate little steps
shared values for shared purpose
convince by example in little steps
getting to know self, context
interplay
Support within
Support out with

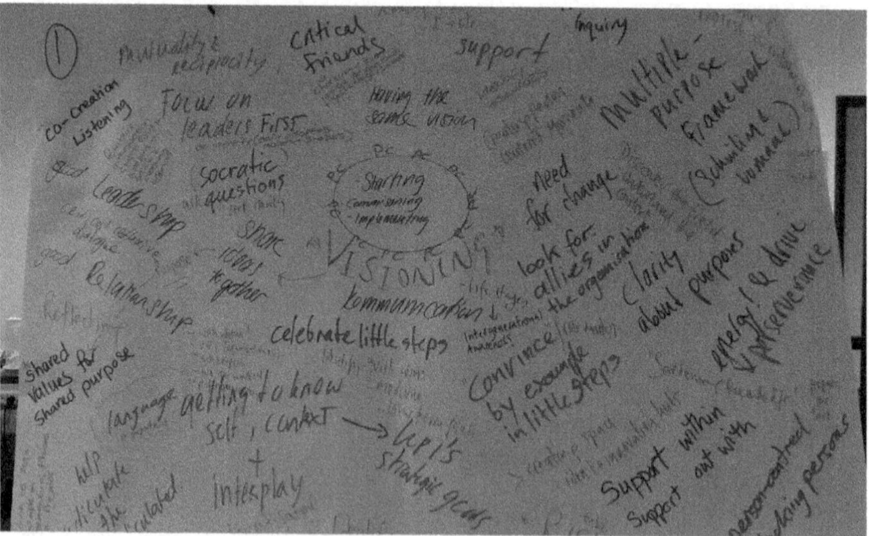

Figure 10.3 Brainstorming how to facilitate starting a PD initiative

Box 10.5 Example day 3 programme

Topic
Managing inner dialogue and working with emotions
Creative approaches to enabling 'stories'
Reflecting on and learning from the collision of heart and mind in the care environment
Linking critical reflection, PD and person-centred approaches
Collecting evidence about facilitation and PD – what, how, extension at micro, meso, macro levels
Role of strategy and leadership in facilitation

individuals and teams at micro, meso and macro levels. This enabled great learning to see the impact of culture on facilitating PD.

Evaluation

Evaluation of courses run to date demonstrates consistent development in participants' knowledge and confidence in relation to their identified learning objectives. Daily programme feedback and in addition qualitative feedback three months after the course identified growth and learning in the following ways:

'I am using [facilitation standards] myself in a very integrated way, the team I lead (52+ educators) are moving their practice significantly towards a facilitative approach and are skilled at identifying features. I will be formally implementing the standards as a next step.' (Australia)

'I move forward.' (Figure 10.4) 'It took my attention that the purposes of integrated facilitation (Martin and Manley 2018) include not only PD but also knowledge translation and inquiry.' (Europe)

'I am less inclined to be tied or determined to reach my designated goal for the session. I am more comfortable letting the conversation go where it needs to and feel more cognitively agile to pull from a variety of skills and theories in order to reach the intent the group need.' (Australia)

The experiences of those participating in the programmes demonstrate how an understanding of the role of critical reflection as an advanced facilitator, participating in the co-design of the programme, being person-centred, achieving learning and development outcomes, and exploring 'new frontiers' of facilitation shaped and contributed to the evolving art and science of facilitation.

'I personally felt immensely grateful for the opportunity to have a body of theoretical work critiqued by the group and to see it brought to life, applied, developed further and invigorated – new realms of possibilities opened in usefulness and practical application.' (Europe)

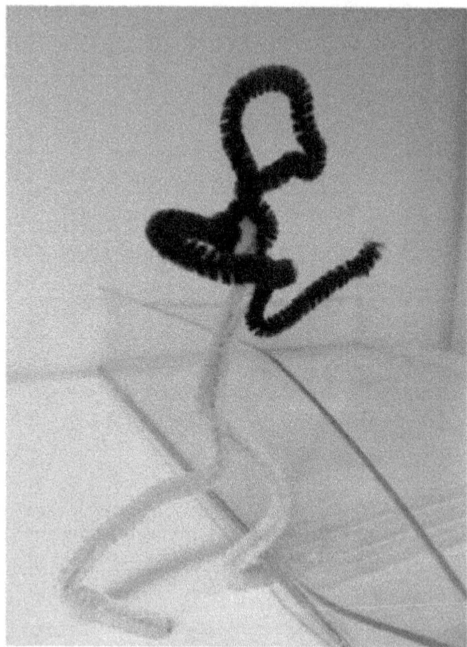

Figure 10.4 Moving forward with facilitation skills

Advanced facilitation take-home message

Facilitating PD-driven change requires a network of support from skilled facilitators and transformational leaders who have capacity and capability of applying theory to practice, developing theory from practice, creating a compelling vision for change, and are reflexive and/or adaptive to the interplay between facilitation and context to connect practitioners at all levels across an organisational system. The international advanced facilitation course helps participants clarify how facilitating PD distinguishes itself from more conventional ways of facilitation and how this could add value in achieving shared (organisational) aims.

'I understand there was an international faculty informing the way it delivered. This is a huge strength as the advanced nature of such a programme benefits from this wider context.' (Australia)

Conclusion

In this chapter we have seen that facilitation at all levels is an essential way of being for practice developers. Facilitation at its core is transformational, but it is a process, a continuum, developing from novice to advanced. In unpacking facilitation, it is a way of being, an embodiment of learning, experiences, values and theory that enable people to be flexible and responsive in varying contexts. How we link our facilitation practice to person-centred principles and approaches is critical to our way of being and doing, to how we engage and embed our practices in the workplace. Extending ourselves is something we should always be striving for; to be more capable, more skilled, more knowledgeable, more applied, reflecting our commitment to growth as practice developers. The two examples outlined in this chapter, a novice and an advanced programme, build on the principles of transformational facilitation and development identified through research. Key to development of facilitators is personal insight and reflection, so that individuals can grow facilitation complexity, integrating theory to practice, be reflexive and adapt. It is a process of being, which enables person-centred language, actions, presence.

References

Crisp, J. and Wilson, V. (2011). How do facilitators of practice development gain the expertise required to support vital transformation of practice and workplace cultures? *Nurse Education in Practice* 11 (3): 173–178.

Dewey, J. (1910). *How We Think*. Boston, MA: D.C. Heath and Company.

Dewing, J. (2010). Moments of movement: active learning and practice development. *Nurse Education in Practice* 10 (1): 22–26.

Dewing, J. and McCormack, B. (2015). Engagement: a critique of the concept and its application to person-centred care. *International Practice Development Journal* 5 (Suppl) [6]. https://www.fons.org/Resources/Documents/Journal/Vol5Suppl/IPDJ_05(suppl)_06.pdf

Dickson, C., Legg, M., Penman, P. et al. (2018). From root to fruit – flourishing in change. Evaluation of a development programme for practice development facilitators in end-of-life care. *International Practice Development Journal* 8 (1) [3]. https://doi.org/10.19043/ipdj81.003

Fay, B. (1987). *Critical Social Science: Liberation and Its Limits*. Ithaca, NY: Cornell University Press.

Guba, E.G. and Lincoln, Y.S. (1989). *Fourth Generation Evaluation*. Newbury Park, CA: Sage.

Hardiman, M. and Dewing, J. (2019). Using two models of workplace facilitation to create conditions for development of a person-centred culture: a participatory action research study. *Journal of Clinical Nursing* 28 (15–16): 2769–2781.

Heron, J. (2001). *Helping the Client: A Creative Practical Guide*. London: Sage.

Kelly, M. (2018). Skilled Facilitation within Transformational Practice Development in Healthcare. *PhD thesis*. University of Technology, Sydney.

Manley, K., Martin, A., Jackson, C. et al. (2015). *Transforming Urgent and Emergency Care Together Phase 2 Report: Developing Standards for Integrated Facilitation in and About the Workplace*. Canterbury: England Centre for Practice Development. December. http://create.canterbury.ac.uk/14241/3/14241.pdf

Martin, A. and Manley, K. (2018). Developing standards for an integrated approach to workplace facilitation for interprofessional teams in health and social care contexts: a Delphi study. *Journal of Interprofessional Care* 32 (1): 41–51.

McCance, T. and McCormack, B. (2017). The Person-centred Practice Framework. In: *Person-centred Practice in Nursing and Health Care* (eds. B. McCormack and T. McCance). Oxford: Wiley Blackwell.

Titchen, A. (2018). Flowing like a river: facilitation in practice development and the evolution of critical-creative companionship. *International Practice Development Journal* 8 (1): 1–23.

Titchen, A., McCormack, B., Wilson, V. et al. (2011). Human flourishing through body, creative imagination and reflection. *International Practice Development Journal* 1 (1): 1-1–1-18.

van Lieshout, F. (2013). *Taking Action for Action: A Study of the Interplay between Contextual and Facilitator Characteristics in Developing an Effective Workplace Culture in a Dutch Hospital Setting, through Action Research*. PhD thesis. University of Ulster, Belfast.

van Lieshout, F. and Cardiff, S. (2015). Reflections on being and becoming a person-centred facilitator. *International Practice Development Journal* 5 (Suppl) [4].

11. *Re-Imagining Participation in Processes of Facilitation: a Case for 'Humble Assertiveness'*

Gudmund Ågotnes, Karen Tuqiri, and Kristin Ådnøy Eriksen

Introduction

The main objective of this chapter is to discuss the process of facilitation of change within organisations in the health and social sectors. We are, in other words, preoccupied with facilitation processes in the context of workplaces within certain sectors. The central theme of this chapter is how within the context of 'participation' we understand facilitation relationships. We will discuss 'participation' in processes of facilitation from a theoretical and analytical standpoint, and present what we believe are significant implications for the facilitator.

Facilitation involves a complex array of activities directed at changing or improving the forms and the practices of organisations (Dahl and Eriksen 2020; Eriksen and Heimestøl 2017). As such, facilitation can be seen as a process of providing means or tools of altering something, which, transferred to a workplace context, would imply working differently and/or more effectively. In the context of the health and social sectors, facilitating change can, for instance, entail the enablement of improving the organisation and provision of care. Furthermore, altering different ways of working, different ways of communication, collaborating or organising is, we believe, particularly relevant in the

International Practice Development in Health and Social Care, Second Edition.
Edited by Kim Manley, Valerie Wilson, and Christine Øye.

health and social sectors, as they are sectors where the primary form of resource is the workforce, and where 'what can be altered' is the practices of workers, as opposed to, for instance, physical and/or digital equipment. Furthermore, facilitation is described as multilayered in the sense of consisting of a continuum of focus and complexity from individual/groups addressing clinical skills and competencies to the opposite end of a spectrum in which the system in its entirety is addressed to enable sustainable innovation (Manley and Jackson 2020). The authors of this chapter have been involved in various forms of facilitation processes linked to health and social services, with an array of different compositions of participants and with different expected aims. Three of these, set in the context of Norway but, we believe, also relevant for other jurisdictions, will be used for illustrative purposes in this chapter and will be presented in the form of extended cases. One of the authors, an experienced Australian facilitator, has enabled the relevance of these cases to be made further explicit.

A common denominator for these cases, as for processes of facilitation in general, is to achieve some form of *change* within organisations and institutions. 'Change', however, has many forms and can be operationalised in many ways. In this chapter, we aim to position facilitation with lasting, transformative change (Manley and Jackson 2020), that is, change that permeates the organisation, that is enshrined in everyday practices and that is incorporated into the institution over time. Lasting, transformative change is the very purpose of the process of facilitation; it is what is to be facilitated.

Lasting, transformative change to any complex social environment, of which we see health and social service organisations as proponents, does not come easy, however. Change of this nature is difficult to achieve, in part because of what we understand as the 'toughness embedded in workplace cultures'. Based on an understanding of 'culture' as both significant and collective, yet implicit and often taken for granted (Bourdieu 1990, 2012), we argue that it sets premises for the interplay and interaction between facilitator and facilitated, with significant implications both for the process of facilitation and for the role of the facilitator in practice development (PD) work. Facilitators cannot escape the fact they must enter, relate to (and as we shall see later, adapt to) a foreign territory, someone else's domain. This domain can have its own customs, systems and organisational peculiarities, to which the facilitator must relate.

In the chapter, we argue that facilitating for change – lasting transformative change in particular – presupposes an approach towards but also *with* those affected by what is to be changed. We propose an approach to facilitation in which mutuality and participatory democracy are central. Within this approach, the facilitator, acknowledging, recognising and responding to the more or less culturally specific context, adapts and surrenders to the contextual framework – a form of situational awareness – and accepts a role of 'humble assertiveness'.

The process of facilitation – case examples

Case 1 Facilitation in an interdisciplinary team – creating a collaborative environment

The participants in this case were an interdisciplinary team, collaborating on a Norwegian development project aimed to evaluate the work in the team as well as to strengthen the team as a working fellowship (Eriksen and Heimestøl 2017). The participants worked collaboratively with pregnant women and parents at risk of substance abuse and/or mental illness. The team was established in order to prevent harm to children caused by parents' poor mental health or substance abuse.

The team members were considered experts in their fields and had different professional backgrounds: child psychologist, pediatrician, midwife, social workers and public health nurses. As this was a newly established team with complex tasks, they realised that it would be very helpful to work systematically in addressing the challenges they faced. Two facilitators, from a research and development department owned by the health services and the university college, led the PD processes and completed an evaluation of the team's work.

From the onset of the processes, the facilitators realised that there was a need to 'prove' to the team that the facilitated workshops and meetings were worthwhile of their time and effort. The team members didn't want to spend time on something that could not be labelled as 'effective' in some way. The facilitators therefore decided the subsequent steps in the process based on the issues identified as important by the team, while at the same time facilitating in a way that gave the team opportunities to bring new issues to the table. The facilitators aimed at developing 'person-centred, safe and effective care and cultures and enabling knowledge translation' (Manley and Jackson 2020, p. 8). Facilitation involved using methods that encouraged all team members to contribute, acknowledging each person's contribution and helping the team to explore whether the services met needs.

Through these facilitated processes, the team decided on the aim for development: to enhance the collaborative work in the interdisciplinary team, both within the team and with external partners, and to explore how the team worked in accordance with their aims. It was important for the facilitated processes that the team remained in charge of priorities, as the facilitators did not have details about the work the team was supposed to do (except from reading the plans and aims for the team). The facilitators were careful to compile an agenda for processes that could be considered relevant for the work and thus for the participants worth spending time exploring.

Based on multistage focus group interviews in three phases (Eriksen and Heimestøl 2017), some experiences from the process can be outlined. Members expressed that the process contributed to the development of the team by being offered what they described as 'new opportunities' provided throughout the facilitated processes. One was scheduling time and space to actively involve oneself in development; it had not been easy prior to this to prioritise time to 'sit down to share and listen'. Part of this was that the sharing became more systematic as the facilitators guided the process of sharing with activities that enhanced involvement from everybody, without spending a lot of time. The facilitator asked questions that opened new agendas for what was worth sharing in the team. They valued opportunities to notice and detect issues and thus became more able to handle them, at the same time getting to know each other better. Being safe and revealing weaknesses made it possible to support each other better. Speaking about their work increased awareness of the strengths of their colleagues, and they reflected that this had resulted in less fear of being left alone with demanding decisions and responsibilities in their work. The team spoke to each other and the facilitators about their work and what they believed were important values in what they were doing, thus building and strengthening the team. This became a narrative about who they were and what they were doing, that made them proud, and, we believe, more likely to see their everyday work as part of a greater picture.

After each session, the facilitators had the opportunity to reflect what they were doing from a meta perspective and to discuss how the different methods were useful for the participants. The facilitators reflected that it was important to be assertive in selling the approach, yet humble and creative to tailor the method and aims to the specific situation. Bringing in an outside perspective on the work in the team, as well as providing tools to make the participants tell the story about who they were and what they wanted to accomplish as a team, was a way of supporting the team in providing safe and effective services.

Case 2 Facilitation among peers – collaboration in the facilitation process

In this case, the task of the facilitators was to create a continuing education component for frontline leaders in Norwegian municipal health and care services (nursing homes, home help care, assisting living) around the overall topic of 'leadership of an increasingly multicultural workforce', connected to the research project 'Multicare' (Tingvold and Fagertun 2020). The programme was envisioned to support frontline leaders, for instance unit or ward managers at a nursing home, in dealing with a significant increase in ethnocultural diversity among their workforce. The continuing educational component was to be created together with representatives in the 'target group': frontline leaders in the sectors. Four municipalities, eight institutions and twelve leaders were involved in the effort to develop what later evolved into a combined online and campus-based education component organised by a university college.

Representatives from the university college functioned as facilitators and adopted an approach in which the participants were given considerable autonomy and responsibility in all phases of development. Such an approach was chosen in part as a strategy because the education component had to be created from scratch. Through a six-month period the group (facilitators and participants) worked on developing the educational component through workshops, online meetings and homework in between, alternating between the different forms. This very process – how content, structure and organisation were made – was developed by the participants. The facilitators, to the surprise of most participants, explained early on that all aspects of what was to be created, including how it was to be made, should be developed together through a form of co-creation process. As such, the facilitators approached the task by presenting themselves as mutual partners and stakeholders, all responsible for what (and how) was to be developed. This approach prompted the facilitators to assume a somewhat detached role in the process and during meetings, while participants from the municipalities were expected to assume responsibility gradually throughout the process.

Based on individual and focus-group interviews with the participants in three phases (beginning, middle, end), we can outline some lessons learned from this process primarily from the perspectives of the participants. The process in general was portrayed as slow and time-consuming. It was described as 'a different way of working', in stark contrast to the immediacy of everyday work life, where results were attained on a daily if not an hour-by-hour basis. This 'slowness' was connected to the form of collaboration, with extended discussions, mutual sharing of ideas and a constant need to compromise, also described as a contrast to everyday work life. The leaders expressed that they were accustomed to a faster pace and a more direct form of communication. In retrospect, the participants also described feelings of frustration and uncertainty in the early phases of PD, particularly concerning uncertain roles among the participants and between participants and facilitators, connected to the absence of a clear hierarchy and a detailed division of roles.

After a period of adjustment, however, a sense of ownership rose among the participants, gradually and exponentially, described as a sense of being a vital part of both the process (how) and the product (what). Several participants described this as an interesting learning experience, realising gradually not only the potential in their own role ('I matter') but also a benefit ('What's in it for me'). When completed, the educational component was described as relevant, interesting and, most importantly for the participants, as adapted and adaptable to their respective contexts and to their various needs. This was attributed to the form of collaboration, where they, albeit slowly, could draw on each other's experience, and, perhaps most importantly, to how the very process was set up: the degree of participation and influence throughout the various stages of development contributed to a 'result' that was made not only for but also with those affected by it. Several participants expressed that such a degree of relevance and adaptability also led to a greater potential of implementation into everyday practices over time, as opposed to yet another project for 'the project graveyard'.

Case 3 Facilitation in a cross-sectorial group – collaboration to achieve system-level collaboration

As part of a larger Norwegian reform of the health and social sectors, called 'the coordination reform' (Ringard et al. 2013), cross-sectoral working groups were established, with the objective of planning how the various sections could work closer together to ensure high-quality patients' paths. This effort made it possible to explore processes of facilitation of collaborative work (Dahl et al. 2019; Dahl and Eriksen 2020).

Several factors inhibited collaboration within the working groups and needed to be addressed in the facilitation process, primarily connected to power imbalances between the participants. First, there is a considerable power imbalance between the specialised services and the municipal services. Second, there is an even stronger power imbalance between patients and patients' representatives and the professionals. Additionally, the services are complex systems, and in-depth knowledge about the systems can be difficult to achieve for patient representatives, making their participation in such working groups challenging.

The main task for the facilitator was to help the group to get an understanding of the other stakeholders' perspectives, to give all groups members an opportunity to participate. One way of doing this was to use 'evoke picture cards' to extend what is considered relevant to say something about. This encouraged people who thought their contribution was less important. It may also have contributed to less 'readymade solutions', as the experts needed to say things in new ways. The pictures on the cards encouraged the use of metaphors and assisted the groups in expressing complex issues, as well as giving a sense of fellowship. The facilitation contributed to the unity of the group by setting the standard for how the process was to transpire: all the voices in the group were acknowledged.

Another way of strengthening the unity of the group and at the same time ensuring that the total competence of the group was utilised was to engage the group in creating a three-dimensional model of the work (Dahl et al. 2019). This way of working together can be enjoyable thanks to trying out variations of explanations and solutions to challenges. Through such moments of joy, the facilitator could enable the group to become aware of underlying thoughts about their understanding of the context by inviting the group to explore emerging issues further. In one group, a participant presented what she experienced as a challenge connected to sectorial collaboration, in the form of a drawing. The facilitator took the opportunity to engage the group by adding to this drawing, opening up for a wider understanding of the challenge in the group and ultimately leading to suggestions about how it could be handled. Most importantly, throughout such creative processes, the formal roles of each person, and the prestige connected to them, seem to become less important.

In this case, the role of the facilitator evolved into that of a neutral but active role in the group. The aim was to help the group to develop a collaborative culture and to build bridges between the participants, placed differently in both a social and a professional hierarchy. The facilitator contributed to this by creating an environment and by offering techniques in which differences between the various positions were less emphasised. In conclusion, the case illustrates a process of facilitation in which finding a common ground and collective understandings across significant differences became possible.

The complexity of facilitation – achieving meaningful participation

As illustrated through these cases, facilitation is a complex and multifaceted process, involving various forms of organisations with various compositions of members; the level of integration of and collaboration among the participants can vary, in other words. Whether or not the participants can be considered a more or less homogenous group is, as such, a variable influencing the process of facilitation. Furthermore, homo/heterogeneity can mean different things in this context. First, the facilitated can vary regarding organisational affinity, as seen in cases 1 and 3, where participants come from different professions, different sectors and have different roles but are still expected to work together. Second, the facilitated can vary in what we can describe as cultural or social affinity, where the participants share a 'position', experience or formal role, as seen in case 2. Here, a common ground exists between the participants – similar work task, similar experience, similar formal education – while they do not necessarily worked together outside the process of facilitation.

Additionally, the very function of the facilitation process can vary, as seen in the cases. The function can involve that of bringing people together across complex organisational hierarchies (which can be comprised of both heterogenous and homogenous collaboratives) and initiating processes of change *within* organisations and institutions already with a high degree of collaboration (which also can be comprised of both heterogenous and homogenous collaboratives). Furthermore, the cases also illustrate that the process of facilitation is indeed a process, something that itself is developing, must be nurtured and has its own life, to which the facilitator must adapt, as illustrated in case 3, where the facilitator introduced different techniques and exercises to change the dynamic in the group. As seen here, the facilitator's adaptability can contribute to the effectiveness of the facilitation process and the degree of engagement that the facilitated demonstrate. The ability of a facilitator to effectively utilise a complex array of activities that focus on purpose, context and effectiveness can, as such, be an essential element to achieve transformative change.

Finally, the cases illustrate that facilitation can occur in different stages in a continuum of complexity (Manley and Jackson 2020), from that of facilitating a common ground/understanding, as seen in case 1, to that of producing instruments of change, as seen in case 2, to that of more overarching organisational change, as seen in case 3, where a main objective was to re-think the ways of how to collaborate and communicate across sectors. An implication of this is that the facilitator will enter the scene at different stages of a process (Martin and Manley 2017) and must adapt accordingly, towards both the goal of the facilitated process and the overarching outcome that is to be achieved. The facilitator should, in other words, exert a degree of adaptability, regarding both the group and its dynamic, and towards the micro-interactions occurring during a meeting. In cases 1 and 3, for instance, the facilitator(s) realised during the process the need for creating an atmosphere of collaboration among the participants. Here the main objective was to create a foundation for further work. To achieve the respective objectives of the groups, an initial focus on 'finding commonalities' was necessary. In case 2, and somewhat contrarily, the participants shared such commonalities and did not need or use time to 'understand each other's positions', prompting the facilitators to prioritise a shared understanding (between the facilitator and the facilitated) of the very process of facilitation.

A commonality: culture

For processes of facilitation within the health and social sectors, the facilitator will need to work with a variety of factors such as who the participants are, their group composition and what they intend to achieve. Still, a commonality is that those about to be facilitated *share something*, a profession, a task, an organisation, a goal, or a workplace. This sharing, or these commonalities, involve, we argue, a cultural component, although on different levels. The facilitated share ways of working, of thinking, of practising or of relating to the tasks at hand, albeit differently from case to case. How 'the outsider' (the facilitator) should understand and relate to such cultures of others (the facilitated) is therefore worth elaborating on.

'Culture' is, from our perspective, difficult to measure or contain, also when transferred to our context, the workplace; it is often non-concrete and becomes, therefore, often unaddressed. We know it is there and we can all experience its effect on everyday work life, but it often remains as something that just is, as a given. Borrowing from Bourdieu (1990, 2012), the intricacies of how things are done, the practices within any given social environment, can to a large degree remain implicit, unchallenged and unreflected. For Bourdieu, *practice* at the workplace, as elsewhere, cannot be reduced to the will or the rationality of the individual agent performing the practice (Bourdieu 2012). Practice is, rather, to a large degree taken for granted, in a form of 'learned ignorance' (Bourdieu 2012, p. 19). Furthermore, the group, the work environment, or the organisation, can be understood as a collective but does not necessarily communicate or articulate a collective intent.

Health and social services or sectors often share characteristics, given that a vital part of the focus is connected to human interaction and guidance, although the work to be performed is of a non-specific and varied form, not to be reduced to easily adaptable scripts for the practitioners. Because of this, regimes of practices (or 'workplace cultures') that by their very definition are local, informal and unique are constructed (Ågotnes 2017). Here, 'how things are done' is embedded in the walls of the organisations, adding to the 'toughness' and slowness of transformative change previously discussed.

An implication of this for processes of facilitation is, we argue, that in any given group, habits, practices and ideas pertaining to the objective of the process of facilitation (regardless of the exact form of the objective) can remain muted or hidden; they can remain taken for granted. This realm of the undiscussed in the form of 'learned ignorance' should, we further argue, be accounted for in the process of facilitation, in an attempt to create an environment of equality of participation, as seen in cases 1 and 3. Creating a venue for discussions beyond the boundaries of what can be considered 'regular workplace interaction' is relevant, regardless of the degree of homogeneity of participants. In facilitation processes where the overarching objective is to create collaboration and change between different organisational entities, as seen in cases 1 and 3, the embeddedness of how things are done can become a hinderance to achieving a collaborative environment. To simplify: one tends to proceed based on one's own (culturally specific) preferences or habits, limiting those of others, without necessarily intending to do so. In processes with a higher degree of homogeneity (as in case 2), meanwhile, 'learned ignorance' takes the form of that which is taken for granted among 'equals', limiting the boundaries of what can be achieved. Despite the variation of group composition and overall objectives discussed, 'culture' therefore becomes an omnipresent aspect in processes of facilitation (Ogrinc et al. 2015); it sets premises for the very process of facilitation and for the more minuscule forms of interaction within it. (See principles of PD, Chapter 8.)

A commonality: participation

Another common theme we believe to be relevant, to processes of facilitation in general, is how one is to understand 'participation', that is, how we consider members are to be involved in the process, with regards both to each other and to the facilitator. We draw inspiration from literature on and practices connected to community work, described broadly as 'the process of assisting people to improve their community by undertaking autonomous collective action, that is, by working together' (Twelvetrees 2017, p. 5). Here, the primary objective is a form of empowerment of those involved in a process of improvement (the facilitated), through an embedded notion of 'participatory democracy' (Ledwith and Springer 2014; Ledwith 2011), relevant, we believe, for 'facilitation' more broadly. Within community work and keeping in mind that it is a broad and varied field, the very idea is that change must be initiated with and most importantly *by* those affected by what is to be changed, achieved by facilitating widespread collaboration and participation with many, on all levels throughout the entire process. Through such a process, the involved (the facilitated) will achieve a sense of ownership not only of the process but also of what is to be produced; of what is supposed to change, gradually 'taking over' the role of the community worker (the facilitator). Case 2 serves as an example of this, also demonstrating a relevance for processes of facilitation within the health and social sectors. Here, an approach emphasising a form of widespread and processual participation led to, according to the participants, a more context-relevant outcome ('it is relevant for us') and to a sense of commitment, to a sense of being part and belonging.

Also, in the other included cases, the form and level of involvement of the participants – what we label as 'degree of participation' (Arnstein, 1969) – were omnipresent, as is the case, we argue, for processes of facilitation in general. The objective of the facilitator will always be to involve and include participants, adapted to the contextual features that apply, but remaining an inescapable 'dilemma' for the facilitator and a primary objective of the process. Achieving this, at least a version of it reminiscent of the core values present in community work, has important and concrete implications for the role of the facilitator, most notably that of removing oneself from a position of authority (Rogers, 1971). This is, we believe, an important aspect of any process of facilitation, but perhaps is particularly important where leaders within an organisation take on a facilitative role to achieve organisation-wide change. Being cognisant of one's position of authority can give leaders an opportunity to take on a more neutral position, consistent with the agreed values of the group, and enable ownership of change to be realised.

An approach towards facilitation: humble assertiveness

Based on an understanding of the influence of culture and of the potential of 're-thinking' participation, we propose an approach towards facilitation in which the facilitator undertakes a role of 'humble assertiveness'. This suggested approach is founded in an understanding of 'participation' in which all involved parties are considered vital and active members of the process, perhaps most strongly illustrated in cases 2 and 3. Within such an approach, the role of the facilitator, as the very function of the facilitator's endeavour, is to enable processes of change without determining a set direction; to be present, to be aware of the concrete situational context, and to allow participants not only formal participation but also a form of control and authority. In this, the process of facilitation is understood as assisting others to approach the process without proposing concrete solutions, and involves the ability to develop learner autonomy as opposed to learner dependency. Such a cooperating approach to facilitation means sharing the power to decide and involve the participants in decisions about the process (Solem and Hermundsgård 2015) and not only the solutions, as exemplified in all three included cases, although in different ways.

For the facilitator, such an approach implies a form of 'controlled surrender', of letting go of authority and of letting go of the often-expected routine of pushing the process forward, of being effective and of delivering tangible results. Such an approach can allow for the utilisation of the resources, traits, practices, strengths and weaknesses of those to be facilitated, both within established collectives (case 2) and within more heterogenous groups (cases 1 and 3), allowing for active participation among all involved. As illustrated in all cases, the role of the facilitator is not that of an expert but rather that of a catalyst for change (Tollyfield 2014), enabling others within a system to work and prosper. Such an approach can often be construed as inefficient, slow and initially unrewarding, from the perspective of both facilitator and facilitated, but remains significant in the pursuit of lasting, transformative change as opposed to short-sighted quick fixes. In other words, facilitators must be able to perceive what is occurring within a 'facilitative space' and demonstrate the ability to be flexible in their approaches to obtain the understanding of the context, remaining neutral yet attentive.

Furthermore, such an approach has the potential of taking into account what can be described as the embeddedness of workplace practices and cultures by allowing for widespread and thorough participation, and by addressing that which often remains muted. Lastly, within such an approach, to adapt to the various contextual features (or cultures) it exists within becomes an integrated part of the process of facilitation, it becomes an objective in itself rather than something one must work around or avoid to achieve results. The facilitator should aim at developing a deeper understanding of the 'embedded culture' (whichever form that might take) by immersing themselves within the contexts of those they facilitate. This enables a greater understanding of the context of the workplace, the known and perceived barriers to change, and informs the direction to be taken for transformative change.

Within this proposed approach, how things are done at the health and social service organisation becomes something more than or something different from its normative qualities; the task in the process of facilitation is not necessarily to isolate good from bad, thriving from toxic work environments, and so on. Rather, the culture at the workplaces is something that a) simply is, and is unescapable, and b) has consequences. Without accounting for the significance of the context at play, by allowing for an overarching approach to participation change will, we believe, most likely be of an illusory nature.

References

Ågotnes, G. (2017). *The institutional Practice: On Nursing Homes and Hospitalizations.* Cappelen Damm Akademisk/NOASP: Nordic Open Access Scholarly Publishing.

Arnstein, S.R. (1969). A ladder of citizen participation. *Journal of the American Planning Association* 35 (4): 216–224.

Bourdieu, P. (1990). *The Logic of Practice.* Cambridge: Polity Press.

Bourdieu, P. (2012). [1977]. *Outline of a Theory of Practice.* Cambridge: Cambridge University Press.

Dahl, H. and Eriksen, K.Å. (2020). Orientation in expected and unexpected landscapes – a case study of a newly established municipal healthcare unit. *International Practice Development Journal* 10 (Suppl): 1–13. https://doi.org/10.19043/ipdj.10Suppl.007

Dahl, H., Eriksen, K.Å., Wennersberg, M.H. et al. (2019). Staying on track in changing landscapes: mapping complex projects in health services. *International Practice Development Journal* 9 (2): 1–20. https://doi.org/10.19043/ipdj.92.003

Eriksen, K.Å. and Heimestøl, S. (2017). Developing a culture of pride, confidence and trust: enhanced collaboration in an interdisciplinary team. *International Practice Development Journal* 7 (Suppl): 1–14. https://doi.org/10.19043/ipdj.7SP.004

Ledwith, M. (2011). *Community Development: A Critical Approach.* Bristol: Policy Press.

Ledwith, M. and Springer, J. (2014). *Participatory Practice, Community-based Action for Transformation Change.* Bristol: Policy Press.

Manley, K. and Jackson, C. (2020). The Venus model for integrating practitioner-led workforce transformation and complex change across the health care system. *Journal of Evaluation in Clinical Practice* 26 (2): 622– 634.

Martin, A. and Manley, K. (2017). Developing standards for an integrated approach to workplace facilitation for interprofessional teams in health and social care contexts: a Delphi study. *Journal of Interprofessional Care* 32 (1): 41–51.

Ogrinc, G., Davies, L., Goodman, D. et al. (2015). SQUIRE 2.0 (Standards for Quality Improvement Reporting Excellence): revised publication guidelines from a detailed consensus process. *American Journal of Critical Care* 24 (6): 466–473.

Ringard, Å., Sagan, A., Saunes, I. et al. (2013). Norway: health system review. *Health Systems in Transition,* 15 (8). World Health Organization. https://apps.who.int/iris/handle/10665/330299

Rogers, C. (1971). Carl Rogers describes his way of facilitating encounter groups. *The American Journal of Nursing* 71 (2): 275–279.

Solem, A. and Hermundsgård, M. (2015). *Fasilitering.* Oslo: Gyldendal.

12. *Leadership Relationships*

Rebekkah Middleton, Shaun Cardiff, Kim Manley, and Belinda Dewar

Introduction

Practice development (PD) is ultimately about developing person-centred cultures that are also experienced as safe and effective by its beneficiaries – those experiencing and those providing care. The main ways that culture at any level can change is through leadership and relationships (Manley et al. 2019a, 2019b). Person-centred leadership values relationships, emphasised through collaborative and authentic engagement (McCormack and McCance 2017). In a complex and dynamic environment, person-centred healthcare leaders are essential to advance and evolve professional roles, influencing and inspiring the clinical, academic, executive and political spheres so that the common goal is excellent person-centred care and flourishing of staff and teams.

This chapter considers how positioning leadership as an explicit relationship process in PD is needed to enable a focus on what matters to people and communities. The chapter commences with an overview of relational leadership drawn from a PhD study (Cardiff 2014) that highlights transformational and person-centred leadership approaches. Five guiding lights for strengthening leadership in all settings are then discussed. The chapter concludes with an example of a person-centred leadership development programme, demonstrating how relational strategies enable and impact effective workplace cultures.

International Practice Development in Health and Social Care, Second Edition.
Edited by Kim Manley, Valerie Wilson, and Christine Øye.

Relational leadership

To support PD work, leaders transform, they work with people to move towards person-centred practices. Leadership should be viewed as a practice exercised in relationships, not hierarchical status, so we have to detach it from any one individual and view it as a process of mutual and reciprocal influence. There is a need for flexible leaders and workforces who are able to respond, often quickly, to changing contexts and needs (Drach-Zahavy and Dagan 2002), including their staff, who 'want to be led – not managed' (Shelton and Darling 2001, p. 264), having strong relationships with their leaders. This is significant in today's healthcare context where many frontline staff are leaving their jobs or indeed the profession.

Relational connectedness

As person-centredness is a core principle of PD (principle 1, see Chapter 8), it means that those engaging in leadership practice should also respect personhood, right of self-determination as well as reciprocal respect and understanding so that the relationship can be considered healthful (cf. McCormack and McCance 2017). The framework of relational processes presented in this first section offers leaders (whether they be practice developers, clinical or hierarchical leaders) meaning, values and essential components to observe and/or reflect on. The relational processes described are core to person-centred leadership; a complex, dynamic, relational and contextualised practice that aims to enable associates and leaders to achieve self-actualisation, empowerment and wellbeing (Cardiff et al. 2018). As is often the case with complex concepts, it is sometimes helpful to visualise it rather than merely describe it in words. Hence, we offer first a metaphor and visualisation of person-centred leadership: that of an Argentine tango danced on a beach, portrayed in Figure 12.1.

We interact and relate with numerous others daily; these relationships are constantly evolving, in a state of 'being' and 'becoming', influenced by ourselves and the context(s) around us. When functioning well, these relationships foster feelings of safety, energise us and offer a sense of belonging and connectedness, even when the other person/people may not physically be present. When weak, the opposite may be felt. However, every relationship is constantly moving along a continuum, and we should strive for strong relationships.

The Argentine tango, like relationships, is in a constant state of flow and movement between an 'open' and a 'closed' embrace (Jensen 2006). In the closed embrace, dancers seem to move as one, while in the open embrace each individual shines. However, the unicity of an individual can be enhanced by the partner's stance. For instance, look at the female dancer in Figure 12.1. She appears elegant, competent, exhilarated and free, but if you look more closely at her partner's feet and pose, he is enabling her to take on the pose without falling. He needs to be attuned to her 'being', ability and capacity; mutual trust is needed if falling is to be avoided, particularly given the context in which they are performing. Others are not in sight, but their presence may be felt. The sand under their

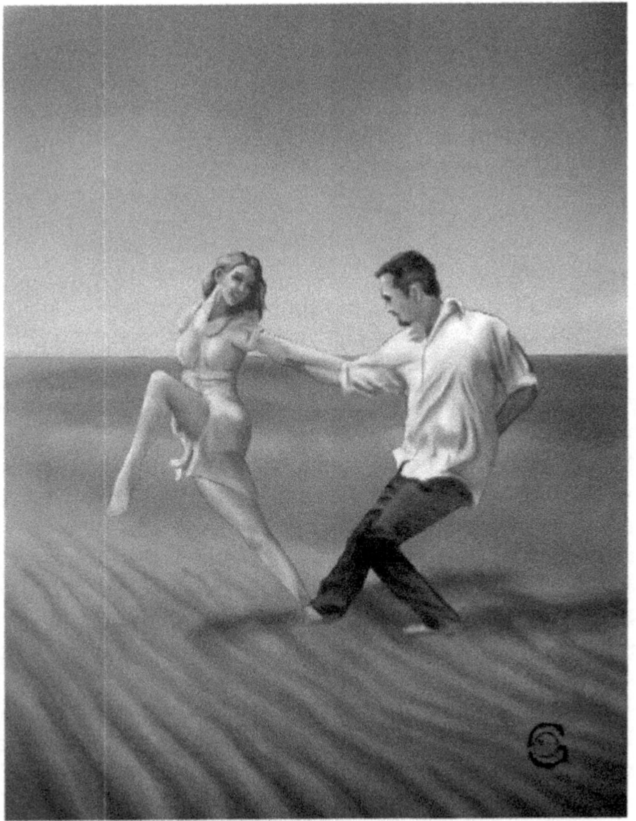

Figure 12.1 The person-centred leadership dance (Artist: George Vink)

feet, alongside a moving shoreline and unpredictable weather, makes dancing here very different to dancing in a studio. Similarly, if they were to change partners and attempt the same dance it would be new as the relationship has changed. Leadership, too, can be viewed as a dance of movement, constant attuning and seeking connectedness between the leader and the associate.[1] Each relationship and 'meeting' is unique, influenced by each person's state of being at that moment in time and the context in which they meet.

Just as it takes two to tango, it takes at least two people for leadership to emerge and/or be practised. The person-centred leader's primary focus is enabling everyone to feel empowered, to experience wellbeing and self-actualisation within the workplace. Leader attributes include being authentically other-centred and caring; intra- and inter-personal intelligence; patience, optimism and openness;

[1] Generally in leadership literature the term 'follower' is used. This conjures images of hierarchy and so we prefer the term 'associate' to better reflect a sense of relational equity.

a willingness to show vulnerability and reflexivity. Such attributes enable the leader to 'be in relation' and to foster relational connectedness (Cardiff 2014).

Feeling connected to leaders is a sign of exemplary leadership (Anonson et al. 2014) and how associates and leaders choose to relate will influence outcomes (Ashman and Lawler 2008). Relationally connected means feeling recognised, safe and a sense of belonging.

Person-centred leadership framework

The person-centred leadership framework from Cardiff's (2014) action research study offers five processes (sensing, contextualising, balancing, presencing, communing), which enable a leader to position self (stancing) in relation to the associate and so enhance the coming into own for both. This is graphically presented in Figure 12.2.

Sensing: a process of constantly assessing where the other person 'is at' – seeing, hearing and feeling their current state of being. Healthcare professionals are usually trained to use all their senses to assess the whole person; leadership development often simplifies/reduces the complex whole into specific aspects deemed relevant for effective leadership.

Aware that what we see is not necessarily all that there is, sensory information may need to be supplemented with data gathered via other resources (personnel files, observations made by others, etc.) and/or interpretations verified by the associate themself. Verification lowers the chance of an inappropriate response. Active listening and inviting the associate to share their narrative also offers the leader insight into associate identity, perceptions, values and beliefs (Holloway and Freshwater 2007; Riessman 2008), to see beyond the observable.

Contextualising: a process of seeing the associate embedded in a greater whole/context. We all 'inhabit' different environments and social roles which can

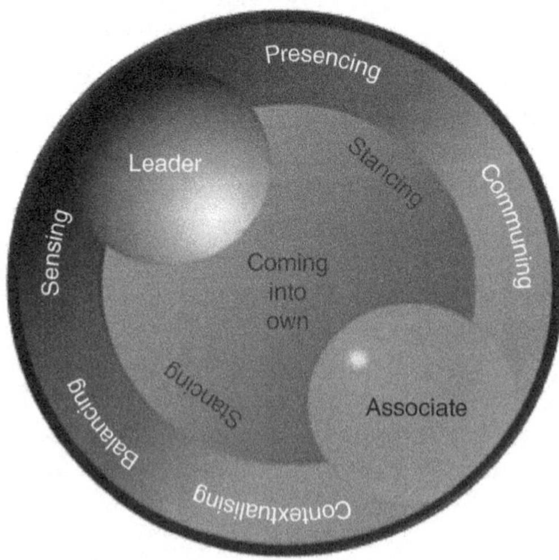

Figure 12.2 The relational domain of person-centred leadership (Cardiff 2014)

influence our state of being in the here and now. Past experiences and future plans can also influence our current being. Seeing and understanding contextual influences enables a leader to better relate and decide on an adequate response given the associate's current situation and future needs, desires, challenges.

Balancing: a process of weighing up a collection of (potentially conflicting) needs. Deciding how to respond adequately often entails taking into account multiple reasons, emotions, practices and social contexts, making leadership a moral activity requiring reflexivity and consideration of consequences.

Communing: a process of action-oriented dialogue. It entails communicating at an intimate level, showing support, seeking understanding, finding common ground, creating shared vision and/or making shared decisions. The reciprocity and mutuality are not always evident in leadership literature, but Groysberg and Slind (2012, p. 78) state that 'smart leaders. . .engage with employees in a way that resembles an ordinary person-to-person conversation more than it does a series of commands from on high. . .[T]alking with employees, rather than simply issuing orders, leaders can retain or recapture. . .operational flexibility, high levels of employee engagement, [and] tight strategic alignment'. While communicating can be mutually beneficial, some healthcare workers may not dare to authentically voice their perspective (Garon 2012) due to perceived power differences (Grill et al. 2011). Leaders can therefore be charged with creating conditions for effective communing, whether it be incidental private conversations or regular structured meetings, but not be solely responsible for the outcome. As it is a relational meeting (Ashman and Lawler 2008), the degree to which associates engage in authentic dialogue will also depend on perceptions of their role, responsibility and status power within the relationship (Reitz 2011).

Presencing: a process of being/thinking with and/or doing for the other person. It is similar to sympathetic presence as described by McCormack and McCance (2017). Baart's (2001) theory of presencing states that it begins with unconditional openness and beneficent attentiveness towards the other with the sole aim of understanding the other's narrative and achieving relational connectedness from which both can decide if and how the other can help (Klaver and Baart 2011). It does not necessarily require technical skills, more the active use of intra- and interpersonal intelligence. In contrast to Senge et al.'s (2004) theory, or Scharmer's (2009) U theory of leading change, 'having presence' here refers less to 'being in context' and 'personal being' and more to 'being in relation with associates'.

Stancing: a process of positioning self in relation to the associate with an intent of fostering coming into own. The assumption here is that when people feel good at work, performance and commitment are more likely to follow. Engaging (continuously) in the relational processes described above gives the leader information and insight into how best to position self and act in a way that is healthful for both. Four basic stances were identified by Cardiff (2014): leading from the front (offering to role model/do for), sideline (offering to instruct), alongside (enabling associate self-action) and behind (observing associate initiative and action, ready to move into a different stance if and when needed). Once embodied, and as expertise develops, leader movement between the four stances becomes fluid like a dance, with an understanding of self, context and domain, with attentiveness to possibilities, congruency and ethical purpose.

It is evident that a relational approach to leadership can help form healthful relationships: good for both leader and those being led. Being present allows leaders to sense the current status of associate being using their senses and other sources to verify interpretations. This contributes to the creation of shared visions and decisions, fostering individual, team and organisational performance. It is crucial, however, to know what works well, why and in what contexts. This next section outlines a project undertaken throughout the United Kingdom (UK) to identify the relational leadership processes and strategies that nurse, midwifery and allied health professional leaders use to achieve and demonstrate impact and to embed innovative practices across different contexts (Manley, Dewar et al. 2019).

Guiding lights of leadership

The guiding lights study aimed to identify how to strengthen nursing, midwifery and allied health professionals' leadership in all contexts (practice, education, research or strategy). The outcome was five 'guiding lights', a metaphor describing the salient features of leadership. The term 'guiding lights' has been coined in preference to 'simple rules' used by other researchers when translating complex insights or findings into principles to remember (Best et al. 2012; Plsek and Wilson 2001). The 'guiding light' metaphor has also been used in research to capture the essence of effective workplace cultures, which resulted in four different guiding lights (see Chapter 15). Further detail is found in Manley, Dewar et al. (2019).

Influenced by realist evaluation and appreciative inquiry, a three-phased approach focused on:

1. interrogating literature to generate tentative insights between contexts, mechanisms and outcomes (the programme theories that explain what works for who and why)
2. using innovative social media strategy to enable nomination of leaders in practice, education, research and strategy contexts, as well as generating other insights about leadership used to refine the programme theories
3. sense-making workshops in each UK country to develop narratives, critique of programme theories arising based on participants' stories, leadership insights and future-orientated ideas about leadership direction.

Programme theory describes the mechanism by which a programme achieves its effects (Davidson 2004). In this study the programme/intervention focused on nurse, midwife and allied health professional leadership.

Five key guiding lights resulted in relation to the complex world of health and social care and were synthesised from context–mechanism–outcome relationships to illuminate how nurses, midwives and allied health professions could strengthen leadership in clinical care, environment of care, social care, education, organisations, communities and interprofessional teams.

These principles were labelled as 'The light between us as interactions in our relationships', 'Seeing people's inner light', 'Kindling the spark of light and keeping it glowing', 'Lighting up the known and the yet to be known' and 'Constellations of connected stars'. These metaphors will be illuminated to illustrate key principles underpinning relationship-based leadership to describe what works, why it works and for whom it works.

Guiding light 1 'The light between us as interactions in our relationships'

The principle underpinning this guiding light emphasises the importance of giving attention to what is happening between us when we are together. It involves being authentic, working towards ensuring a space of civility and careful listening. Listening enables what is important to people to be heard and is the starting point for reflection, stretching our current thinking and innovating together. Two outcomes result for all who are touched by this aspect of leadership – it is experienced as compassionate and credible, and authentic, caring, appreciative with respectful relationships and communication.

Guiding light 2 'Seeing people's inner light'

Seeing people's inner light is a metaphor for seeing each person's worth (including own) and cherishing the varied ways people connect, contribute and bring about change. It is manifested through working with others, creating experiences of being safe to be authentic and share ideas and emotions. Guiding light 2 is closely linked to guiding light 3 in terms of the outcomes achieved.

Guiding light 3 'Kindling the spark of light and keeping it glowing'

The metaphor for guiding light 3 builds on 'seeing the inner light'. 'Kindling the spark' and then 'keeping it glowing' both demonstrate different subtleties. Kindling involves generating shared understanding of what lights people's fire and finding ways for people to get energy from each other's different light sources (priorities, values, beliefs, enabling them to come into their own – as described above). Keeping the light glowing when the light flickers involves helping ourselves and others to take risk and to harness learning from disappointments alongside delights.

Guiding lights 2 and 3 are intertwined and so are their outcomes. Leadership is experienced as inclusive, collective, shared and distributive by all who are touched by it, thereby dispersing traditional views of leadership as something practised only by hierarchical leaders. Additionally, there are outcomes for staff and teams. Staff feel valued, supported, involved and heard, which leads to:

- improved morale, commitment, wellbeing, satisfaction and retention, with reduced burnout, stress and exhaustion
- improved confidence to speak up, self-awareness and empowerment, contributing to increased skills, improved relationships and career development.

Teams are recognised as healthy, effective and empowered with cultures of active learning, engagement, reflection and adaptation. This results in a strong team commitment to better practice, creativity, innovation and improving performance.

Guiding light 4 'Lighting up the known and the yet to be known'

This guiding light is illustrated by the metaphor of a lighthouse with its rotating light beam. It reveals features illuminated by the beam, before plunging them into darkness as the beam passes by. The light beam represents our aspiration to be a source of steadiness during change by sharing information on what is known and stable. This may include shared foundation values, purpose and ways of working. Leadership in this guiding light involves showing a level of comfort when engaging with uncertainty – the unpredictability of the darkness, and valuing that which lights the way forward to be found in relationships that facilitate flexible and creative approaches. These approaches may differ from action plans, risk aversion strategies and hierarchical rules due to the relational aspect.

The outcomes of guiding light 4 are for people and organisations. People experience better healthcare outcomes, quality and satisfaction. Organisations demonstrate improvement in services, performance, safety and quality with healthy teams. These organisational outcomes further the positive outcomes for patients, clients and service users, and also for staff through improved retention, stability and commitment aligned with the qualities of a learning organisation.

Guiding light 5 'Constellations of connected stars'

Stars are individually brilliant sources of energy. When connected invisibly through electromagnetic forces holding them in constellations, they are awesome. This metaphor accentuates the power of collective leadership and collective action through tuning into local resources, networks and communities, and recognising where there is potential for enhanced futures.

The guiding light is about fostering ways of connecting to maximise possibilities for collective action. This requires responding to the unique nature of local context and practising adaptability in order to tap into the distinctive riches on offer. Such an approach benefits the system and society through building social capital, identified as a resource for system change; increasing resources available to people, organisations and communities for change; and ultimately improving population health.

The five guiding lights aim to provide simple metaphors based on researching the complexity of leadership in every context and setting, whether that be practice, education, research, strategy or combinations. For PD it provides essential principles for leadership and leaders nurturing and achieving relationship-centred, safe and effective cultures in any context at every level. To achieve these principles requires development of individuals (see the following example) who can then influence teams and organisations.

Leadership development strategies that enable effective workplace cultures

It is evident, then, that 'culture is informed by the nature of its leadership' (Francis 2013, p. 66). Leadership in healthcare can promote a culture that ensures staff are committed to and capable of living organisational values and standards, and ultimately providing evidence-based, compassionate care to patients (Debono et al. 2016; Gierlinger et al. 2019). In PD we are conscious of the need for active involvement in creation of standards and values so that they are 'shared' and more readily upheld and lived by all. With an aim of developing workplace cultures that imbue person-centred approaches to practice, relational leadership is the conduit for the facilitation of PD methods to transform people and cultures.

Roles and titles do not make a leader; rather, it is behaviours that reflect leadership qualities, which can be learned and developed. Current leadership practices in healthcare focus on theories and models that are transformational, authentic, adaptive, collaborative and innovative (Careau et al. 2014; Boamah 2018). In PD and person-centred practices and work, these tend to merge to form the person-centred leader. We have seen Cardiff's work that explores person-centred leadership as a dynamic relationship where the leader enables others to come into their own, focusing on wellbeing and empowerment to enable flourishing.

Leadership in health requires integration of interdisciplinary knowledge, skills, vision and innovation for effective and collaborative healthcare practice (Figueroa et al. 2019). By harnessing leadership potential in healthcare professionals across disciplines, leadership capacity increases and a sharing of power enhances more effective, successful outcomes that are responsive to organisational needs. This can be attributed to the multiple voices and perspectives that emerge when disciplines learn together, thereby deepening and broadening individuals' concepts and approaches to leadership and to its application in practice (Bloomquist et al. 2018). This enables individuals to give and receive energy necessary for reciprocal healthful relationships, thereby enabling people to thrive (Dewing and McCormack 2017). A flourishing organisation ensues, one guided by person-centred leaders who invest in people so that positive energy is established and positive practices are implemented and evident throughout the organisation. This can be challenging in current health systems (public and private) with difficult business dynamisms, complexities of systems and pressures of managing various aspects of care, including pandemics.

This final section considers what a person-centred leader might look like and how we can develop person-centred leaders who enable flourishing person-centred workplace cultures. An example is given below where a postgraduate university subject (Effective Leadership in Health) was delivered to healthcare professionals in three health districts in New South Wales, Australia. Using qualitative methodology, 15 participants were invited to share stories that uncovered the impact of their learning and leadership on their own practice and relationships one year after subject completion.

'Effective Leadership in Health' subject

This subject gives participants the opportunity to work with other disciplines, enabling networking and diversity in expertise and opinion – a highly valued aspect of leadership programmes outlined in the literature (Careau et al. 2014), particularly in terms of contributing to skill development and knowledge that builds, supports and sustains current interprofessional models of care in practice (Sebastian et al. 2018). This enables participants to apply leadership principles to their everyday practice, a commonly noted absence in formal leadership programmes (Figueroa et al. 2019).

The subject focuses on awareness and understanding of self as a leader, promoting understanding, exploration and analysis of leadership to create climates in which people work together to achieve successful outcomes, along with application to interpersonal relationships, processes and systems. The subject particularly focuses on supporting individuals to develop authentic relationships with others (principle 7, see Chapter 8), concentrating on person-centred practice to develop effective workplace cultures where people can flourish (principle 1), using creativity (principle 3) and evidence (principle 6) to enable participants to explore their own antecedent leadership characteristics and to translate theory and learning into their context (principle 4), thereby transforming contexts.

Reflection is a skill featured prominently in the subject – on self, others and the organisation. How to incorporate leadership, and be strategic, in each of these levels is explored in a variety of creative ways that aim to promote engagement and contribution from participants, so that authentic understanding and articulation of learning occur (Busari et al. 2018).

The participant stories highlighted their understanding of leadership and how being deliberate and attentive to person-centred leadership principles has transformed their approach to their practice, to their teams and more widely. These were particularly around learning approaches, translation and articulation of learning to practice.

Learning approaches

Leadership development programmes often target nurses solely, neglecting to include allied health, medical and administrative professionals, who all contribute to healthcare processes and organisations and who share the same leadership development needs. The value of interdisciplinary learning cannot be understated:

> *'I really like how [the subject] is open to people in health, more than just nurses. Learning together so we can work together and make a difference together. And that work we did about making connections more broadly, made me think about how I could work on fitting those principles into my work.'* (Gabby, Social Worker)

Partnership between academia and local health districts and co-production of material are important and prioritised in the subject to bring theory and application into the same space, a crucial practice to enabling transformative learning and implementation of evidence into the workplace (Busari et al. 2018). In addition, this practice promotes strong emphasis on person-centredness through collaborative and authentic engagement, placing value on relationships (McCormack and McCance 2017). An example of how these practices facilitate flourishing environments for learners is seen in Chapter 6 in relation to an undergraduate curriculum.

> *'The shared facilitation impacted me, it inspired passion in me about leadership. The shared approach between university and practice facilitators helped to resonate partnership.'* (Olivia, Physiotherapist)

Translation of learning

The subject and associated assessment focused on the theory and practices of leadership and how an individual can have impact at micro, meso and macro levels. Cognisant of the challenge to enable leaders to move easily between education, theory and the practice environment, focus is translation to personal practice. Translation of leadership knowledge into practice is key for healthcare improvement, giving voice to inform and influence healthcare policy and practice (Harvey et al. 2019).

> *'Since completing the subject, I've had opportunities to speak to the organisation's executive team around change – which was terrifying! But... the subject taught me how to use evidence in conversations and this has made me believable and helped my confidence. It taught me to look beyond self.'* (Xavier, Nurse Manager)

Articulation of learning to practice

Articulation of learning into practice occurred in multiple ways, expressed by participants in relation to the following:

> Incorporating patients into decisions... *'I'm always bringing the patient back into decisions now, which I really had never thought of doing beforehand.'* (Jesse, Occupational Therapist)
>
> Learning from facilitators' actions... *'The clear tools that were modelled and then we could practise were terrific. I've been using ones like values clarification and change management in my practice and the staff are surprisingly responsive.'* (Simone, Nurse Educator)
>
> Being proactively positive in approaches... *'And then the positive working environment, that's my whole business now. I only focus on the positive now... and it's worked amazingly.'* (Moira, Nurse Manager)
>
> Intentionally listening to others... *'I learned to listen, to back off, to use enabling questions... It was the slowing down, the stopping and then "what about this, have you tried this..." rather than "this is what you're doing". I'm more articulate and value people's opinions, including them in conversations, actions and processes.'* (Sally, Clinical Nurse)

> Conscious reflection. . . *'I've been continuing to journal and reflect – and I hated that before. I used to think it was self-indulgent, but it helped me understand myself and why I react to things and people. I'm being more mindful, more intentional, suspend and not react.'* (Renae, Nurse Manager)

> Personal challenge and risk taking. . . *'The subject made me think so much more deeply. So much so that I found confidence to take a risk and move into a new role to try and influence success more broadly – hospital-wide success, using the principles I had learned. I would never have done that or thought I could do that before.'* (Keith, Executive)

> Influence on others. . . *'People have said to me, "there's been a culture shift since you took over". Not only have there been conversations with each other, but more with our clients. People are telling me they are having more meaningful conversations with each other based on my interactions with them. And that blows my mind.'* (Angela, Social Worker)

This approach to leadership development, based on the CIP principles and values underpinning person-centred practice, emphasises the importance of *being* what we espouse leadership to be. This enables mutuality, reciprocity and trustworthiness/credibility, evident through these participant stories. Learning with other disciplines formally and focusing translation of leadership principles and theory to personal practice reveals how people can transform themselves as leaders and influence their context. Developing leadership in healthcare professionals using person-centred approaches aligns to emancipatory PD. It is a sustainable means of moving forward to develop leaders who focus on enabling inclusion, who use collaborative methods and processes, and who, through relationship, are able to positively influence others' values towards person-centredness.

Conclusion

Leadership as a practice manifests in relationships within PD work, moving it away from traditional views of it being an attribute or task of hierarchical leaders. It is essential to enable focus on what matters to people and communities. Leadership models and programmes that promote leadership have been reported on widely (Bloomquist et al. 2018; Busari et al. 2018; Debono et al. 2016; Careau et al. 2014), but this chapter has demonstrated that transformational and person-centred leadership approaches are necessary to influence and develop person-centred cultures. Using the image of the dance and metaphors of the guiding lights helps leaders to see and remember principles that can be applied to strengthen leadership in any context and at any level, and the relational processes enable persons to come into their own. When leadership is developed in healthcare professionals and opportunity exists to learn together, then workplace cultures that are safe, person-centred and flourishing are grown.

References

Anonson, J., Walker, M., Arries, E. et al. (2014). Qualities of exemplary nurse leaders: perspectives of frontline nurses. *Journal of Nursing Management* 22 (1): 127–136.

Ashman, I. and Lawler, J. (2008). Existential communication and leadership. *Leadership* 4 (3): 253–269.

Baart, A. (2001). *Een theorie van de presentie*. Den Haag: Lemma.

Best, A., Greenhalgh, T., Lewis, S. et al. (2012). Large-system transformation in healthcare: a realist review. *The Milbank Quarterly* 90 (3): 421–456.

Bloomquist, C.D., Georges, L., Ford, D.J. et al. (2018). Interdisciplinary leadership practices in graduate leadership education programs. *Journal of Leadership Studies* 12 (2): 60–63.

Boamah, S. (2018). Linking nurses' clinical leadership to patient care quality: the role of transformational leadership and workplace empowerment. *Canadian Journal of Nursing Research* 50 (1): 9–19.

Busari, J., Chan, M.K., Dath, D. et al. (2018). Sanokondu: The birth of a multinational network for the development of healthcare leadership education. *Leadership in Health Services* 31 (2): 254–264.

Cardiff, S. (2014). *Person-centred leadership: a critical participatory action research study exploring and developing a new style of (clinical) nurse leadership*. PhD. University of Ulster, Belfast.

Cardiff, S., McCormack, B. and McCance, T. (2018). Person-centred leadership: a relational approach to leadership derived through action research. *Journal of Clinical Nursing* 27 (15–16): 3056–3069.

Careau, E., Biba, G., Brander, R. et al. (2014). Health leadership education programs, best practices, and impact on learners' knowledge, skills, attitudes, and behaviors and system change: a literature review. *Journal of Healthcare Leadership* 6: 39–50.

Davidson, E.J. (2004). The 'baggaging' of theory-based evaluation. *Journal of Multi-Disciplinary Evaluation* 3 (4): iii–xiii.

Debono, D., Travaglia, J.F., Dunn, A.G. et al. (2016). Strengthening the capacity of nursing leaders through multifaceted professional development initiatives: a mixed method evaluation of the 'Take The Lead' program. *Collegian* 23 (1): 19–28.

Dewing, J. and McCormack, B. (2017). Creating flourishing workplaces. In: *Person-centred Practice in Nursing and Health Care. Theory and Practice* (eds. B. McCormack and T. McCance), 150–161. West Sussex: Wiley Blackwell.

Drach-Zahavy, A. and Dagan, E. (2002). From caring to managing and beyond: an examination of the head nurse's role. *Journal of Advanced Nursing* 38 (1): 19–28.

Figueroa, C.A., Harrison, R., Chauhan, A. et al. (2019). Priorities and challenges for health leadership and workforce management globally: a rapid review. *BMC Health Services Research* 19: 239.

Francis, R. (2013). *Report of the Mid Staffordshire NHS Foundation Trust Public Inquiry*. London: The Stationery Office. https://www.gov.uk/government/uploads/system/uploads/attachment_data/file/279124/0947.pdf (accessed 14 March 2020).

Garon, M. (2012). Speaking up, being heard: registered nurses' perceptions of workplace communication. *Journal of Nursing Management* 20 (3): 361–371.

Gierlinger, S., Barden, A. and Giammarinaro, N. (2019). Impact of a patient experience leadership structure on performance and engagement. *Journal of Patient Experience* 7 (2). https://doi.org/10.1177/2374373519831079

Grill, C., Ahlborg, G. and Lindgren, E. (2011). Valuation and handling of dialogue in leadership: a grounded theory study in Swedish hospitals. *Journal of Health Organization and Management* 25 (1): 34–54.

Groysberg, B. and Slind, M. (2012). Leadership is a conversation. *Harvard Business Review* 90 (6): 76–84.

Harvey, G., Gifford, W., Cummings, G. et al. (2019). Mobilising evidence to improve nursing practice: a qualitative study of leadership roles and processes in four countries. *International Journal of Nursing Studies* 90: 21–30.

Holloway, I. and Freshwater, D. (2007). *Narrative Research in Nursing*. Oxford: Blackwell Publishing.

Jensen, M. (2006). *Sensuous and Gendered Embraces: An Investigation into Tango Dance Practices*. MA Dance Anthropology. Roehampton University.

Klaver, K. and Baart, A. (2011). Attentiveness in care: towards a theoretical framework. *Nursing Ethics* 18 (5): 686–693.

Manley, K., Dewar, B., Jackson, C. et al. (2019a). Strengthening Nurse, Midwifery and Allied Health Professional Leadership. Final Report 11 March. Funded by Burdett Trust.

Manley, K., Jackson, C. and McKenzie, C. (2019b). Microsystems culture change – a refined theory for developing person centred, safe and effective workplaces based on strategies that embed a safety culture. *International Journal of Practice Development* 9 (2) [4]. https://doi.org/10.19043/ipdj.92.004

McCormack, B. and McCance, T. (2017). Underpinning principles of person-centred practice. In: *Person-centred Practice in Nursing and Health Care. Theory and Practice. 2nd Edition* (eds. B. McCormack and T. McCance), 13–35. West Sussex: Wiley Blackwell.

Plsek, P.E. and Wilson, T. (2001). Complexity, leadership and management in healthcare organisations. *British Medical Journal* 323 (7315): 746–749.

Reitz, M. (2011). Dialogue: possible in a leadership context? Paper presented at the International Studying Leadership Conference, University of West England, Bristol, UK (12 December 2011).

Riessman, C. (2008). *Narrative Methods for the Human Sciences*. Los Angeles, CA: Sage Publications.

Scharmer, C. (2009). *Theory U: Learning from the Future as It Emerges*. San Francisco, CA: Berrett-Koehler Publishers.

Sebastian, J.G., Breslin, E.T., Trautman, D.E. et al. (2018). Leadership by collaboration: nursing's bold new vision for academic-practice partnerships. *Journal of Professional Nursing* 34 (2): 110–116.

Senge, P., Scharmer, O., Jaworski, J. et al. (2004). *Presence: Human Purpose and the Field of the Future*. Cambridge, MA: SoL Press.

Shelton, C. and Darling, J. (2001). The quantum skills model in management: a new paradigm to enhance effective leadership. *Leadership & Organization Development Journal* 22 (6): 264–273.

13. *From Fractured to Flourishing: Developing Clinical Leadership for Frontline Culture Change*

Duncan McKellar, Helen Stanley, Kim Manley, Selena Moore, Tyler Lloyd, Clare Hardwick, and Julia Ronder

Introduction

This chapter explores leading for culture change in frontline teams, through five first-person narrative accounts of clinical leaders from diverse disciplines and service contexts, who found themselves confronted by cultural dysfunction and service ineffectiveness. Their journeys, from fractured to flourishing teams, are unified by transformative clinical leadership as a key enabler of culture change, integrating values into ways of working that deliver person-centred care, resulting in human flourishing (Manley et al. 2011; Manley and Jackson 2019). Not all were appointed to managerial roles. Irrespective of role or discipline, all encountered the challenge of influencing others to move individuals and teams towards more positive and effective workplaces, through 'ground up', rather than 'top down' change. All grappled with their function and agency as leaders while drawing on processes and resources to support the work of leading change. Reflecting on what worked and why offers insight to empower other clinical leaders on their own journeys of culture change.

Background

Clinical leaders contributing to this chapter represent nursing, allied health, medicine and biomedical science, emphasising the notion that clinical leadership promoting culture change is an interdisciplinary concern. Traditionally,

International Practice Development in Health and Social Care, Second Edition.
Edited by Kim Manley, Valerie Wilson, and Christine Øye.

healthcare organisations have been characterised by discipline silos and hierarchical relationships, impeding development of positive and effective service culture (van Rossum et al. 2016; Laloo et al. 2019). The narratives here reflect the role of clinical leaders reimagining workplace relationships and power differentials, contributing to counter-cultural change and delivering empowered workforces.

An important question is: what are the features of effective clinical leadership that facilitate culture change? In response, it is helpful to consider several leadership models, providing a frame of reference for the narratives.

Transformational leadership is characterised by ability to motivate others through appealing to shared values and inspiring teams to place the greater good above personal self-interest. Transformational leadership contrasts with traditional compliance-based cultures, instead inspiring curiosity, innovation, learning and sharing of ideas (Weberg 2010; Doody and Doody 2012; Hewitt-Taylor 2015). It supports improved workplace engagement, increased staff satisfaction and reduced burnout (Nielsen et al. 2008; Weberg 2010).

Adaptive and complexity leadership models acknowledge uncertainty and flux as ubiquitous in contemporary systems, generating anxiety and resistance to change (Heifetz et al. 2009; Porter-O'Grady 2020). This is highly relevant to stressful clinical environments. To successfully lead culture change, clinical leaders will manage complexity through adaptive challenges where technical application of existing knowledge, skills and processes is insufficient to support frontline teams to tolerate uncertainty, question beliefs and habits, and experiment with new ways of working (Heifetz et al. 2009). Authentic leadership is characterised by self-awareness, balanced processing, moral self-identity and relational transparency (Hewitt-Taylor 2015). Authentic leaders demonstrate consistency between values and behaviours. Rather than building through personal charisma, authentic leaders build enduring relationships, demonstrating commitment to purpose, meaning and hard work (Harter 2002; Luthans and Avolio 2003; Cooper et al. 2005; Diddams and Chang 2012).

Relevant to the relational component of leadership emerging from these models is the concept of psychological safety, in which the workplace is seen as safe for interpersonal risk taking (Edmondson and Lei 2014; Edmondson 2019). Psychological safety supports 'bottom up' transformation, where team members are safe to contribute, ask for help and admit failures without fear of punitive responses (Edmondson 2019, pp. 3–24). In achieving culture change, clinical leaders manage complex relationships, modelling vulnerability and promoting psychological safety, collaborating with others to move towards shared purpose for common good. Davidson (2020, p. 101) expresses this, observing that 'leadership then, is not command and control; not tools and techniques; it is at its core noticing and co-creating meaning about how we are working together and talking about what matters to us'.

The following five narratives reflect aspects of the leadership models acknowledged above. In each case, the clinical leader utilised a framework, resources and practices, consistent with practice development (PD), enabling

Case study 1 Stepping up to unexpected expansion – a hospital medical ward

Sometimes life throws unexpected 'curve balls' that turn out as opportunities for growth. In 2012, I was managing an 18-bed trauma ward. I was also part way through the Clinical Leadership Programme (CLP) run by our NHS Trust. Preparing to leave work one Friday afternoon, I received a call from my service director informing me that when I returned on Monday, I would additionally be leading the adjacent 25-bed medical ward. This was a critical point in my leadership journey.

them to adaptively deliver sustainable transformation in real-world environments (Akhtar et al. 2016).

The case studies

The previous manager had been removed from their role with immediate effect. Several staff had been issued conduct warnings. Staff were bewildered and anxious. The combined service instantaneously became 43 inpatient beds across two clinical areas. I felt overwhelmed and did not know where to begin. It was evident that the 'inherited' ward was characterised by entrenched dysfunction. Some staff were complicit in perpetuating a toxic culture. One of my first concerns was for staff from my original ward and how change would impact them. I was also concerned about delivering safe and effective care to our patients.

As a developing clinical leader, I drew on multiple resources and relationships to support my steep learning curve. The CLP provided access to action learning sessions with colleagues, where I was able to debrief and gain support working through the many adaptive challenges I faced. The CLP facilitated a 360-degree leadership assessment, helping me develop insight regarding my leadership style, identifying strengths and vulnerabilities. While both encouraging and confronting, this feedback informed my development. Reflecting on the question 'What does it feel like to be on the end of me?' became an important part of my leadership journey.

The first two years following the amalgamation were the most challenging. Holding closely to core values of integrity, honesty, being person-centred towards patients and staff and being committed to making a positive difference kept me grounded. I progressively developed a greater sense of clarity around my role and was able to articulate direction for the ward. A shared vision for the new, combined ward emerged as I grew into my role and developed relationships across the service.

A number of staff left the service completely. While this was difficult in the short term, I recognised this was part of their journey of change and an opportunity for us to shape our growth. I was able to lead the recruitment of new staff, embedding values that were important to our developing team.

I first encountered claims, concerns and issues (CCIs) as a strategy in the CLP, reflecting a PD approach (Akhtar et al. 2016). CCIs is a collaborative meeting between stakeholders, supporting solution-focused, shared decision-making. Conversation is facilitated around *claims*, which are positive statements a participant makes about a subject; *concerns*, which are negative statements regarding the same subject; and an *issue*, which is a question drawing insight from both claim and concern, providing a way forward (McCormack and Manley 2004). (See Chapter 5 for further information on CCIs.) Using this process, our team facilitated conversations between different disciplines and levels of staff, sharing perspectives and building relationships. Also important was 'closing the loop' where I was able to demonstrate action on areas which could be changed or, alternatively, communicate about things that could not.

Since those early years of service transformation, I have continued my personal journey of leadership growth. I have undertaken other leadership programmes, gaining new insights. As I reflect on these opportunities, what stands out about the rapid growth I encountered in the early years after the formation of our ward and through engagement in the CLP was how leadership training came together with my practical experience. The greatest resonance has occurred when training has been integrated with the frontline clinical context.

Today our ward is flourishing. A person-centred culture is embedded. We do our best work caring for vulnerable people. Leadership is shared across a number of nurses who collectively ensure high-quality care is delivered. We remain committed to values-based recruitment. We create innovative roles to develop team members. There are inherent clinical and non-clinical leaders within the team, who influence culture and practice despite not having formal leadership roles. In 2019, our team received a gold award in the NHS Achieving and Celebrating Excellence Recognition scheme (ACER) (EKHUFT, 2020). Celebrating achievement maintains motivation to continue pursuing excellence, supporting the team to achieve, lead, flourish and succeed.

Case study 2 Transformation from the ground up – a public pathology service

During my career, I have experienced a number of 'top down' change approaches, with change mandated by executives, implemented by middle managers and met by frontline staff with anxiety and resistance. Transformation has been costly: high attrition rates, decreased productivity and toxic cultures contributing to and resulting from these drivers.

Newly promoted to a managerial role in the Cellular Pathology Service, I was tasked with leading change in a department struggling to deliver services, with a high vacancy rate and demotivated team. I felt a directive approach would not bring positive change. I was curious to see how we could collaboratively define vision and expectations, agreeing collectively on accountabilities.

To commence this process, focus groups were used with frontline staff. Key areas for improvement included quality, communication, career development, connection to the patient, staff sick leave, training and competency standards and discipline-specific performance data tracking, relating to performance trending beyond results turnaround times. Focus group themes provided insight regarding issues staff regarded as relevant to them and impacting on success.

One year into my role, I participated in a CLP that introduced me to the ACER scheme. This provided a framework to think about developing effective workplace culture. It supported a structured process for visualising and documenting success. We had a number of early achievements in culture and performance transformation. The ACER framework facilitated the team articulating gaps in practice, taking ownership to co-create an improvement plan to deliver sustainable services.

From a team of 80 staff, 20 volunteered to participate in ACER working groups, disseminating information to the team using weekly huddles, keeping staff informed, engaged and able to provide feedback. Working group membership was mixed, comprising different disciplines and levels of experience, providing balanced and holistic perspectives. Smaller sub-groups were established, breaking down tasks and supporting transparent conversations. Recognising the NHS as a large and complex hierarchy, a senior staff member joined each smaller group, so issues could be escalated effectively.

The ACER framework had originally been written for patient-facing clinical staff. With some critical thinking, the team adapted the framework to better suit a healthcare laboratory, prompting reconsideration of day-to-day routines. Laboratory-based staff came to appreciate the experiences of patient-facing staff and, through better appreciating the whole patient journey, experienced greater validation of their role. There were some 'lightbulb moments' where groups discovered that the service had already been meeting goals within the framework, but without visibility around this. Focused, easy-to-implement goals were prioritised and provided 'quick wins', fostering confidence.

Framework areas, such as staff wellbeing, were addressed by providing stress management training, expanding service roles to include mental health link workers and establishing a mentoring system for new staff. Redesigning service roles enabled creative reallocation of funds to support training and education. Taking a growth-oriented, fair and transparent approach to individual career development, underpinned with enhanced appraisal processes, combined with more flexible rostering arrangements, further supported staff wellbeing. Improved staff wellbeing correlated with a decrease in staff sick leave rates, reducing from 3.55% to 2.14%, reflecting a reduction of 263 days per annum. Vacancy rates, which had varied between 27% and 33% reduced to 12–13.5%.

Leading and participating in this change process has been personally transformative. Experientially, I am now part of a much more engaged workforce. Tasks are completed on time. Our leadership team does not end up micro-managing staff. There is a flow of team discussion, leading to active processes of continuous improvement. Our team is characterised by being accountable, responsible and self-motivated.

Case study 3 Integrating values and vision for change – a hospital-based allied health service

I took on the leadership of the Speech and Language Therapy Team (SLTT) in October 2016, after two restructures in two years. The workforce was fractured. Teams worked in silos across three hospital sites. Staff experienced change fatigue without confidence of being heard as stakeholders. My leadership goal was to develop an effective workplace culture, providing high-quality, safe and efficient services. My challenge was achieving this in a complex and disjointed service environment.

My experience taught me that top-heavy management styles do not build collaborative teams. I needed to engage the team to understand our challenges so we could more meaningfully contribute within the high-pressured hospital environment. We had an opportunity to undertake ordinary tasks, extraordinarily well, and if we could embrace this, we could achieve excellence. I needed to work with the team to reconsider everyday practices and processes and at the same time think about how we worked together as a team. I aspired to build a culture where everyone's contributions were valued. I believed that listening responsively to staff would promote motivation, commitment and positive investment in change.

I used the ACER framework to plan, implement and assess our growth goals. By describing criteria for us to work towards, the ACER framework enabled us to build a body of evidence about how we were working. We used the ACER self-assessment tool to track our progress and then invited the ACER external assessment team to provide objective review, validating our achievements and making recommendations for further action. This approach provided support and enabled us to showcase achievements.

We commenced with facilitated conversations regarding values and how we would embed these in practice. Emerging from this, we co-created a team vision. The vision guided service objectives to support shared decision-making. These processes and outcomes cascaded through the department. We established new individual appraisal and personal development processes that kept values as a central focus. We created opportunities for individuals to participate in and lead projects, providing visibility around outcomes, in line with the vision and agreed service objectives. This resulted in more inclusive working, where staff felt part of something meaningful.

Forums facilitated team members debriefing and learning in a safe, no-blame environment. We considered how to translate reflections into practice. We implemented work-based and university-based training opportunities. Active learning promoted a competency-based approach from basic to specialist skills. Staff were empowered to lead quality improvement projects within the SLTT and in Trust-wide projects. More transparent quality monitoring processes promoted increased quality improvement initiatives.

Commitment and courage have been important within our change process. This has been paramount for me personally but has also been crucial for other clinical leaders within the team. Culture change is shared work. No one can achieve it alone. The dedication of values-based individuals has resulted in a team who work together effectively, guided by mutual respect and purpose.

Celebrating achievements along the way has also been important. Recognition of commitment, loyalty and hard work of team members is self-perpetuating, promoting continued drive towards improvement. Members of our team are now regularly nominated for awards for innovation, leadership and clinical excellence.

Using the ACER framework and resources was an important part of our journey. While needing to be adaptable and customising strategies to our specific context, having an evidence-based framework supported confident direction for me as a clinical leader and provided a common language regarding our transformation experience.

Our team is now committed to delivering compassionate, safe and effective person-centred care. We promote active learning and translation to practice. With a more effective workplace culture, the dividends include greater staff satisfaction, successful recruitment and retention, and better care for our community. From my perspective, definitely worth the effort.

Case study 4 Utilising strategies and tools for growth that works – a community child and adolescent service

As a consultant psychiatrist in a combined community paediatrics and child and adolescent mental health service, I did not have a formal managerial role. I attended, and later became a facilitator in, our NHS Trust CLP and was struck by the idea that we can all be leaders, profoundly influencing our teams. Inspired by my learning in the CLP, I became convinced that investing in the development of high-quality clinical leadership is essential to providing safe, compassionate and person-centred care.

I was keen to influence culture within my workplace and across community paediatrics as a whole. Seeking to initiate change within an already stretched system, I collaborated with two consultant paediatricians. We submitted an application for ACER accreditation focusing on developing and evaluating person-centred culture across our three teams: the ADHD service, outpatient community paediatrics and child audiology. The standards we wanted to demonstrate were improving patient experience, making sure that people feel cared for, and having all people – both patients and staff – feel that teamwork, trust and respect are at the heart of everything we do.

We wanted a robust culture change process and chose tools we believed would work for us. We used CCIs as a structure for team meetings. We used child-friendly feedback forms to gather feedback from children and their families. We developed emotional touchpoints, where we interviewed clinical and non-clinical colleagues and service users about what was important to them. We used observations of practice, where we visited other services to observe their culture. We also obtained non-anonymous feedback for our own 360-degree appraisals by interviewing colleagues or receiving written feedback, asking for honest feedback about our performance.

Most tools and strategies were easily integrated within a 'business as usual' model. The tool which required extra time, beyond our usual roles, was emotional touchpoints. I managed the emotional touchpoints by conducting one interview each week over several weeks, building data incrementally. Our project leadership team also met monthly, ensuring we were communicating, connecting, debriefing and planning.

Two years on from the project, all three project leads continue to build positive culture within our teams. A number of foundational tools are still being used. We continue to use CCIs, which has enhanced efficient and transparent communication, identifying problems and celebrating achievements. We still use child-friendly feedback forms to authentically capture the voice of children and families as stakeholders.

We discontinued using emotional touchpoints interviews. While feedback was powerfully insightful, we could not identify the human resource required to continue using this tool. This underlines the need for change processes to have sustainable investment. Despite letting go of emotional touchpoints, the overarching result of our project was sustained culture growth across all teams, resulting in more person-centred services.

Using non-anonymous 360-degree feedback supported our leadership development. While challenging, insight provided through constructive feedback became an important aspect of leadership growth. One colleague reflected that feedback 'made me a better team leader'.

Our team was awarded gold and silver NHS ACER awards. An independent review by the Royal College of Paediatrics and Child Health found 'enthusiastic, dedicated, happy teams' and the community doctors and admin staff were given an 'outstanding contribution' Trust award.

For me personally, the tools we used kept me motivated and appreciative of our team through the change journey. I learned that it is possible to lead and achieve workplace culture change, working within existing budgets and time constraints, through being deliberate, reflective and adaptable, enabling us to flourish.

Case study 5 The culture club story of change after trauma – an extended care older persons' mental health service

My life changed when, in January 2017, I joined an interdisciplinary panel undertaking a review of the Oakden Older Persons' Mental Health Service, a state-run specialist service in Adelaide, South Australia, providing 64 extended places-of-care for people with complex needs resulting from severe to extreme behaviours and psychological symptoms of dementia or mental illness. We found failures in governance, poor nursing practices, high levels of restraint, neglect of older people and toxic culture.

The Oakden Report (Groves et al. 2017) was released in April 2017 and became a landmark in Australian health and aged care history. A nationwide scandal erupted, with significant media attention. There was a leadership crisis and I was recruited to the health network responsible for service reform. Work began on local and state-wide levels. An oversight committee was established, and stakeholder working groups were formed to respond to recommendations. A culture reform working group co-designed a culture framework, articulating a central philosophy of compassionate person and family-centred care, supported by four priorities: (1) developing a values-based workforce; (2) cultivating psychological safety; (3) facilitating excellence in care; and (4) providing transparent accountability (McKellar and Hanson 2019).

There was a time of disruptive change. The service at Oakden was decommissioned. Organisational responses were punitive. There were industrial and human resource challenges. Numerous staff were stood down and some reported to police and registration authorities. Remaining staff were traumatised by organisational reactivity and intense public outrage, driven by a dramatic media narrative. Within this context, a new specialist service called Northgate House was established.

By early 2018, the new service was functional, with robust governance arrangements. Nevertheless, old and new staff had not integrated. Many staff remained wounded. Trust in management remained low.

This time coalesced with the release of the co-designed culture framework. A pilot project to operationalise the framework was established, also informed by concepts from the Deliberately Developmental Organisation (DDO) (Kegan and Lahey 2016). A project board was established and leadership consultants engaged as facilitators. A key idea was that rather than taking staff out of the service to attend training programmes, leadership and culture development should be grounded locally, involving everyone as equals. As skills and knowledge were handed over from visiting facilitators to embedded staff, the work became independent and sustainable.

The work involved underpinning principles, emerging from DDO literature, operationalised through customisable and repeatable practices. Key principles included 'everyone can grow', reflecting commitment to adult development; 'rank does not have its usual privileges', referring to shared responsibility for engagement in growth; 'the bottom line is the same thing', reflecting the interdependence of quality, efficiency and investment in staff; and 'everyone builds the culture', recognising the importance of teamwork (Kegan and Lahey 2016, p. 86).

Practices included 'check ins' and 'check outs', which were used in clinical handovers and team meetings. These were opportunities for team members to talk about what was happening for them as people, promoting vulnerability and psychological safety. A key to success was modelling by leaders within the team.

Another practice was regular 'forums' which evolved into our 'culture club' meetings, a quarantined time for the team to talk about how we work together, rather than what we do. Being counter-cultural, early meetings were awkward as we learnt to communicate across traditional boundaries. As medical head of unit, a position of traditional privilege, I sat with hotel services staff and learnt to listen, modelling the principle that 'rank does not have its usual privileges'. Over time, this transformed team relationships.

As practices became 'rituals', psychological safety improved. Mentoring relationships were established, supporting personal growth. Creativity and innovation increased. During the project period, we achieved a 59% reduction in staff sick leave. The team transformed to a high-performing, award-winning unit, with staff proud of the 'Northgate House way' where 'we deliver exceptional, innovative and compassionate person and family-centred care through teamwork where everyone matters; everyone contributes; everyone grows'.

Learning informed change across the whole of the Older Persons' Mental Health Service. The culture framework was implemented through service-wide values-based recruitment and by rolling out piloted principles and practices.

Reflecting on the journey, I am reminded of a 'check out' from one of our hotel services staff who quietly stated, 'I like what we're becoming'. This captures the dynamic nature of frontline workplace culture change. We are not a finished piece of work but continue moving forward, becoming a better version of ourselves.

Discussion

This chapter asked the question: What are the features of effective clinical leadership that facilitate culture change? Clinical leadership has a key role in person-centred care and quality improvement, but there is limited evidence regarding how clinical leadership programmes translate into transformed organisational cultures (West et al. 2015). The five narratives can be considered through the lens of programme theories emerging from research undertaken at the UK Centre for Practice Development and Canterbury Christchurch University, using realist evaluation to explore the impact of CLPs on workplace culture and person-centred practice. Realist evaluation asks, 'what works in which circumstances and for whom?' and explores context, mechanism and outcome in order to understand interventions and activities (Pawson and Tilley 1997).

Two programme theories described how CLPs contribute to flourishing workplace cultures and person-centred practice. First, CLPs responded to *contexts* promoting effective workplace cultures, combined with *mechanisms* that invest time and support, promote interdisciplinary activity and provide expert facilitation, achieving culture change *outcomes*. Second, CLPs responded to *contexts* promoting clinical leadership development, combined with *mechanisms* that embed person-centredness and enable clinicians to drive change locally through customised programmes, enhancing person-centred practice *outcomes*. These theories were synthesised into 'simple rules', consistent with PD, that can be mapped against features of clinical leadership evident in the narratives presented in this chapter (Box 13.1).

Living values and beliefs was evident across all cases. Clinical leaders were supported to explore values and beliefs, fostering self-awareness and optimism, valuing leadership roles and contributing to organisational vision, practice development and culture change (cases 1-5). This aligns closely with authentic leadership (Hewitt-Taylor 2015).

Box 13.1 Simple rules: CLP and clinical leadership leading to flourishing workplace cultures

1. **Living values and beliefs**
2. **Focusing on building interdisciplinary relationships**
3. **Enabling learning in the workplace**
4. **Fostering change and quality improvement**
5. **Focusing on transformational leadership**
6. **Linking to organisational objectives**

(*Source:* Helen Stanley)

Building interdisciplinary relationships was illustrated through engagement in action learning groups (case 1) and through 'culture club' (case 5). All cases reflected collaboration, interpersonal relationship building and interdisciplinary learning. PD strategies such as claims, concerns and issues (case 1), emotional touchpoints and observations of practice (case 3), alongside expert facilitation (case 5), *enabled learning in the workplace*. Clinical leaders focused on their own and their teams' personal and professional development, empowering effectiveness (cases 1-5).

Through the emphasis on *fostering change and quality improvement*, clinical leaders were able to drive change and gain recognition for their teams' evidenced improvements (cases 1-5). The *focus on transformational leadership* re-energised the clinical leaders, clarifying roles and supporting values-based leadership development, impacting workplace motivation, recruitment and retention (cases 1-5). This aligns with the relevance of transformational, adaptive and authentic leadership models (Heifetz et. al 2009; Hewitt-Taylor 2015).

In each case, *linking to organisational objectives* facilitated clinical leaders applying learning in localised contexts. This supported sustainability of outcomes from the ACER projects (cases 1-4) and the culture framework pilot in the older persons' mental health service (case 5).

The identification of six simple rules should not be an indication that clinical leadership in frontline teams is straightforward. As described in the narratives, clinical leaders encounter numerous challenges, conflicts and contradictions. The realist evaluation captured leadership paradoxes, identifying that, on the one hand, clinical leaders work to achieve flourishing frontline microsystems, while on the other hand, they struggle with disconnected or unsupportive organisational cultures at meso and macro levels. Clinical leaders aspire to 'leadership' as a noble pursuit, applying principles of PD and transformational leadership while potentially getting caught in the 'dark side' of leadership, with hubris and hierarchical power differentials, where dissenting opinions may be marginalised, undermining psychological safety, and where upward communication becomes flattery rather than critical decision-making (Tourish 2013, p. 77; Edmondson 2019, p. 14). Consciousness of these paradoxes and pitfalls, addressed through self-awareness and commitment to values-based and democratic leadership, is part of the journey towards flourishing frontline teams. These paradoxes are illustrated in Figure 13.1.

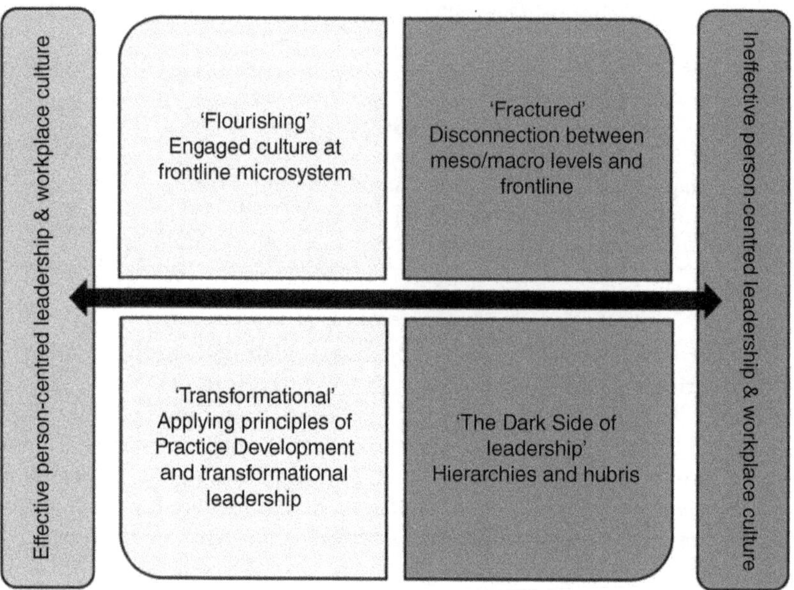

Figure 13.1 Paradoxes of clinical leadership (*Source:* Helen Stanley)

Conclusion

This chapter has explored features of effective clinical leadership facilitating culture change through five narrative accounts of clinical leaders on their journeys from fractured to flourishing teams. Six 'simple rules' provide insight regarding the impact of clinical leadership and CLPs on culture transformation. These 'simple rules' align with PD and with aspects of transformational, adaptive and authentic leadership models. Leadership aspirations should be balanced by recognition of ever-present challenges and the paradox of the 'dark side' of leadership, prompting reflection, self-awareness and tenacity within the leadership journey. The insights emerging from these narratives may inform future developments in CLPs and personal leadership experiences, with implications for practice development, effective workplace culture and person-centred clinical leadership (Eide and Cardiff 2017).

References

Akhtar, M., Casha, J., Ronder, J. et al. (2016). Leading the health service into the future: transforming the NHS through transforming ourselves. *International Practice Development Journal* 6 (2). https://doi.org/10.19043/ipdj.62.005

Cooper, C., Scandura, T. and Schriesheim, C. (2005). Looking forward but learning from our past: potential challenges to developing authentic leadership theory and authentic leaders. *The Leadership Quarterly* 16 (3): 475–493.

Davidson, S. (2020). Hard science and 'soft' skills: complex relational leading. *Nursing Administration Quarterly* 44 (2): 101–108.

Diddams, M. and Chang, G. (2012). Only human: exploring the nature of weakness in authentic leadership. *The Leadership Quarterly* 23 (3): 593–603.

Doody, O. and Doody, C. (2012). Transformational leadership in nursing practice. *British Journal of Nursing* 21 (20): 1212–1218.

East Kent Hospitals University NHS Foundation Trust (EKHUFT) (2020). Achieving and Celebrating Excellence Recognition (ACER): Workplace teams/services/departments that demonstrate person-centred, safe and effective workplace cultures that are also good places to work. Handbook. Version 5. In collaboration with England Centre for Practice Development, Canterbury Christ Church University, Kent.

Edmondson, A. (2019). *The Fearless Organization.* Hoboken: John Wiley and Sons.

Edmondson, A. and Lei, Z. (2014). Psychological safety: the history, renaissance, and future of an interpersonal construct. *Annual Review of Organizational Psychology and Organizational Behavior* 1 (1): 23–43.

Eide, H. and Cardiff, S. (2017). Leadership research: a person-centred agenda. In: *Person-Centred Healthcare Research* (eds. B. McCormack et al.), 95–115. Hoboken, NJ: Wiley Blackwell.

Groves, A., Thomson, D., McKellar, D. et al. (2017). *The Oakden Report.* Adelaide: South Australian Department of Health.

Harter, S. (2002). Authenticity. In: *Handbook of Positive Psychology* (eds. C. Snyder and S. Lopez), 382–394. New York;: Oxford University Press.

Heifetz, R., Grashow, A. and Linksy, M. (2009). *The Practice of Adaptive Leadership: Tools and Tactics for Changing Your Organization and the World.* Boston, MA: Harvard Business Press.

Hewitt-Taylor, J. (2015). *Developing Person-Centred Practice: A Practical Approach to Quality Healthcare.* London: Palgrave Macmillan.

Kegan, R. and Lahey, L. (2016). *An Everyone Culture: Becoming a Deliberately Developmental Organization.* Boston, MA: Harvard Business Review Press.

Laloo, E., Bakand, S., Hanley, N. et al. (2019). Reflections on group power differentials across one safety professional's career: in search of an optimal psychosocial safety climate. *International Practice Development Journal* 9 (2): 9.

Luthans, F. and Avolio, B. (2003). Authentic leadership: a positive development approach. In: *Positive Organizational Scholarship: Foundations of a New Discipline* (eds. K. Cameron et al.), 241–261. San Francisco, CA: Berrett-Koehler.

Manley, K. and Jackson, C. (2019). Microsystems culture change: a refined theory for developing person-centred, safe and effective workplaces based on strategies that embed a safety culture. *International Practice Development Journal* 9 (2) [4]. https://doi.org/10.19043/ipdj.92.004

Manley, K., Sanders, K., Cardiff, S. et al. (2011). Effective workplace culture: the attributes, enabling factors and consequences of a new concept. *International Practice Development Journal* 1 (2) [1]. https://www.fons.org/library/journal/volume1-issue2/article1

McCormack, B. and Manley, K. (2004). Evaluating practice developments. In: *Practice Development in Nursing* (eds. B. McCormack et al.), 83–117. Oxford: Blackwell Publishing.

McKellar, D. and Hanson, J. (2019). Codesigned framework for organisational culture reform in South Australian older persons' mental health services after the Oakden Report. *Australian Health Review.* https://doi.org/10.1071/AH18211

Nielsen, K., Randall, R., Yarker, J. et al. (2008). The effects of transformational leadership on followers' perceived work characteristics and psychological well-being: a longitudinal study. *Work Stress* 22 (1): 15–32.

Pawson, R. and Tilley, N. (1997). *Realist Evaluation*. London: Sage.

Porter-O'Grady, T. (2020). Complexity leadership: constructing 21st-century health care. *Nursing Administration Quarterly* 44 (2): 92–100.

Tourish, D. (2013). *The Dark Side of Transformational Leadership: A Critical Perspective*. London: Routledge.

van Rossum, L., Aij, K., Simons, F. et al. (2016). Lean healthcare from a change management perspective: the role of leadership and workforce flexibility in an operating theatre. *Journal of Health Organization and Management* 30 (3): 475–493.

Weberg, W. (2010). Transformational leadership and staff retention: an evidence review with implications for healthcare systems. *Nursing Administration Quarterly* 34 (3): 246–258.

West, M., Armit, L., Loewenthal, L. et al. (2015). *Leadership and Leadership Development in Health Care: The Evidence Base*. London: The King's Fund.

14. *Systems Leadership Enablement of Collaborative Healthcare Practices*

Annette Solman, Kim Manley, and Jane Christie

Introduction

This chapter focuses on work undertaken in the United Kingdom (UK) and Australia regarding leading system change utilising practice development (PD) principles and approaches. The purpose is to share approaches and outcomes to inform contemporary education and workforce development strategy essential to shaping health system reform (see Chapter 4). Reform requires people to be the enablers of system change for practice improvement in patient-centred care. Examples of reform pieces are described within the chapter to support the reader in contextualising how practice improvement was implemented using PD methods.

Developing systems leadership and management capability using facilitated learning

One approach to contemporary education strategy being undertaken in New South Wales (NSW), Australia is the focus on systems leadership and management capability development by the Health Education and Training Institute (HETI). NSW has a population of 7.95 million residents, the largest within

International Practice Development in Health and Social Care, Second Edition.
Edited by Kim Manley, Valerie Wilson, and Christine Øye.

Australia[1]. HETI was established following a Royal Commission into Healthcare by the Office of Australian Commissioner, Garling SC (2008), to ensure consistency of education and training across NSW Health, Australia. It is an agency of NSW Health, responsible for system-wide education and training of the workforce including clinical practice, leadership and management capability development. HETI has a range of governance functions for NSW Health. HETI places the learner, partners, consumers and better patient outcomes at the centre of its work.

HETI uses facilitated learning as a strategic intent drawing on knowledge, experience and evidence to inform staff practices and ways of working. This approach ensures consistency of practice and knowledge opportunity across healthcare. Facilitation is used to unpack traditions, the known and the unknown of practice, upon which to challenge assumptions, establish new ways of working and knowledge acquisition in support of best practice. A participatory approach to curriculum design through engagement of stakeholders, experts in the field of study and extensive literature review, is essential.

The Australian National Health Leadership framework, Health LEADS Australia (Shannon 2015), is reflected in leadership programmes with facilitative learning as a core approach to delivery. The patient experience, person-centredness and new ways of learning with and from each other are central to all programme design.

A key programme developed by HETI is the NSW Health Leadership Programme (Table 14.1). The programme brings together executives, senior managers, clinicians and corporate staff to work on understanding wicked problems within the health organisation.[2] The programme incorporates facilitative processes within programme design, delivery of individualised development and a strong focus on collective learning. Participants work on enhancing patient care planning, delivery, engagement and performance, at the same time building trustful and effective working relationships between the executive and clinicians for the enhancement of patient care.

Table 14.1 NSW Health Leadership Programme

Programme Title	Target Group	Focus Area	Duration
• NSW Health Leadership Programme	• Executives • Clinical leaders • Corporate service staff	• Person-centred practice for clinician engagement in decision-making with the executive regarding strategy to positively impact on patient care for those issues that have no known or one answer	• Initially 9 months; followed by further cohorts to establish a critical mass of staff who have completed the programme and can utilise these approaches in their work

[1] www.nsw.gov.au/about-nsw/key-facts-about-nsw

[2] https://www.wickedproblems.com/1_wicked_problems.php

Capabilities of leadership, facilitation, learning with and from others, the giving and receiving of feedback, the importance of stakeholder engagement including the consumer healthcare voice are built into this programme. The programme challenges self, assumptions and cultural norms that are impeding work practices and encourages participants not to rush to a solution but rather to work through different approaches in addressing any proposed change.

> At the heart of effective person-centred systems leadership and management is a facilitative approach to enable progress of programmes of work. Facilitation capability is essential to developing the health workforce to lead and manage with key skills and mindsets necessary to allow and to shape person-centred practice health system reform.

Recently HETI has developed facilitation standards and an assessment process for those seeking to understand their current level of capability and those seeking to further their capability to another level. These standards require the candidate to write a minimum of two reflective journal entries (critical reflection log (CRL)) about two different facilitation experiences. Each of the 25 key performance descriptors (KPDs) that constitute the standards must be referenced and accepted as demonstrable evidence of capability at least once.

- At least one of the entries must be supplemented with a facilitation activity plan (FAP), a facilitation evaluation plan (FEP), and a facilitator development action plan (FDAP). Each of these is required by specific KPDs.
- One of the journal entries must represent an observed facilitation session (by our two independent assessors). This is to provide a more well-rounded perspective of the candidate's facilitation capability and self-awareness (i.e. what is observed should be reflected in the journal entry).
- The observed session is followed by an interview with the two assessors. The focus is on underlying theory and self-awareness. Theory knowledge is required by specific KPDs.
- The purpose of the above requirements is to both support direct assessment of KPDs and get at a more general sense of self-awareness.

This programme was established from an identified need for staff development in the area of facilitating reasonable and challenging conversations regarding practice improvement and teamwork as enablers of change within the PD framework. The programme draws on the international facilitation standards work, grounded in PD theory, from the UK (Martin and Manley 2018) contextualised to the Australian environment. Staff are assessed against a category band of facilitation attainment and have the opportunity for further facilitation development (see Figure 14.1).

The HETI facilitation standards inform development for effective facilitation of individuals, teams and organisations to improving person-centred cultures and health outcomes.

To be effective in their work, leaders and managers must engage in systems leadership, foster life-long learning for individuals, themselves, target groups

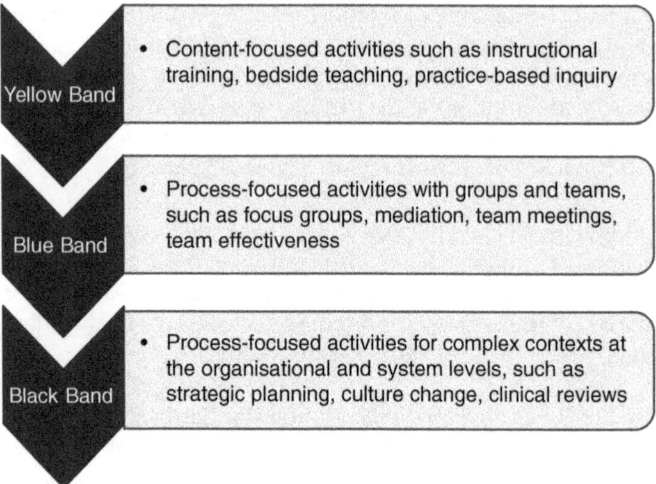

Figure 14.1 Facilitator training model

and organisations, and role model person-centred and evidence-based practice. The importance of facilitation capability for leaders is in managing rigorous discussion, challenging the norms and having respectful conversations that lead to purposeful outcomes for the healthcare systems in which they work.

Keeping people focused with increasingly complex healthcare systems

Healthcare systems are generally large and complex. They necessarily have a focus on people, the patient experience, their significant others, with a lens also on staff who provide both direct and indirect patient care, and systems, processes, policies and outcome measures. Understanding this complexity and these areas of focus is important to inform the work of supporting staff engaged in person-centred practice, 'an approach to practice established through formation and fostering healthful relationships between all healthcare providers, service users, and others significant to them in their lives' (McCormack and McCance 2017, p. 2).

Globally, health services are moving towards coordinated, integrated, people-centred systems as these are associated with better health outcomes and experiences (World Health Organization, Europe 2014). Care in these systems, instead of being focused on disease, is organised around the health needs and expectations of people and communities. The distinguishing features are:

- focusing on health needs
- enduring personal relationships
- comprehensive, continuous and person-centred care

- responsibility for the health of all in the community along the life cycle; responsibility for tackling determinants of ill-health and maintaining health
- working with people as partners in managing their own health and that of their community. Their preferences and motivations are integrated into care planning.

(World Health Organization, Europe 2013).

Achieving this vision necessitates dismantling historical boundaries across healthcare systems, with large-scale transformation programmes and leadership approaches that support such transformation (Dreier et al. 2019a, 2019b). The COVID-19 pandemic required large-scale transformation and highlights such an approach. This challenge necessitated a system view of cross-government agencies, private providers, staff and innovators to come together to understand the challenge from multiple perspectives. Collaboration in problem-solving was necessary to inform planning, prevention, treatment and reduction of transmission, alongside monitoring the impact while making changes as new evidence came to light.

Systems leadership and workforce factors influencing transformation

Best et al. (2012), through a rapid realist review, identified five simple rules that need to be applied differently in varied contexts to capture those factors more likely to enhance success in large-scale transformation. The first of these emphasise the need to blend designated and distributive leadership. 'Designated' leadership is recognised through formal accountability for a transformation programme and 'distributed leadership' as engaging individuals, partner organisations and teams at all levels in leading the change efforts to meet global challenges (Best et al. 2012). Both designated and distributed leadership approaches include underpinning of values and ways of working when applied to the system level reflect the concept of systems leadership, the focus of this chapter.

> *'Systems leadership is a set of skills and capacities that any individual or organization can use to catalyze, enable and support the process of systems-level change. It combines collaborative leadership, coalition-building and systems insight to mobilize innovation and action across a large, decentralized network.'* (Dreier et al. 2019b, p. 13)

In a study to answer the question of how to transform urgent and emergency care across the health economy using a whole-systems approach, systems leadership, enhanced by clinical expertise, was identified as one of three essential workforce enablers for supporting transformation (Manley et al. 2016) (Table 14.2).

The enablers, attributes and activities that characterise systems leaders are distilled from the literature linked to their consequences (see Appendix 14.1 unpublished concept analysis Setchfield and Manley, 2020).

Table 14.2 Specific workforce enablers for transformation

Specific workforce enablers	Workforce strategies for transformation
Clinical systems leadership across the health economy enables: • integration to happen and silos to be broken down; • workforce development; • dissemination of expertise • evaluation of impact. **A single career and competence framework** identifies the composite competences required from the multiprofessional team to wrap person-centred, safe and effective care around people's needs rather than around the professional. **Work-based facilitators are required** to use the workplace as the main resource for learning, development and improvement.	• To develop clinical systems leadership across the health economy to break down silos and achieve integrated whole-systems approaches. • To enable whole-systems working informed by values-based care. • To align integrated career and competence frameworks with the health needs of people. • To grow facilitators with the skills to use the workplace as a key resource for learning, developing and improving.

Enablers interplay between those individual qualities and skills required of a systems leader and those of the system needed to achieve the system's values and purpose (McHardy and McCann 2015; Turnet et al. 2016).

Individually, personal qualities and many skills are no different from those required by all relationship-based leaders in any setting – for example, striving to live values authentically (Storey and Holti 2013; Vize 2017), developing person-centred cultures and using appreciative approaches (Senge et al. 2015). Chapter 11 focuses on leadership approaches that enable effective workplace cultures while Chapter 12 describes the qualities and approaches that characterise relationship-based leadership in depth.

Specific individual enablers include the ability to:

- be collaborative, creative, reflective and transformational (Storey and Holti 2013; Caro 2016; Manley and Titchen 2016)
- translate theory into action (Marchildon and Fletcher 2016)
- co-create direction and solutions in partnership with others (Goss 2015; The King's Fund 2017).

Clinical credibility is essential to the work as it ensures a focus on bottom-up approaches, driving integration and breaking down silos for this work (Manley et al. 2016).

System enablers (Table 14.3) encompass structures, processes and patterns of behaviours across interdependent partners and organisations in keeping with the concepts of systems theory. Person-centred and place-based approaches embrace shared values, local objectives that meet local needs and what matters

Table 14.3 System enablers that support systems leadership

- Development of systems leadership (Senge et al. 2015; McHardy and McCann 2015).
- Authority to act (Turnet et al. 2016).
- Integrated approaches to workforce development with workforce capabilities structured around the person and their pathway rather than the professional (Manley et al. 2016).
- Measures and governance systems that enable progress to be demonstrated to guide service improvement (Perkins 2016) – for example, shared governance approaches (Perkins 2016), investment in information technology (Vize 2017), e.g. social media to galvanise the workforce.

to stakeholders (Turnet et al. 2016). Systems enablers are matched by financial models (Perkins 2016).

The attributes of systems leadership are emphasised as 'leadership' rather than 'management' and are focused in their function towards achieving the systems purpose of care centred around people and place (Manley et al. 2016; Vize 2017). The activities that describe what systems leaders do (Setchfield and Manley 2020 – see Appendix 14.1) have been synthesised to describe essential systems leadership functions:

Stimulating and facilitating high engagement.
Yielding in practice co-created values, purpose, goals, vision, principles.
System challenge to navigate complexity towards the future.
Testing assumptions, fostering reflection.
Enabling system improvement.
Modelling and facilitating learning in and about work.

Three intermediate/process outcomes arise from effective systems leadership and act as a foundation for more sustained impact. These intermediate and ultimate outcomes of systems leadership are presented in Table 14.4. While similar impact is common to good leadership in any context, in systems leadership this is experienced across the system; it involves all interdependent partners, sectors and organisations.

Clinical systems leadership embraces compassionate and collective leadership with the skills, values and qualities required to achieve transformation, which impacts on health outcomes and performance (Dawson 2014; National Health Service, England 2018). Systems leadership is based on 'developing shared values that focus on being person-centred, delivering care that is both safe and effective, embracing continuous learning, improvement and development' (Manley and Jackson 2020).

Clinical systems leadership is defined as:

'the leadership approach that drives integration across boundaries based on specialized clinical credibility working with shared purposes to break down silos and deliver person-centred, safe and effective care with continuity.' (Manley et al. 2016, p. 5)

Table 14.4 Intermediate and ultimate outcomes of systems leadership

Intermediate outcomes	Ultimate outcomes
• An ethos of shared ownership, risk, responsibility and accountability across the system (Vize 2017; Perkins 2016; Young et al. 2015) combined with the use of better information technology to underpin shared partnerships (Perkins 2016). • Committed, high-performing teams that are effective and innovative (Goss 2015; Manley et al. 2016; Storey and Holti 2013; Manley and Titchen 2016; Welbourn et al. 2012) • Integrated systematic learning, improvement and adaptability to meet system need (Perkins 2016; Caro 2016). • Workforce aligned with shared vision, purpose and cultures that are person-centred, population focused with place-based systems and patients involved in service design (Manley et al. 2016; Vize 2017; Senge et al. 2015; Caro 2016). • Employees experiencing high-quality support (Storey and Holti 2013; Senge et al. 2015).	• Improved patient experience (Welbourn et al. 2012; Fealy et al. 2013). • Timely and appropriate care (The King's Fund 2017). • Population-focused change (Caro 2016). • People taking greater responsibility for their own health and wellbeing (The King's Fund 2017; Vize 2017). • Reduced staff turnover (Young et al. 2015).

Systems leaders need:

- skills in sustainable cultural change, required to break down silos, enabling others to be empowered, especially at the microsystems level;
- a strong focus on enabling and developing the workforce and its talent system-wide;
- research and inquiry skills to monitor and evaluate subsequent impact;
- key consultancy models that disseminate evidence and expertise rapidly. (Manley et al. 2016)

System leadership achieves its goals through:

- integrated ways of working and effective teamwork across partner organisations;
- the dissemination of expertise to as many people across the system through advanced consultancy approaches;
- creating a learning culture that uses the workplace as the main resource for learning, development and improvement;
- growing the workforce competences across the system, evaluating effectiveness and fostering inquiry and curiosity (Manley et al. 2016).

Distributive leadership focuses on the practices and relationships involved in leadership and developing shared and evolving leadership through intentional mentoring strategies (Best et al. 2012). This insight endorses the importance of systems leaders having the facilitation skills required to work with multiple purposes, levels, stakeholders and complexity (Martin and Manley 2017). Complex layering of both the system and multiple levels of professionalised, autonomous practice in healthcare systems creates a case for distributive leadership as the optimal leadership approach necessary to support large-scale transformative change (Best et al. 2012).

While systems leadership has been recognised as a key enabler of systems change, the interdependent skills required for engaging and developing the workforce in the achievement of purpose, informed by shared values, merits highlighting facilitation skills as a key skillset (Martin and Manley 2017). In an action research and stakeholder evaluation that focused on a programme of support for consultant and aspiring consultant practitioners in nursing and midwifery, facilitation skills were identified as the key catalyst that enabled others at different levels to become more effective (Manley and Titchen 2016). This research has subsequently underpinned an emerging focus on the development of multi-professional consultant practice aligned with systems leadership in England through the development of a capability and impact framework (England Centre for Practice Development 2019) that makes explicit the capabilities required (see Figure 14.2).

System leadership approaches deliver capabilities for collective leadership essential for transformation of healthcare services aligned to the World Health Organization aspirations. These capabilities and their intended impact are closely aligned with the values, ways of working and purpose of PD. It inspires and develops the workforce through collaboration, inclusion and participation, enabling ways of working that keep the person and communities at the heart of care and services, using human and health resources effectively, avoiding duplication but maintaining continuity to meet population needs.

1. Expert practice[3]	2. Strategic, enabling leadership	3. Learning, developing, improving across the system	4. Research and innovation
5. Consultancy for embedding expertise across systems			

Figure 14.2 Four pillars and consultancy foundation of consultant practice across systems

[3] Expert practice refers to the primary profession of consultant e.g. allied health professional, bio-medical scientist, nurse, midwife, orthodontist, pharmacist;psychological professions, therapist. These roles will be generally patient-facing, but others, such as bio-medical scientists may be indirect in terms of service provision. This has been captured underneath the paragraph that follows the figure.

The role of facilitative leadership in improving care for older people across the system

The following study carried out in Scotland, UK is an example of how facilitative leadership enabled a multidisciplinary clinical team to improve the care of older people who had sustained a hip fracture (Christie et al. 2015). Hip fracture care delivery is vigorously supported by international clinical guidance, audit and performance targets that aim to incentivise and improve practice. Evidence-based practice was driving the agenda and expected targets were being met; however, the feedback from older people and carers indicated that the experience was far from satisfactory. This was of great discomfort and concern to the organisation and the clinical team involved.

A multidisciplinary group of clinical leaders working in different services along the older persons' care journey was invited to participate in a series of action meetings. The aims were to create a safe space, to demonstrate genuine understanding and expertise, to enable the group to reflect on their experiences and actions, and to consider the collective way forward that would improve the experience of care. Clear ground rules based on trust, respect and a commitment to working together were negotiated and agreed. Evidence-based PD methods were applied to facilitate the development of a shared vision, clarification of values, sharing clinical experiences, auditing records and reflecting on older people's and caregivers' experience of care.

Initial findings identified the priorities for care to be the evidence-based guidelines that focused on functional recovery. Meeting the older people's personal and psychosocial needs appeared to be hidden or ignored. Services along the care pathway were disjointed and care was delivered by disparate subgroups of specialist healthcare professionals, working independently and each keeping separate records. This evidence-based, target-driven culture was stressful for practitioners, who were managing the conflicting values of efficiency and compassion inherent in the system, as well as their professional expectations and the needs of older people and caregivers. Defence mechanisms were used to rationalise their actions.

Accepting the situation as it was and facilitating a collaborative, participatory process in a psychologically safe environment afforded the multidisciplinary team time to work together across the traditional management boundaries and to see the whole experience of care. At each stage the data recorded was verified by those participating through a process of checking interpretation, clarifying understanding and agreeing action. The team valued the opportunity to share different perspectives and to be involved in exploring different ways to deliver and evaluate person-centred, safe, effective practice.

Findings of the study were validated through a series of participatory, person-centred workshops involving corporate and clinical managers. Creating a safe space and the time to reflect on the findings, these designated leaders acknowledged the risks inherent in the present ways of working, identified the actions required by all to enable teams to work together effectively across boundaries and realised the shared outcomes of person-centred, safe, effective practice.

Table 14.5 Key learning from facilitating this collaborative development process

Key learning
Expertise in the field of practice and in the application of adult learning principles in the workplace is essential.
Gaining access and permission to work with the multidisciplinary group of clinical leaders [distributive leaders] across traditional workplace boundaries required the support of those who know the whole system and see the need for different disciplines to work together to develop a shared understanding of a troubling dilemma.
Academic supervision and support are required from those who know and understand the challenges of participatory, collaborative action research.
Actions agreed during the collaborative process involved returning to the ethics committee for approval.
Making positive use of professional networking by starting small, using learning time creatively to collect data and seeking out safe spaces to work with others to validate ideas proved to be invaluable.
Involving, listening, hearing and taking heed of the 'voices' of practitioners and the people that we support and care for improves relationships, values expertise and promotes equity, inclusion and wellbeing.
Sharing issues with the managers [designated leaders] in an experiential way promoted listening, like-mindedness, positive feedback and better understanding between professional groups along with an acceptance of the findings from the study.
Valuing diverse perspectives and facilitating the transition from a 'clashing to collective' ethos raised awareness of the battle between different paradigms [worldviews] that is played out inadvertently in day-to-day health and social care practice.

Applying facilitative leadership skills (Table 14.5) across the system enabled a multidisciplinary team of clinical leaders to show that they cared about the service they provided and were unhappy when the care delivered was not as good as it could otherwise be. Ownership and sustainability were achieved by having dedicated time to work across service delivery boundaries, to learn together in a safe, supportive workplace environment and to agree collective action. Promoting a culture of psychological safety, collaboration, learning and wellbeing enabled the multidisciplinary team to get to know each other, to understand each other's professional perspective, to realise that they had shared aspirations and to agree collectively how to deliver and evaluate evidence-based practice that improved the experience for those in which they were caring.

Conclusion

This chapter presented international practice evidence examples of contemporary PD systems leadership as essential for enabling sustained transformation to evidence-based, patient-focused and informed healthcare practices. Staff development in the area of facilitation capability is recognised as an enabler to effective collaboration in the challenging of assumptions, seeking out evidence, enabling and supporting patient engagement. To successfully maximise clinical partnering with patients requires staff who are highly skilled in facilitative approaches and understand the importance of systems thinking, learning with and from each other and using a strong evidence base. Clinical partnering is achieved by breaking down the silos through active collaboration to bring about enhanced systems approaches to patient care. To achieve this a systems lens is required to focus on the contributing factors to the set of circumstances from multiple perspectives. In the review of current practices, supporting clinicians and managers to review their practice in light of evidence and the use of research to inform work practice are enablers of person-centred, evidence-based care. The process of engagement using a strategic lens coupled with person-centred facilitation creates an environment of safety for high-challenge and high-support conversations to occur in critically analysing practice with and for patients to achieve best practice and to inform policymakers.

References

Best, A., Green, T. and Lewis, S. (2012). Large-system transformation in health care: a realist review. *Millbank Quarterly* 90 (3): 421–456.

Caro, D. (2016). Towards transformational leadership: the nexus of emergency management systems in Canada. *International Journal of Emergency Management* 12 (2): 113–135.

Christie, J., Macmillan, M., Currie, C. et al. (2015). Improving the experience of hip fracture care: a multidisciplinary collaborative approach to implementing evidence-based, person-centred practice. *International Journal of Orthopaedic and Trauma Nursing* 19 (1): 24–35.

Dawson, J. (2014). Staff experience and patient outcomes: what do we know? A report commissioned by NHS Employers, July 2014. https://www.nhsemployers.org/-/media/Employers/Publications/Research-report-Staff-experience-and-patient-outcomes.pdf (accessed 23 April 2020).

Dreier, L., Nabarro, D. and Nelson, J. (2019a). Systems leadership can change the world – but what exactly is it? *World Economic Forum* 24 September 2019. https://www.weforum.org/agenda/2019/09/systems-leadership-can-change-the-world-but-what-does-it-mean/ (accessed 01 May 2020).

Dreier, L., Nabarro, D. and Nelson, J. (2019b). *Systems Leadership for Sustainable Development: Strategies for Achieving Systemic Change*. Harvard Kennedy School. https://www.hks.harvard.edu/sites/default/files/centers/mrcbg/files/Systems%20Leadership.pdf

England Centre for Practice Development [ECPD]. (2019). Multi-professional Consultant Practice Capability and Impact Framework. Unpublished report. Co-badged with Health Education England, *ECPD*. Canterbury: Christ Church University.

Fealy, G.M., McNamara, M., Casey, M. et al. (2013). Service impact of a national clinical leadership development programme: findings from a qualitative study. *Journal of Nursing Management* 23 (3): 1–9.

Garling, P. (2008). Final Report of the Special Commission of Inquiry: Acute Care Services in New South Wales Public Hospitals. https://www.dpc.nsw.gov.au/assets/dpc-nsw-gov-au/publications/Acute-Care-Services-in-NSW-hospitals-listing-437/7d979f4786/Overview-Special-Commission-of-Inquiry-into-Acute-Care-Services-in-NSW.pdf (accessed 23 April 2020).

Goss, S. (2015). Systems leadership: a view from the bridge. An OPM Paper. https://traverse.ltd/application/files/4915/3062/4273/Systems-Leadership-A-view-from-the-bridge.pdf

The King's Fund. (2017). *Leading across the Health and Care System: Lessons from Experience*. London: The King's Fund.

Manley, K., Martin, A., Jackson, C. et al. (2016). Using systems thinking to identify workforce enablers for a whole systems approach to urgent and emergency care delivery: a multiple case study. *BMC Health Services Research* 16 (a): 368.

Manley, K. and Jackson, C. (2020). The Venus model for integrating practitioner-led workforce transformation and complex change across the health care system. *Journal of Evaluation in Clinical Practice* 26 (2): 622–634.

Manley, K. and Titchen, A. (2016). Facilitation skills – the catalyst for increased effectiveness in consultant practice and clinical systems leadership. *Educational Action Research* 24 (2): 1–24.

Marchildon, G.P. and Fletcher, A.J. (2016). Systems thinking and the leadership conundrum in health care. *Evidence and Policy* 12 (4): 559–573.

Martin, A. and Manley, K. (2017). Developing standards for an integrated approach to workplace facilitation for interprofessional teams in health and social care contexts: a Delphi study. *Journal of Interprofessional Care* 32 (1): 41–51.

Martin, A. and Manley, K. (2018). Developing standards for an integrated approach to workplace facilitation for interprofessional teams in health and social care contexts: a Delphi study. *Journal of Interprofessional Care* 32 (1): 41–51.

McCormack, B. and McCance, T. eds. (2017). *Person-Centred Practice in Nursing and Health Care: Theory and Practice. 2nd Edition*. Chichester: John Wiley and Sons Ltd.

McHardy, K. and McCann, L. (2015). Shortfalls in clinical and health system leadership. *Internal Medicine Journal. Royal Australasian College of Physicians*. DOI: 10.1111/imj.12901

National Health Service [NHS] England. (2018). *Links between NHS staff experience and patient satisfaction: analysis of surveys from 2014 and 2015*. Leeds: NHS England.

Perkins, D. (2016). One size fits all . . . or not! *The Australian Journal of Rural Health* 24 (2): 71–72.

Senge, P., Hamilton, H. and Kania, J. (2015). The dawn of system leadership. *Stanford Social Innovation Review. Winter* 2015. https://networkpeninsula.org/wp-content/uploads/2014/12/The_Dawn_of_System_Leadership-1.pdf

Setchfield, I. and Manley, K. (2020). *Concept analysis of systems leadership*. East Kent Hospitals University NHS Foundation Trust. Unpublished Framework.

Shannon, E.A. (2015). Health LEADS Australia: implementation and integration into theory and practice. *Asia Pacific Journal of Health Management* 10 (1): 56–62.

Storey, J. and Holti, R. (2013). *Towards a New Model of Leadership for the NHS*. The Open University Business School. London: NHS Leadership Academy.

Turnet, S., Ramsey, A., Perry, C. et al. (2016). Lessons for major system change: centralization of stroke services in two metropolitan areas in England. *Journal of Health Services Research & Policy* 2 (3): 156–165.

Vize, R. (2017). *Swimming Together or Sinking Alone: Health, Care and the Art of Systems Leadership*. London: Institute of Healthcare Management.

Welbourn, D., Warwick, R., Carnall, C. et al. (2012). *Leadership of whole systems*. London: The King's Fund. http://eprints.chi.ac.uk/id/eprint/1231/1/Kings%20Fund%20Whole%20Systems%20Leadership.pdf

World Health Organization. Regional Office for Europe & Health Services Delivery Programme, Division of Health Systems and Public Health. (2013). *ROADMAP. Strengthening People–centred Health Systems in the WHO European Region: A Framework for Action towards Coordinated/Integrated Health Services Delivery (CIHSD)* Copenhagen: WHO Regional Office for Europe. https://apps.who.int/iris/bitstream/handle/10665/108628/e96929.pdf?sequence=1&isAllowed=y

World Health Organization [WHO] Europe (2014). *Strengthening People-centred Health Services Delivery in the WHO European Region: Concept Note*. Health Services Delivery Programme, Division of Health Services and Public Health, Copenhagen: WHO Regional Office for Europe.

Young, J., Lanstrom, G., Rosenberger, S. et al. (2015). Leading nursing into the future. Development of a strategic nursing platform on a system level. *Nursing Administration Quarterly* 39 (3): 239–246.

Appendix 14.1

ENABLERS INDIVIDUAL	ATTRIBUTES CLINICAL SYSTEMS LEADERSHIP	CONSEQUENCES
Personal qualities • Values driven (Goss 2015; The King's Fund 2017), authentic with integrity (Storey and Holti 2013; Vize 2017; Caro 2016; Welbourn et al. 2012) • Calm, creative (Goss 2015) with an open mind set (Welbourn et al. 2012), responsive and flexible (Goss 2015) • Emotional intelligence (Caro 2016) • Think outside of the box (Caro 2016) **Collective and transformational leadership skills** • Collaborative and partnership working (Goss 2015; The King's Fund 2017; Welbourn et al. 2012; McLellan 2015); who can co-produce (Goss 2015) and use appreciative inquiry to foster co-creation (Senge et al. 2015) • Motivate and encourage teams and individuals to work effectively (Storey and Holti 2013); inspire and motivate others (Caro 2016; Manley and Titchen 2016) • Effective communication (Caro 2016), conflict resolution (Perkins 2016) and transformational leadership skills (Caro 2016; Manley and Titchen 2016) • Develop others as transformational leaders (Storey and Holti 2013) • Ability to translate theory into action (Marchildon and Fletcher 2016) • Have an entrepreneurial attitude (Welbourn et al. 2012) and can take risks (Manley and Titchen 2016) • Requirement for leaders to have skills across different leadership styles (McLellan 2015)	**Collaborative/collective/distributive leadership** that is participative and facilitative (Goss 2015; The King's Fund 2017; Manley et al. 2016; Vize 2017; Senge et al. 2015; McHardy and McCann 2015; Manley and Titchen 2016; Welbourn et al. 2012) and inclusive (Manley et al. 2016) across different sectors (Caro 2016) **Co-created values, purpose, goals, vision, principles: place and people based** • Co-create shared endeavour/shared purpose/vision/framework of values and goals (Goss 2015; The King's Fund 2017; Manley et al. 2016; Storey and Holti 2013; Perkins 2016; Manley and Titchen 2016; Welbourn et al. 2012) – compelling to partners and safety and systems principles (Goss 2015; The King's Fund 2017; Manley et al. 2016) • Purpose is place based, not the organisation (Caro 2016) • Doing the right thing for people we serve (Vize 2017) • Promotes values and recognises link between values and behaviours (Welbourn et al. 2012) **Public engagement and involvement** • Public and patient engagement (Vize 2017) • Support from patients and public to support implementations (Turnet et al. 2016) • Involvement of patients in system service design essential (McLellan 2015) • Focus on needs and experiences of service users (Vize 2017)	**Joint shared risk, responsibility, accountability across system** • Joint risk and shared responsibility (Perkins 2016) • Shared ownership of problems and solutions (Vize 2017) • Shared leadership partnership (incl HEIs) and accountability (Young et al. 2015) **Committed, high-performing teams (effective and innovative) aligned with shared vision and purpose** • Take people with them (Goss 2015); commitment from followers (Welbourn et al. 2012) • Alignment of workforce with shared vision and purpose (McLellan 2015) • Gives permission for staff to be innovative (The King's Fund 2017) • High-performing teams who meet and evaluate effectiveness (Storey and Holti 2013); higher performance (Welbourn et al. 2012) • Positive impact on individual effectiveness (Manley and Titchen 2016; Fealy et al. 2013) **Employees experience high-quality support** • Value created by satisfied, loyal and productive employees stems from high-quality support (Storey and Holti 2013; Senge et al. 2015) • Reduced staff turnover (Young et al. 2015)

(Conti.)

Appendix 14.1 *(conti.)*

Clinical credibility and system leadership • Clinical expertise drives integration and provides credibility (Manley et al. 2016; Caro 2016; Manley and Titchen 2016) • Strong clinical leaders (Manley et al. 2016) • Empowered leadership close to the frontline (McLellan 2015) • Engaged clinicians who have power to influence (Turnet et al. 2016) • Bottom-up approach (McLellan 2015; Turnet et al. 2016; Marchildon and Fletcher 2016) • Leadership aligned to purpose of health system (McHardy and McCann 2015) and transformational goals (Turnet et al. 2016) **ENABLERS: SYSTEM, INTERDEPENDENT PARTNERS AND ORGANISATIONS** **Strong values, supportive cultures and local objectives** • Strong values (McHardy and McCann 2015) with supportive organisational cultures (Fealy et al. 2013) • Local objectives that reflect local need (Perkins 2016), focusing on outcomes that matter to stakeholders (Turnet et al. 2016) matched by financial models (Perkins 2016) **Integrated workforce models** • Integrated career and competence framework to align workforce and meet changing healthcare needs (Manley et al. 2016) **Systems leadership authority** • Bottom-up approach to leadership and top-down coordination (Marchildon and Fletcher 2016); clinically led services (McLellan 2015) • System leadership with authority (Turnet et al. 2016)	**High engagement across boundaries and networks vertically and horizontally** • Frequent personal contact (The King's Fund 2017); High engagement (Storey and Holti 2013) • Engage/work across boundaries (Senge et al. 2015; Perkins 2016) • Develop and maintain networks vertically and horizontally (Caro 2016) • Invests in relationships and values behaviours (Welbourn et al. 2012) **Clinical leadership focused rather than management** • Clinical leadership – less management (Manley et al. 2016) • Clinically led rather than management (Vize 2017) **Challenges system, navigates complexity, future orientated with clear goals and time for planning** • Enables navigation of complex processes (Turnet et al. 2016) • Clear and challenging goals (Storey and Holti 2013) • Future focused rather than reactive (Senge et al. 2015) • Create space for change and discussing plans (Senge et al. 2015) **Challenges and tests assumptions, fostering reflection and enabling time and support for staff to think differently** • Challenges system and enables transformation stakeholders (Turnet et al. 2016) • Challenging assumption and patterns of behaviour (Storey and Holti 2013; Senge et al. 2015) • Testing assumptions, unpacking beliefs (reflective elements) (Goss 2015); fostering reflection (Senge et al. 2015; Manley and Titchen 2016)	**High-performing systems that integrate systematic learning, improvement and adaptability to meet system need** • High-performing systems that integrate systemic learning, improvement and adaptability (Caro 2016) • Meet service need through reduced duplication (Perkins 2016) • All elements of system paid attention to (Goss 2015) • Systems networks and social movements (Welbourn et al. 2012) • Systems embrace uncertainty rather than linearity (Caro 2016) • Career and competence frameworks aligned to patient pathways in any context (Manley et al. 2016) • Enables multiple organisations to align at scale (Turnet et al. 2016) **Systems alignment for person centred place based/population sustainable transformation** • Robust sustainable system change (Senge et al. 2015) • Person centred place-based system and service design (Vize 2017) • Transformed practice towards a culture that is person centred (Manley and Titchen 2016) • Change in culture (Young et al. 2015) Organisational culture change (Caro 2016) • Organisation and political strategy alignment (Young et al. 2015) • Sustained systems change (Young et al. 2015), more likely to achieve sustained change (Manley et al. 2016) **Population-focused change** • Population-focused change (Caro 2016) • Addresses complexity of healthcare population needs (Manley et al. 2016)

<table>
<tr>
<td></td>
<td>• Create a climate where everyone feels empowered to think and work differently (Vize 2017)
• Time for staff to undertake transformation not bolted on to job (Vize 2017)</td>
<td></td>
</tr>
<tr>
<td>Systems leadership development
• Investment in leadership training that reflects the needs of the clinical workplace (McHardy and McCann 2015)
• Development of systems leaders (Senge et al. 2015)
• Need to grow leaders by talent management/mentoring/coaching (McHardy and McCann 2015; McLellan 2015; Fealy et al. 2013)

Measures for progress and improvement
• Measures to enable progress to be Identified and to identify further system improvement (Perkins 2016)

Governance structures
• Shared governance (Perkins 2016)
• Appropriate governance structure (Perkins 2016)

Information technology and social media
• Investment in IT (Vize 2017)
• Social media technology (Welbourn et al. 2012) to galvanise the workforce (McLellan 2015)</td>
<td>Facilitating and modelling learning in and about work, enabling action and workforce development
• Facilitate work-based learning (Manley and Titchen 2016)
• Focus on learning and actions (Goss 2015)
• Model learning behaviours (Storey and Holti 2013)
• Facilitators learning in workplace to enable role clarity and team approach (Manley et al. 2016)
• Learning that leads to action (Goss 2015)
• Lifelong commitment to learn on the job (Senge et al. 2015)
• Enabling workforce development (Manley et al. 2016)

Improving systems performance
• Focus on improving systems performance (Storey and Holti 2013)
• Build services around place – looking at patients' journey and connections between services rather than system architecture (Vize 2017)</td>
<td>Improved patient experience, timely appropriate care
• Clinical leadership makes a difference to patient's experience (Fealy et al. 2013)
• Improved patient experiences (Welbourn et al. 2012)
• Timely and appropriate care (The King's Fund 2017)

Greater responsibility for own health and wellbeing
• People take responsibility for own wellbeing (The King's Fund 2017)
• Patients take an active role in managing own health (Vize 2017)

Network of collaborative leaders
• Network of leaders (Goss 2015)
• Collaborative networks (Senge et al. 2015)
• Organisational systems leaders who feel valued and supported (McLellan 2015)
• Collective leadership and work with other systems leaders (Senge et al. 2015)
• New connections (Welbourn et al. 2012)

Better use of IT
• Better use of IT (Perkins 2016)
• Increased use of technology (Perkins 2016)</td>
</tr>
</table>

Concept analysis of systems leadership. East Kent Hospitals University NHS Foundation Trust. Unpublished Framework. (Source: Setchfield and Manley 2020)

References

Caro, D. (2016). Towards transformational leadership: the nexus of emergency management systems in Canada. *International Journal of Emergency Management* 12 (2): 113–135.

Fealy, G.M., McNamara, M., Casey. M. et al. (2013). Service impact of a national clinical leadership development programme: findings from a qualitative study. *Journal of Nursing Management* 23 (3): 1–9.

Goss, S. (2015). Systems leadership: a view from the bridge. An OPM Paper. https://traverse.ltd/application/files/4915/3062/4273/Systems-Leadership-A-view-from-the-bridge.pdf

The King's Fund. (2017). *Leading across the Health and Care System: Lessons from Experience*. London: The King's Fund.

Manley, K., Martin, A., Jackson, C. et al. (2016). Using systems thinking to identify workforce enablers for a whole systems approach to urgent and emergency care delivery: a multiple case study. *BMC Health Services Research* 16 (a): 368.

Manley, K. and Titchen, A. (2016). Facilitation skills – the catalyst for increased effectiveness in consultant practice and clinical systems leadership. *Educational Action Research* 24 (2): 1–24.

Marchildon, G.P. and Fletcher, A.J. (2016). Systems thinking and the leadership conundrum in health care. *Evidence and Policy* 12 (4): 559–573.

McHardy, K. and McCann, L. (2015). Shortfalls in clinical and health system leadership. *Internal Medicine Journal*. Royal Australasian College of Physicians. DOI: 10.1111/imj.12901

McLellan, M. (2015). Future of NHS Leadership. Hospital Service Journal. Ending the crisis in NHS Leadership: A Plan for Renewal. June 2015. https://www.hsj.co.uk/Journals/2015/06/12/y/m/e/HSJ-Future-of-NHS-Leadership-inquiry-report-June-2015.pdf (accessed 19 July 2020).

Perkins, D. (2016). One size fits all . . . or not! *The Australian Journal of Rural Health* 24 (2): 71–72.

Senge, P., Hamilton, H. and Kania, J. (2015). The dawn of system leadership. *Stanford Social Innovation Review*. Winter 2015. https://networkpeninsula.org/wp-content/uploads/2014/12/The_Dawn_of_System_Leadership-1.pdf

Setchfield, I. and Manley, K. (2020). *Concept analysis of systems leadership*. East Kent Hospitals University NHS Foundation Trust. Unpublished Framework.

Storey, J. and Holti, R. (2013). *Towards a New Model of Leadership for the NHS. The Open University Business School*. London: NHS Leadership Academy.

Turnet, S., Ramsey, A., Perry, C. et al. (2016). Lessons for major system change: centralization of stroke services in two metropolitan areas in England. *Journal of Health Services Research & Policy* 2 (3): 156–165.

Vize, R. (2017). *Swimming Together or Sinking Alone: Health, Care and the Art of Systems Leadership*. London: Institute of Healthcare Management.

Welbourn, D., Warwick, R., Carnall, C. et al. (2012). *Leadership of whole systems*. London: The King's Fund. http://eprints.chi.ac.uk/id/eprint/1231/1/Kings%20Fund%20Whole%20Systems%20Leadership.pdf

Young, J., Lanstrom, G., Rosenberger, S. et al. (2015). Leading nursing into the future. Development of a strategic nursing platform on a system level. *Nursing Administration Quarterly* 39 (3): 239–246.

15. *Recognising and Developing Effective Workplace Cultures Across Health and Social Care that are Also Good Places to Work*

Kate Sanders, Jonathan Webster, Kim Manley, and Shaun Cardiff

What is workplace culture and why is it important?

At its simplest, culture is defined as 'how things are done around here' (Drennan 1992, p. 9). It is the patterns, habits and behaviours that become established over time as social norms. These embedded ways of working reflect the assumptions, values and beliefs that exist within particular settings (Schein 1990). As such, these practices may go unnoticed and unchallenged (Plsek no date) as essentially they become taken for granted.

Interest in culture within health and social care organisations has increased over the last two decades. Reports have highlighted significant failings in care, identifying the need for cultural change in the UK, for example Patterson (2011), Francis (2013) and Kirkup (2018). Greatest attention has been given to organisational and corporate cultures (Mannion and Davies 2018), yet organisations are made up of many cultures at a micro-systems level – for example, wards, units, and health and care teams. We call these workplace cultures (Manley et al. 2011), the place where care is given, received and experienced. Because these cultures have an immediate and lasting influence on service user and care worker experiences, Manley et al. (2011) argue that significant consideration should be given to enabling change and transformation at this level, acknowledging the interdependency with the corporate culture of the organisation. While demonstrating

International Practice Development in Health and Social Care, Second Edition.
Edited by Kim Manley, Valerie Wilson, and Christine Øye.

relevance across all levels of the system, practice development (PD) primarily focuses on this micro-systems level (McCormack et al. 2013).

Background to collaborative inquiry

Because of our shared interest in workplace cultures and the impact on care over a decade (2000–2010), we engaged in a four-phased approach to developing a framework of an effective workplace culture, defined as:

> *'The most immediate culture experienced and/or perceived by staff, patients, users and other key stakeholders. This is the culture that impacts directly on the delivery of care. It both influences and is influenced by the organisational and corporate cultures with which it interfaces as well as other idiocultures through staff relationships and movement.'* (Manley et al. 2011, p. 4)

This work culminated in the publication of a concept analysis that identifies the enablers, attributes and consequences of effective workplace cultures in care settings (Manley et al. 2011). The resulting framework suggests that three sets of values are shared and realised in practice. These focus on providing care that is person-centred, safe and effective by working and learning in ways that are collaborative, inclusive and participatory. Staff and stakeholders are encouraged to be creative and innovative, adapting and making changes in response to the needs of service users. This is supported by formal systems of evaluation, learning and development. Factors that enable effective workplace cultures include transformational leaders, skilled facilitation, role clarity, organisational readiness, a flat and transparent management structure as well as a supportive human resource department.

Subsequently, a refinement of this theory of culture change at the micro-systems level has been offered, drawing on the findings of the Safety Culture Quality Improvement Realist Evaluation (SCQIRE) project (Manley et al. 2017, 2019a). Combining realist evaluation and practice development methodology, this regional project across four acute NHS hospital sites in the South-East of England aimed to embed safety culture and grow quality improvement and leadership capability in ten frontline teams.

The refined theory proposes a more explicit and integrated relationship between the values of an effective workplace culture, contending that a safety culture can be created only if staff and patients establish and experience person-centred relationships. Subtle changes to two of the values are also offered, including the recognition of the importance of appreciative and active ways of learning and a greater emphasis on the 'being' of person-centredness. The key enabling factors identified are quality clinical leadership and skilled facilitation at both the workplace and corporate organisational levels. While other organisational enablers relating to the characteristics of a learning organisation were found to be helpful, Manley et al. (2019a) argue that change in workplace cultures will not be achieved without the workplace enablers.

Developing 'guiding lights' through collaborative inquiry

We recognise that our understanding of workplace cultures continues to develop based on our collective experiences, but also that the related theories are complex. This complexity reflects the nature of health and social care and the individuals and systems (processes, structures and patterns of thinking and behaviour) that make up our workplaces and organisations. Such complexity might dissuade some practitioners from trying to evaluate their workplace cultures, impacting on their understanding of what might be working well and how this could happen more often, but also what needs to be improved and what support might be needed to achieve this.

With this in mind, we engaged in a collaborative inquiry to develop a guiding theory with and for health and social care practitioners about how to recognise and develop effective workplace cultures that are also good places to work. The inquiry drew on principles from appreciative inquiry and realist evaluation. Full details of the methodology and methods are published elsewhere (Cardiff et al. 2020), but the four resulting guiding lights – collective leadership, living shared values, safe, critical, creative, learning environments and change for good that makes a difference – are introduced in Table 15.1.

Guiding light 1 Collective leadership

Leadership has traditionally been seen as a practice exercised by those in formal, hierarchical positions. As the landscape of healthcare has structurally changed due to rising demand with fewer resources, so have interpretations of leadership. There is increasing emphasis on developing capacity recognising that everyone can be a leader of something, and also leadership as a phenomenon that manifests in relationships, focusing on 'power with' rather than 'power over'. In an action research study on person-centred leadership, Cardiff (2014) described how such a transition, although not free of challenges, enabled hierarchical leaders (nurse manager and charge nurses) and those they were leading to become more empowered and to experience wellbeing at work.

Manley et al. (2019b) first used the term 'guiding lights' as a metaphor for what Best et al. (2012) described as 'simple rules'. The outcomes of their project, which focused on relational leadership processes, is presented in Chapter 12. The guiding lights generated are complementary to those outlined in this chapter. Essentially, guiding lights are cues that are easy to use and remember and also flexible enough for adaptation in different contexts. Each guiding light describes which contexts combined with which mechanisms result in which outcomes. There are specific intermediate outcomes for the individual guiding lights but in combination they give rise to a number of ultimate outcomes.

The leader journey started by gathering stories and observing practice. With the best of intentions the protective and directive stance of charge nurses had created dependency among staff and service users missed continuity, coordination

Table 15.1 The four guiding lights for recognising and developing an effective workplace culture that is also a good place to work

Guiding light	Descriptor	Intermediate outcomes	Ultimate outcomes
1. **Collective leadership**	In contexts (with formal opportunities) that support and develop visible, authentic, credible, relational and collective leadership. Leaders are able to: • role model trust and confidence in each other, mutual respect, collaboration and participation • engage in and foster dialogue • balance needs with skills • respectfully and constructively challenge each other • focus on staff health and wellbeing • build on quick wins towards sustainable change.	Staff: • feel valued, respected, listened to and heard • have a sense of mutual/shared understanding • are empowered to speak out and lead.	
2. **Living shared values**	In contexts where the following is fundamental to the way things are done: • compassionate care • positivity • learning • teamwork (interprofessional) and • celebrating change for good. Caring teams: • co-construct shared values with patients, service users, communities and staff at all levels • regularly revisit values to create collective goals • build person-centred relationships • live their values authentically by 'doing what they say they will do' • set the mood for what good workplace cultures look and feel like.	Staff: • feel valued and supported • have a voice • are empowered • enjoy being at work • have a sense of belonging and connectedness. Patients, relatives and others sense: • enthusiastic staff • a warm, authentic, caring atmosphere • an environment that is clean, tidy and welcoming.	• Strong, high-performing teams. • Staff retention and low sickness rates. • Staff flourish, blossom and grow their potential. • Quality care: person- and relationship- centred, safe and effective. • Sustained positive, improving workplace cultures which are not dependent on specific individuals. • Building effective partnership within and across settings.

3. **Safe, critical, creative, learning environments**	In contexts where: • practice is caring, safe and effective • mutual learning relationships value openness, difference, curiosity and creativity • there are space and structures to stop, think, reflect, share ideas and plan together as a team. People: • feel respected, free from fear to question and explore • feel supported and enabled to take risks • exchange knowledge and actively notice and learn from what is working well • are courageous and self-aware.	Staff: • build on what works well • focus on solutions, not blame. Service users experience an environment that: • is safe (clean and tidy) • values their feedback about what works and what can be improved.	
4. **Change for good that makes a difference**	In contexts that focus on: • what matters to people (staff, patients and service users) and change for good • having a collective purpose • external influences • navigating complexity. Staff are able to: • care for patients, service users and each other with compassion • actively seek feedback from different groups • use positivity to enable innovation, feel energised and know that they can make a difference both individually and collectively • work with different sources of knowledge to generate evidence both from and in practice.	• Staff experience 'joy' in their work and are energised for development, innovation and changes for good. • Staff spread what works. • There is effective service delivery with ongoing, sustained improvement and innovation.	

and person-centredness. Transformation manifested when the leadership team worked with staff to review and change the nursing system, and leaders critically and creatively reflected on the leadership they aspired to and practised. The transformations ensured that they were still visible and credible but also more relationship orientated and authentic as they discovered how to achieve what they themselves found most rewarding: enabling others to come into their own (Cardiff 2014).

These changes were a developmental process, inviting and encouraging participation and collaboration. The appointment of two primary nurses required respectful and constructive challenging of traditional views on how things should be done. The primary nurses joined the charge nurses on a journey of exploring the meaning and enactment of person-centredness in daily care and leadership. Role modelling person-centredness was not limited to care relationships. Attending to peer relationships enhanced reciprocal understanding, respect and support. A more collective culture emerged and leader stories demonstrated growing collaboration and inquiry within the team, with less immediate resistance to proposed changes. Staff reported a better atmosphere on the unit, continuity and coordination of care and student mentoring. While bed occupancy, turnover and complexity of care remained unchanged, the unit was more tranquil as more people began to take the lead in solving issues and/or working in collaboration. New staff also contrasted how leadership was enacted, compared with what they were accustomed to elsewhere. They expressed feeling of equal value to everyone else within the team (including the hierarchical leaders), free to offer their talents and skills at appropriate times, and able to share how they would like to grow and develop. Initial staff reservations that their scope of nursing practice would be restricted proved to be unfounded. This was attributed to how the primary and charge nurses exercised clinical leadership, negotiating how to work together in ways that were healthful for themselves, those they worked with and service users.

Collective leadership could conjure images of ideological democracy with everyone involved in all decisions, or self-directed teams, and be criticised as unrealistic or unobtainable, particularly in the current healthcare climate. Since the success of Buurtzorg in The Netherlands, an approach that 'starts from the client perspective and works outwards to assemble solutions that bring independence and improved quality of life' (https://www.buurtzorg.com/about-us/buurtzorgmodel/), the 'implementation' of self-directing/organising teams has been widespread, particularly in community and long-term care organisations. However, problems have arisen when little attention is paid to the cultural changes needed for successful implementation. PD theory and research teach us the importance of working collaboratively to create shared visions/purposes before moving on to participatory processes to planning, acting, observing and reflecting on changes. Such processes are characteristic of collective leadership (Friedrich et al. 2009), becoming a dynamic, emergent and interactive process of influence based on core values such as person-centredness. Strong internal relationships are required to ensure team members experience mutual support and feel valued, respected and heard (Carson et al. 2007; Akhtar et al. 2016). At the same time, in workplaces where people and contexts are dynamic, Carson et al. (2007) state that (hierarchical) leadership external to the team should be responsive: active and high when support is needed and present (rather than active) but observant when the team is leading itself effectively. This was observed in the action research study described above.

Guiding light 2 Living shared values

This guiding light is illustrated through blogs written by Deb Smith (2019) and Joanne Mohammed (2019) during their involvement in a year-long development programme for clinical nurse leaders. Their stories reflect the need for shared values in the workplace and the requirement for these values to be realised in practice, reaffirming two of the five attributes of an effective workplace culture as identified by Manley et al. (2011). They also demonstrate the potential outcomes.

Key learning for both leaders was the acknowledged need to work in different ways. As a consequence, they began to have different conversations with their team, asking: 'What is it like to work here? How are things done around here? What values do you hold as part of a team and about care?' They used one-to-one and small-group discussions, stimulated by picture cards, creative activities and questionnaires. These methods helped staff to think about what is important to them and the people they care for. Developing an awareness of the values, beliefs and assumptions that staff hold and how they impact on the care is one of the fundamental methods associated with PD as a methodology for transforming individuals and cultures of care (McCormack et al. 2013) and is key to the delivery of person-centred practice (McCormack and McCance 2017).

The stories reflect how the leaders enabled individuals to consider their values, then use a collective approach to co-construct shared values and ultimately collective goals and actions. West and Dawson (2012) argue that this is key for effective teamworking. Deb's team used a values clarification exercise (Warfield and Manley 1990) to facilitate individual contributions towards the creation of a shared purpose, recognising the need to create a safe space (see guiding light 3) to enable staff to have a voice. Joanne used picture cards to help staff to explore what is important to them and acknowledged the benefit of the team 'really listening to each other'. Working in this way ensures that all voices are heard and valued, in line with a key principle of PD, 'collaboration, inclusion and participation' (McCormack et al. 2013). These examples reflect staff engagement, which West (2018) contends is an important predictor of outcomes across health and social care. While these stories primarily focus on working with values at a team level, the guiding light suggests that this process should involve patients, service users, communities and staff, working together from the bottom up and the top down, to facilitate support and 'buy-in' at all levels.

Joanne's story shows how creating a shared vision provides purpose and meaning for teams, motivating them around agreed actions (Martin et al. 2014). She used 'claims, concerns and issues' (Guba and Lincoln 1989) to enable staff to identify the key issues facing them and to develop appropriate action plans. This helped them to concentrate 'on what [they] were going to do on a daily basis to ensure that [they] provided the best care [they] could for... patients whilst respecting each other as valued members of a team' (Mohammed 2019). Deb shared how her team worked explicitly with values on a daily basis. At handover, with 'word' cards as prompts, staff identified how they wanted to work together during the shift. Team members referred to these words during the day, should they want to draw attention to what was shared and expected, ensuring that there was congruence between what is said and what is done, i.e. living shared values. Reflecting on the vision can help teams to identify any gaps between the vision and the reality of practice. However, as Deb describes: 'Putting yourself and your team under a microscope and really hearing your staff can lead to uncomfortable self-reflection but also amazing unseen development opportunities for staff' (Smith 2019).

The stories provide examples of both the intermediate and ultimate outcomes, arising from the change in the 'way things were done'. Staff reported that they felt valued and that their voice had been heard. They identified areas for improvement and led on developing and implementing action plans. Staff offered support and challenge to each other and celebrated success. Joanne reports how this has impacted team performance. She started from a point where staff morale was low and inspections identified that care was not at the required standard. This has all changed – care has improved, and staff reported that they feel positive and enjoy coming to work. As highlighted in the guiding light, continuous reflection on the values and goals is needed to ensure that teams are 'doing what they say they will do' (Manley et al. 2011) and that they remain inclusive of the perspective of those both giving and receiving care.

Guiding light 3 Safe, critical, creative, learning environments

The achievement of guiding light 3 relies on the leadership and facilitation skills needed to build cultures through embedding values about learning, safety and being person-centred. This enables psychological safety, which facilitates collaborative critique – the prerequisites for creativity and innovation. Teams that reflect this guiding light demonstrate evidence across four characteristics, illustrated by data from the Safety Culture, Quality Improvement, Realist Evaluation (SCQIRE) project (Manley et al. 2017). This project set out to identify strategies that embed a safety culture in ten frontline teams across four large acute hospital providers in South-East England and led to refinements in culture change theory at the micro-systems level (Manley et al. 2019a).

Teams that actively develop a culture of psychological safety for staff show equal value both to being person-centred and to holistic safety. This relies on developing relationships and patterns of behaviours that create safe spaces to talk about expectations:

> *'In my role I need to develop relationships with staff which enables me to challenge behaviours. . . this has an impact and makes a difference to both staff and patients'.* (Emotional Touchpoints with Team Facilitator)

The impact of creating psychological safety, the ability to speak up and be courageous, is illustrated below:

> *'The pharmacy technician reviews medication interaction and highlights to senior doctor the two drugs prescribed by Dr should not be given together. Dr responded, "thank you for pointing this out", demonstrating respectful exchange'.* (Observations of practice)

Other observations in the project showed a similar relationship between being person-centred and safety:

> *'The Dr on the ward round praises the registered nurse for detecting the deteriorating condition in the patient which meant that patient needed to be transferred elsewhere.'* (Observations of practice)

Similarly, the impact on patients and families was also observed:

> *'Patient looks unkempt, he needs to take some medication and requests bottle water as can't take tap water which the team gracefully accommodate without making a judgement – nurse comes back with bottled water for the patient from his own supplies.'* (Observations of practice)

Teams with a learning culture support everyone to learn from each other, using the workplace as a key resource for learning, developing and improving, building appreciatively on what works. This was illustrated in a team where contributions were mutually respected and the ability to speak up courageously for the patient was observed:

> *'The team sharing and listening to each other, jointly making decisions regarding how to take things forward. The occupational therapist states the patient has "really been trying and he needs our support now" in response to the team who are not sure how to use the finite resources available to them.'* (Observations of practice)

Communication and information systems support learning and enable everyone to know what is happening. This was evidenced in the use of safety huddles across different teams. Safety huddles were identified as particularly powerful when enabling frontline teams to feel valued and empowered to focus on safety issues in real time. When well led and implemented, through transformative and collective leadership, huddles help to identify what works, find solutions collectively and learn how to improve practice for the benefit of staff and patient wellbeing.

> *'Each team member was given the opportunity to speak up in urgent care. They remind each other of the current waiting time, talk about concerns, reference patients, confirm doctors' roster so know who is available, and maintain notes. . . They work together to resolve issues. Creating solutions as a team, exploring problems from all sides.'* (Observations of practice)

Teams collectively review different sources of evidence to evaluate team function and culture with regards to whether this is safe, caring, effective and evidence informed. The PD methods used within the SCQIRE project included qualitative 360-degree analysis (RCN 2007b); emotional touchpoints with patients, service users, staff and students – focusing on what matters (Dewar et al. 2009); collaborative observations of practice teams (RCN 2007a); and claims, concerns and issues (Guba and Lincoln 1989). Three of the four hospital sites were unfamiliar with the methods used and reviewed this evidence collectively with staff. Subsequently these methods were continued, complementing key quality and safety performance processes and indicators. Drawing on a range of evidence sources and using a collective review approach with team members, focusing on what matters to those providing and experiencing care, is a key feature when providing evidence related to this guiding light.

Teams foster creative, innovative and solution-focused approaches through nurturing curiosity and trying out new ideas in the workplace, enabling staff to be creative and innovative. Psychological safety helps teams to challenge the status quo and experiment with different ideas. Kessel et al. (2012) demonstrate that a high level of team psychological safety, mediated by sharing information and know-how, is a significant predictor of creative team performance.

Guiding light 4 Change for good that makes a difference

Within the world of PD, culture and context are intrinsically linked. Transforming care environments requires skill, understanding (McCormack et al. 2013), expertise (Hardy et al. 2009) and evidence-based care that directly links research to practice (Williamson et al. 2012). Grappling with the complexity of day-to-day practice, competing priorities and constant pressures, while forging strong and sustainable, collaborative person-centred relationships, requires skill, understanding and a true belief that change can make a difference, across all points of care (giving, receiving and experiencing).

In many cases complexity is taken for granted, as it is the real world of practice. Practice can be uncertain and unpredictable; the 'tectonic' plates of organisational change and leadership can suddenly move, leaving what was certain less so. Despite this, practitioners dive into this uncertainty, knowing that transformational change that is centred on enabling the development of person-centred relationships and change for good will make a difference.

The following reflective conversation with 'Sue' aims to illustrate what 'change for good that makes a difference' looked like in her role as a senior nurse involved in commissioning a leadership development programme for care home managers:

'There were many complex drivers that were multifaceted which needed skilled understanding and navigation stretching across a large health and care system. Having worked with the care home sector for a number of years I knew how important "leadership" was to enable practice development and transformation. I was keen to focus on supporting care home managers by developing this programme as I knew how important their role is in

leading and setting standards of care. I also recognised how isolating their role could be and that care homes were central to delivering many of our strategic priorities from a health and care perspective.

What were the drivers for improvement?

Working with, supporting and enabling care homes to develop quality was important, fundamentally making a difference to care through supporting them to develop practice, which was recognised, celebrated, valued and made a positive difference to people experiencing care and staff working as part of their teams. Balanced against this was the need to work with and deliver agreed key performance indicators related to contractual performance and activity. Previously I had led an appreciative inquiry, which showed a direct correlation between 'good' nursing leadership in care homes and the quality of care delivered. I was keen to optimise this learning by working collaboratively across the health and care system.

What were the outcomes?

In evaluating outcomes, participants expressed increased confidence in their professional skills, they identified improvement in the quality of engagement with their staff and reported improved quality of interaction between staff and residents. The design of the programme facilitated a strong sense of ongoing, continuous sustained improvement that was being led by the care homes.

By learning together through reflection, peer support and access to education specialists, the participating care home managers were able to collectively develop and grow their leadership potential. Embedding learning in practice was key; this was achieved through workplace programmes of development, which were owned and led by the participating care homes.

The outcomes from the programme were really positive and the learning immensely "rich" in building sustainable relationships along with practice and service transformation across the health and care system.

What did you learn?

I knew the system in which care homes function was complex, with many different drivers and requirements, but I hadn't necessarily realised how complex and what this really felt and looked like through the lens of a care home. What I started to see and understand was that at times what is measured from a quality assurance and contract management perspective does not always capture the multidimensional elements that enable us to better understand quality of care. It struck me also that we all see care homes "differently" depending on where we stand. Working with and not "doing to" the care home sector is really important – care homes must be equal partners in system transformation and development.

What would you do differently in the future?

Although we worked with care home managers to shape the programme, stronger involvement at the outset in co-design and development would have helped strengthen the value of working together. Understanding early on the world through the lens of care homes and their drivers from a quality perspective would have helped lay a stronger foundation to build upon.'

In this reflective conversation, Sue captured many of the elements that appear in guiding light 4. Organisations and systems are not homogeneous as there can be many different micro-cultures. 'Bottom-up' transformation supported and enabled by collaborative approaches is crucial as they have a far greater likelihood of being owned, lived and sustained. This enables authentic change and transformation for good that makes a difference for services and cultures of care within and across systems (Manley and Jackson 2020).

Conclusion

Delivering health and social care services across different settings is complex, multifaceted and constantly changing and evolving. The culture in which care is experienced by all at the point of contact is fundamental to the development of person-centred relationships. Within this complexity, organisations and practitioners are required to navigate multiple needs, interests and demands, both external and internal (Hannah 2014). At the start of this chapter we defined culture, drawing from the work of Drennan (1992, p. 9), as 'how things are done around here'. In its most simplistic form that is the case; however, we know that making sense of workplace culture in the world of practice and ever-changing organisations is complex – at its best a 'calmness'; at its most it is challenging, 'stormy' and unpredictable. We also highlighted numerous reports that have brought to the fore significant failings in care, all identifying the need for cultural change and learning.

Understanding and making sense of a workplace culture, what it feels and looks like, is critical to enabling care and systems to grow, thrive and transform. The guiding lights developed as part of our collaborative inquiry build upon our previous work (Manley et al. 2011) and the subsequent theory of culture change and transformation (Manley et al. 2019a). The guiding lights – collective leadership, living shared values, safe, critical, creative, learning environments and change for good that makes a difference – are interwoven and interdependent. In combination they enable strong teams to flourish in delivering quality care, ultimately enabling effective workplace cultures to grow and thrive, creating 'good places to work'.

Inspired by Tweet 113, November 2019, generated during the collaborative inquiry, we suggest that '. . . a constant presence of the rule [guiding lights] will anchor us in the storms' that form a familiar part of our health and social care systems:

'The Storm rages around me,
I stay anchored,
The turbulence, tosses and throws me,
I stay anchored,

I taste the salt on my lips,
I stay anchored,
The wind bellows in my ears,
I stay anchored,
I'm pulled and thrown in different directions,
I stay anchored,
My senses are assailed,
I stay anchored,
Darkness fades and I see light,
The calm after the Storm has arrived.'
(*Source:* Jonathan Webster)

References

Akhtar, M., Casha, J., Ronder, J. et al. (2016). Transforming the NHS through transforming ourselves. *International Practice Development Journal* 6 (2). https://doi.org/10.19043/ipdj.62.005.

Best, A., Greenhalgh, T., Lewis, S. et al. (2012). Large-system transformation in health care: a realist review. *The Milbank Quarterly* 90 (3): 421–456.

Cardiff, S. (2014). Person-centred Leadership: A Critical Participatory Action Research Study Exploring and Developing a New Style of (Clinical) Nurse Leadership. PhD thesis. Ulster University.

Cardiff, S., Sanders, K., Webster, J. et al. (2020). Guiding lights for effective workplace cultures that are also good places to work. *International Practice Development Journal.* https://doi.org/10.19043/ipdj.102.002

Carson, J., Tesluk, P. and Marrone, J. (2007). Shared leadership in teams: an investigation of antecedent conditions and performance. *Academy of Management Journal* 50 (5): 1217–1234.

Dewar, B., Mackay, R., Smith, S. et al. (2009). Use of emotional touchpoints as a method of tapping into the experience of receiving compassionate care in a hospital setting. *Journal of Research in Nursing* 15 (1): 29–41.

Drennan, D. (1992). *Transforming Company Culture.* London: McGraw-Hill.

Francis, R. (2013). *Report of the Mid Staffordshire NHS Foundation Trust Public Inquiry.* London: HMSO.

Friedrich, T., Vessey, W., Schuelke, M. et al. (2009). A framework for understanding collective leadership: the selective utilization of leader and team expertise within networks. *The Leadership Quarterly* 20 (6): 933–958.

Guba, E.G. and Lincoln, Y.S. (1989). *Fourth Generation Evaluation.* Newbury Park, CA: Sage.

Hannah, M. (2014). *Humanising Healthcare: Patterns of Hope for a System under Strain.* Axminster: Triarchy Press.

Hardy, S., Titchen, A., McCormack, B. et al. (2009). *Revealing Nursing Expertise Through Practitioner Inquiry.* Chichester: Wiley-Blackwell.

Kessel, M., Kratzer, J. and Schultz, C. (2012). Psychological safety, knowledge sharing and creative performance in healthcare teams. *Creativity and Innovation Management* 21 (2): 147–157.

Kirkup, B. (2018). *Report of the Liverpool Community Health Independent Review*. London: NHS.

Manley, K. and Jackson, C. (2020). The Venus model for integrating practitioner-led workforce transformation and complex change across the health care system. *Journal of Evaluation in Clinical Practice – International Journal of Public Health Policy and Health Services Research* 26 (2): 622–634.

Manley, K., Jackson, C. and McKenzie C. (2019a). Microsystems culture change – a refined theory for developing person-centred, safe and effective workplaces based on strategies that embed a safety culture. *International Practice Development Journal* 9 (2). https://doi.org/10.19043/ipdj.92.004

Manley, K., Dewar, B., Jackson, C. et al. (2019b). *Strengthening Nurse, Midwifery and Allied Health Professional Leadership*. Final Report March 2019. London: Burdett Trust.

Manley, K., Jackson, C., McKenzie, C. et al. (2017). *Safety Culture, Quality Improvement, Realist Evaluation (SCQIRE). Evaluating the impact of the Patient Safety Collaborative Initiative developed by Kent Surrey and Sussex Academic Health Science Network (KSSAHSN) on Safety Culture, Leadership and Quality Improvement Capability*. ISBN 978-1-909067-79-0 (accessed 20 April 2020).

Manley, K., Sanders, K., Cardiff, S. et al. (2011). Effective workplace culture: the attributes, enabling factors and consequences of a new concept. *International Practice Development Journal* 1 (2): Art 1.

Mannion, R. and Davies, H. (2018). Understanding organisational culture for healthcare quality improvement. *British Medical Journal* 363 (k907). https://doi.org/10.1136/bmj.k4907

Martin, J., McCormack, B., Fitzsimons, D. et al. (2014). The importance of inspiring a shared vision. *International Practice Development Journal*. https://www.fons.org/Resources/Documents/Journal/Vol4No2/IPDJ_0402_04.pdf (accessed 19 March 2020).

McCormack, B. and McCance, T. (2017) *Person-centred Practice in Nursing and Healthcare: Theory and Practice*. Chichester: Wiley-Blackwell.

McCormack, B., Manley, K. and Titchen, A. (2013). *Practice Development in Nursing and Healthcare, 2nd Edition*. Chichester: Wiley-Blackwell.

Mohammed, J. (2019). Changing how i work as a ward manager. https://www.fons.org/common-room/blogs?year=2019&month=7#blg5340 (accessed 20 April 2020).

Patterson, M. (2011). *From Metrics to Meaning: Culture Change and Quality of Acute Hospital Care for Older People*. London: HMSO.

Plsek, P. (no date). Structures, processes and patterns: key to understanding and transforming. http://www.directedcreativity.com/pages/PatternsOnePage.pdf (accessed 19 March 2020).

Royal College of Nursing (RCN). (2007a). RCN and Cambridge University Hospitals observations of practice research protocol. *RCN Workplace Resources for Practice Development*. London: RCN.

Royal College of Nursing (RCN). (2007b). RCN and Cambridge University Hospitals Qualitative 360 Degree Feedback Research Protocol. *RCN Workplace Resources for Practice Development*. London: RCN.

Schein, E.H. (1990). Organizational culture. *American Psychologist* 45: 109–119.

Smith, D. (2019). Providing a safe space for people to grow and develop. https://www.fons.org/common-room/blogs?year=2019&month=9#blg5382 (accessed 20 April 2020).

Warfield, C. and Manley, K. (1990). Developing a new philosophy in the NDU. *Nursing Standard* 4 (41): 27–30.

West, M. (2018). How teams improve staff engagement and why it matters. https://www.youtube.com/watch?v=Gmw7EsfUfNg (accessed 20 January 2020).

West, M. and Dawson, J. (2012). *Employee engagement and NHS performance*. London: The King's Fund. https://www.kingsfund.org.uk/sites/default/files/employee-engagement-nhs-performance-west-dawson-leadership-review2012-paper.pdf (accessed 20 January 2020).

Williamson, G., Bellman, L. and Webster, J. (2012). *Action Research in Nursing and Healthcare*. London: Sage Publications.

16. *Wellbeing at Work*

Tristi Brownett, Valerie Wilson, and Alera Bowden

Introduction

Staff wellbeing is an indicator of a flourishing workplace culture that impacts on staff commitment, resilience and retention, and in healthcare it results in an experience of quality, person-centred care (Maben et al. 2012). This chapter examines staff wellbeing in the context of workplaces with links to practice development (PD) concepts. The chapter will discuss what wellbeing is, and why it is important in health and social care workplaces and wider work environments. Two case studies are presented showing how PD as an approach strives to develop person-centred workplaces that enable workplace wellbeing to flourish. The chapter concludes with key insights drawn from the case studies, summarising how workplaces can support staff wellbeing, enabling staff teams and their care recipients to benefit fully from the potential that staff have to offer.

What is wellbeing?

Our understanding of wellbeing is influenced by our beliefs and experience. Ultimately, our own experience is about whether we feel we are floundering or flourishing, sometimes referred to as feeling good and functioning well

International Practice Development in Health and Social Care, Second Edition.
Edited by Kim Manley, Valerie Wilson, and Christine Øye.

(Keyes and Annas 2009). Wellbeing is a concept that is studied within many different professional and academic disciplines; for example, researchers focus on the physical or psychological and medical sociology concepts (de Chavez et al. 2005), or community and social aspects (Wiseman and Brasher 2008). It is studied extensively because it is well recognised that well-being influences the perception of good health and affects mood and behaviours (Steptoe et al. 2015).

The ancient Greeks utilised terms describing wellbeing, still used today: 'hedonic' and 'eudaimonic' wellbeing. Hedonic wellbeing is likened to the pursuit of happiness and gratification; eudaimonic wellbeing recognises that wellbeing extends beyond happiness, connecting to a perception of inner peace, life well lived and the consequent satisfaction derived (Phillip 2010). Taking the eudaimonic view recognises the value of communal life and connects to a sense of life fulfilled, leading to states of flourishing and growth (Ryff and Singer 2006). Flourishing is critical to the state of wellbeing; it contributes a sense of having personal meaning, purpose and active engagement in all aspects of life (Ryan and Deci 2001).

Flourishing

PD aspires to human flourishing as an outcome of person-centred transformative work (Dewing and McCormack 2017). The art of person-centred PD is recognising both the uniqueness and agency of the person(s) that the practice developer works with, supporting what Aristole might have regarded as the actualisation of human potential. Critically, the conditions for flourishing must be created for the experience and action that accompany it (Titchen et al. 2011). Flourishing therefore is not passive, transporting a person beyond their usual norm or boundary. The opportunity for moral dilemma here must be recognised; in supporting others to flourish, recognition of their autonomy, beliefs and values is essential along with the importance of authenticity, mutuality, co-creation and safety within the space (Titchen et al. 2011).

Utilising an 'asset-based' approach, where the competencies and strengths of the workforce are recognised and drawn upon, supports and creates opportunities for staff to flourish. Person-centred practice therefore nurtures pre-existing or embryonic skillsets rather than focusing on deficits to both acknowledge and enable competencies and experiences learned from life (Gaffney 2012).

Embracing how we develop workplaces that enable people to flourish is central to the achievement of workplace wellbeing. Flourishing may in some respects be a clearer concept than wellbeing to define and to experience. However, as outlined later, in the course of our practice we came to understand that the culture and language used in the workplace is one where 'wellbeing' is the term that is used universally. Many large global and national organisations have wellbeing high on their business agenda, where often the word wellbeing is used with a varied number of meanings.

Why wellbeing matters at work

Wellbeing matters because it impacts our quality of life and our physical health (Diner and Chan 2011). Wellbeing at work matters, as the places where we work influence health and wellbeing, having long been recognised to provide income, networks, social and psychological support (Waddell and Burton 2006). To benefit from employment, a person's work should be 'good work', where the individual is not harmed by workplace activities and has a say in how the work is done, ultimately resulting in a sense of self-worth (Waddell and Burton 2006, pp. vii–ix).[1]

A range of interrelated social factors influences individual thought and behaviour at work. Workplace culture influences these factors. Workplace culture is often implicit, underpinned by the collective beliefs and actions within teams, manifested in collective behaviours and values (Braithwaite et al. 2017). In short, culture can be described as 'the way we all do things here' (Balogun and Hailey 2004, p. 50).

Workplace culture combines other factors such as a perceived ability to fulfil role tasks affecting subjective wellbeing (Health and Safety Executive 2000). Attention to wellbeing through practices that support workers is vital; this support includes learning and development opportunities, feedback to improve motivation and excellent communication (Ogbonnaya and Daniels 2017). As the case studies below will show, safe and effective cultures contribute to flourishing workplaces.

The case studies highlight two very different workplaces and approaches to wellbeing at work. The first, a healthcare setting in Australia, illustrates responses to staff survey results that identified that staff felt stressed. The second, an English manufacturing workplace, focuses on a desire to catalyse change for wellbeing. These case studies have been chosen to highlight diverse approaches to addressing the challenge of achieving wellbeing in workplaces.

Case study 1 IMAGINE – a wellbeing programme for healthcare staff

The catalyst of the 'IMAGINE' study began with a conversation. This conversation was a feedback session run by the Bulli hospital leadership team exploring staff survey results about workplace experiences and practices. Bulli Hospital is a 52-bed sub-acute aged-care hospital within the Illawarra Shoalhaven Local Health District (ISLHD). Bulli staff expressed that they were stressed and wanted an initiative that helped with their wellbeing. This ignited the creative ideas of the then director of nursing (DON), who on seeing a sign in a local homewares store titled 'IMAGINE', took this as a literal sign of imagining a future workplace culture of happy and engaged staff.

---

[1] Internationally, 'good work' is comparable to 'decent work' (International Labour Organization 2015) and Sustainable Development Goal 8 (United Nations Development Programme 2015).

A multidisciplinary working party of hospital staff (nurses, allied health and support services) was formed to help co-design IMAGINE. From these discussions the idea for 'Wellness Wednesdays' emerged, a programme designed by staff for staff. The CIP (collaborative, inclusive, participative) PD principle was used in the development and suitability of this programme. Other staff were invited to participate in the working party, including those with PD, research and wellbeing expertise from the ISLHD and the University of Wollongong (UOW). Together they worked to provide guidance on the programme structure, measurements of success and potential funding sources to support the programme launch.

A review of the wellbeing literature provided programme insights and supported taking an empirical approach to the implementation and evaluation of the programme. This enabled the successful application for funding of the IMAGINE pilot research study, through the New South Wales (NSW) Ministry of Health. The working party then transitioned into a research advisory group to oversee the study. Ethical approval was successful and a part-time programme coordinator was recruited to assist with the implementation and evaluation of the study.

Using the initial programme ideas as a starting point, the research advisory group worked in partnership with staff to develop an eight-week 'Wellness Wednesdays' programme, designed to deliver a one-hour weekly session on a Wednesday afternoon during staff shift crossover time. This day and time were thought to be the most conducive to releasing staff to attend and ensured easy access for all participants. All sessions were built on the foundations of mindfulness and meditation activities, while each weekly session introduced a different theme. Sessions were facilitated by research advisory group members with no specific expertise in the topic (see Table 16.1) and for the final two weeks participants decided the topics.

Table 16.1 (C = core, E = elective)

	Focus for each week (all sessions included meditation and mindfulness)
1 C	Developing personal portraits – staff were able to connect with each other on a personal level, sharing common interests
2 C	Gratitude – this was the opportunity to share what staff valued and what they were grateful of on a daily basis
3 C	Yoga – delivered by a local company, this session was designed to be inclusive of all fitness types, from chair-based gentle exercises to more advanced yoga poses
4 C	Understanding triggers – in this thought-provoking session, staff explored how they were triggered by different aspects of home and work life
5 E	Reflexology and hand massage – staff were guided by the facilitator in a practical session on basic massage techniques, exploring the benefits of this type of relaxation
6 E	Identifying strengths – this was a self-exploration session on staff strengths
7 E	Mindful walking (outdoors, e.g. at the local beach)
8 E	Nutrition

Staff members were recruited to the programme via 'expressions of interest' and word of mouth from the original working party staff. The beauty of staff promoting a programme for staff meant there were plenty of volunteers and the programme slots were filled quickly. In 2018, the pilot study commenced. Two programmes ran back to back over 16 weeks. Staff members involved in the programme were given a welcome pack (Figure 16.1) in their first weekly session.

It was hoped that the programme objectives would result in staff reporting an increased sense of wellbeing and job satisfaction, and a decrease in stress levels and intention to quit their job. These were measured through surveys collected prior to the first session and at programme completion. Additionally, participants completed a weekly session evaluation using anonymous sticky notes to identify what they liked best and to suggest changes and takeaway learnings.

Collated responses influenced changes within the current and in future programmes. Participants were also invited to participate in post-programme focus

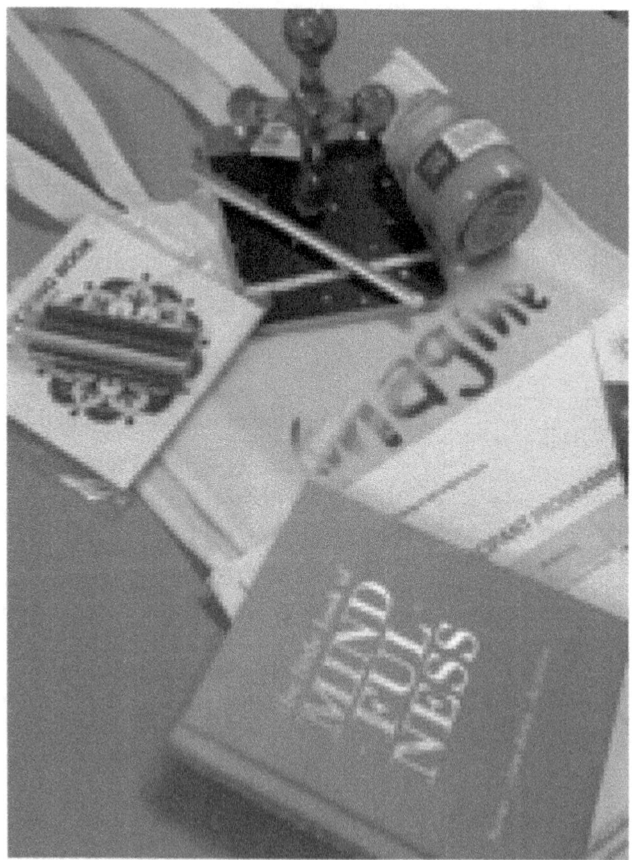

Figure 16.1 IMAGINE welcome pack

groups to share their overall thoughts, impressions of meeting objectives and recommendations for the future.

The programme was well received and feedback was overwhelmingly positive (see Figure 16.2). Participants expressed gratitude for a programme designed specifically for their wellbeing and for the opportunity to interact with their colleagues on a personal level. The practical sessions were engaging, and participants easily applied learnt techniques for work and home life. One participant shared her experiences of how using programme techniques helped to reduce her blood pressure and relaxed her energetic son. Overall, pilot study results demonstrated positive trends in the data and a strong sense of human flourishing, but a greater number of participants were needed to establish statistical significance. The research advisory group shared the results and were able to secure further funding to expand the study across other hospitals in the district.

To build sustainability, interested staff were invited to register to be trained as programme facilitators. Eighteen multidisciplinary staff attended a one-day train-the-trainer day prior to establishing the programme in their hospital. Facilitators were given a pack that included individual session outlines and resources to successfully roll out the programme.

All eight ISLHD hospitals and community services hosted at least one programme, with 232 staff attendees and 27 programmes completed over the study timeframe. Programmes were reduced to six one-hour weekly sessions and included four core sessions from the original programme and four elective sessions from which each group chose two (see Table 16.1). Participants included nursing, midwifery, allied health, management and support services.

Programme data was collected using surveys and statistical tests showed that the programme met its objectives. Staff workplace engagement (increased 6.11%), workplace wellbeing (increased 5.6%) and job satisfaction (increased 4.12%) all significantly improved following the IMAGINE programme (Almeida et al. 2020). Three main themes emerged from the focus group data (see Figure 16.3). Staff had looked forward to the programme, it was 'a bit of brightness' in their week, they actioned what they had learnt for themselves with what they described as a 'wellbeing toolkit'. They also paid this forward, sharing with other staff, 'we do a little two-minute meditation before we get into meetings', and at home – one participant outlined she 'shared the breathing [techniques] with my husband'. It was easy to see from this data that staff who participated flourished and were able to share their learning and wellbeing strategies with other people in their work team and at home.

Dissemination and sustainability

The outcomes of the IMAGINE programme have been shared at local, state, national and international levels. The programme is being introduced to other NSW health services and interstate.

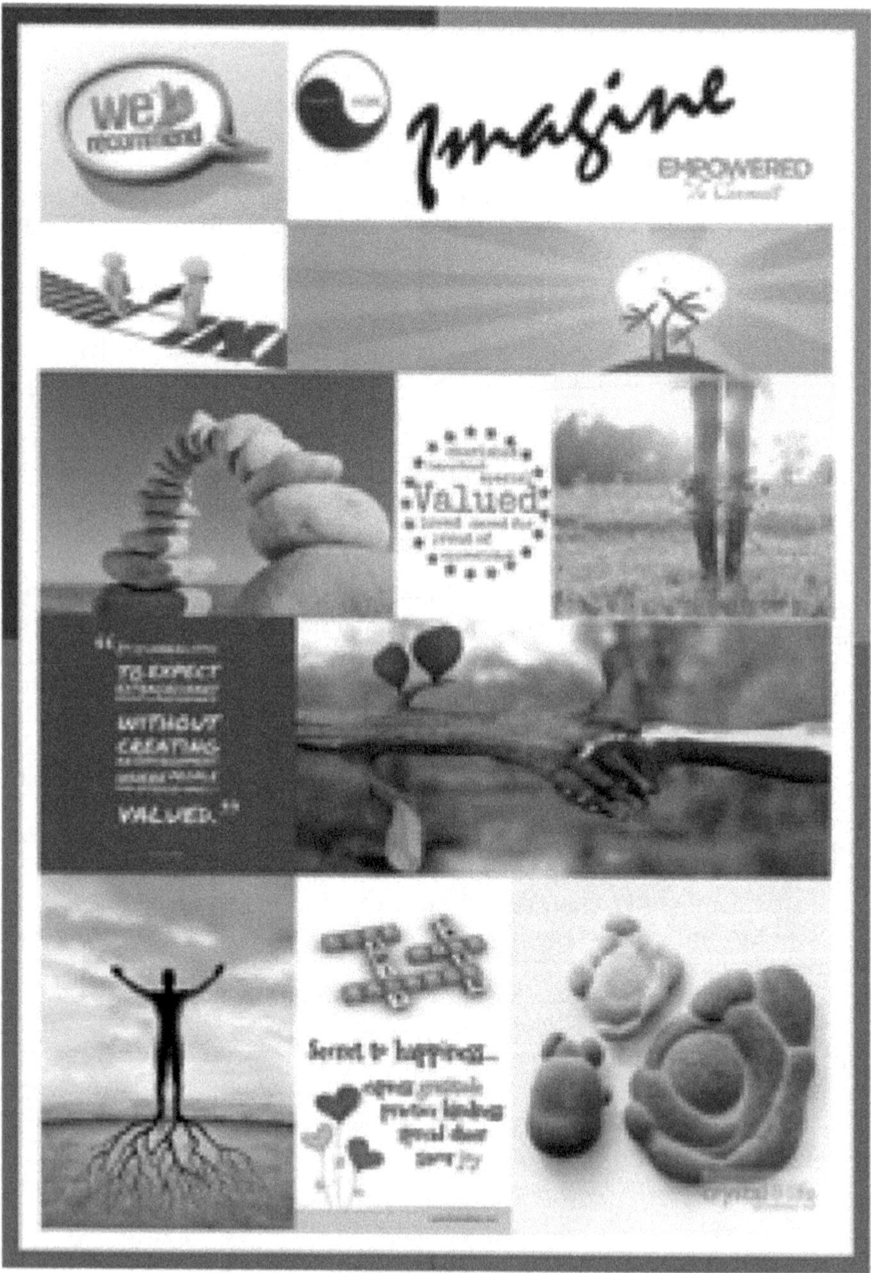

Figure 16.2 Themes from the IMAGINE pilot study

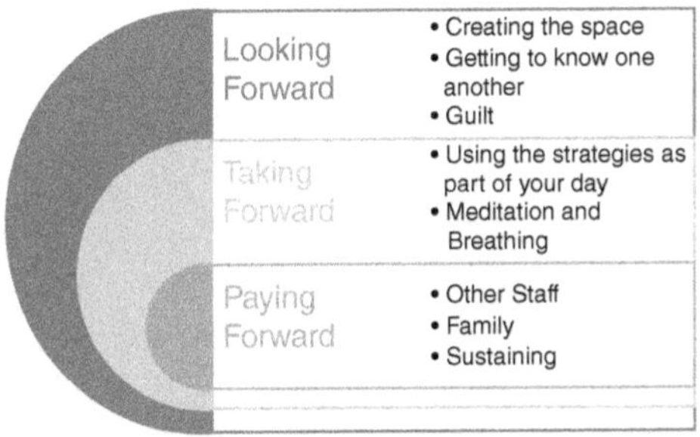

Figure 16.3 Themes from the IMAGINE study

At a local level, programme components continue across various hospitals adapted to fit with local contexts and competing demands. For example, the IMAGINE programme was used in a wellbeing programme (SEED) at Milton-Ulladulla Hospital, developed in response to the bushfire tragedy (2019/20920) which resulted in a number of staff losing their homes and all staff being impacted in some way. Bulli Hospital continues with a Wellness Wednesdays session once a month using the various sessions developed from IMAGINE. The Bulli Hospital DON shared her personal experience:

> *'I recalled a little note that I had received which read, "Thank you for taking the time to come onto the wards, even though you have a demanding job. We appreciate your warm smile. Thank you." I recall the absolute lift this gave me. I know others had been receiving these messages as well and it was making a difference to their day. It struck me how kind and compassionate this was as there was no expectation from the giver that they would be recognised or thanked for what they were doing – it was just perfect kindness acting from perfect kindness. It is truly amazing the ripple effect that the IMAGINE programme has had on our staff.'* (Orinda Jones, Director of Nursing, Bulli Hospital)

The IMAGINE wellbeing programme has been a success not only in the outcomes achieved but also in the way staff have been engaged in the process throughout, including such aspects as using a collaborative, inclusive and participative approach, co-design model and supporting facilitator development to lead the programme across all hospitals (three key PD principles – see Chapter 8). We believe that the programme will have ongoing success within our organisation and beyond.[2]

The second, very different, case study offers an overview of a wellbeing programme run within the food industry that sought to change workplace culture to create a place that was safe, supportive and nurtured wellbeing.

---

[2] *We would like to acknowledge the work, dedication and commitment of the IMAGINE research team, the facilitators of the programme and all the staff who attended the programme.*

Case study 2 A better place

Salco, a company in the South-East of England, produces fresh supermarket products. Its 700 regular staff represent 26 countries; many speak more than one language but almost half speak little or no English. The director of human resources (HR) wanted employees to feel that Salco was 'a great place to work' and this would be evident by the way that people greeted each other in the corridors. However, other members of the senior management team indicated clearer measures, such as a reduction in the annual turnover of staff leaving the business and reduced absenteeism. Conversations with senior managers revealed they interpreted wellbeing in very different ways, from an absence of stress in their own lives to a place of flourishing for others.

A pilot survey revealed that wellbeing was not directly translatable in some languages. Four statements were subsequently identified as common lay beliefs about wellbeing that were most relatable:

- a contented state of being happy, healthy and prosperous
- physical fitness
- something different to health
- in the workplace it is how we 'work better together'.

The survey results showed that each statement was equally valued by respondents. The survey helped to identify what mattered to staff (Box 16.1) and subsequently informed the three-year strategy (Box 16.2).

A high number of the workforce engaged in the survey, more so than in any other previous survey. Follow-up conversations revealed that the translated survey enabled participation, signalling the importance of everyone's opinions for the first time. Communication and the recognition of need for the spirit of true partnership were championed. Management agreed that for wellbeing to be

Box 16.1 What mattered to staff

- Enhanced communication opportunities
- Access to education
- Health-promoting initiatives and advice
- Improved career prospects
- Consistency in management practice

Box 16.2 Overview of the strategy

- Supporting our people in poor health and preventing future ill health
- Promoting good health and wellbeing through attention to work organisation, good work and access to services
- Taking challenges and making them opportunities
- Finding innovative ways to involve and value our staff

achieved, it was necessary that voices were not only heard and understood but respected; employees were to be recognised as trusted partners and leadership should be collective.

Key moments on the journey

- It is not possible here to discuss the 30 or so integrated initiatives that comprised the strategy; we have therefore focused on elements that demonstrate how key moments on the journey to workplace wellbeing mapped against core features of PD (Box 16.3).

Launching the Wellbeing Strategy

The organisation committed to the strategy and the occupational health and HR team championed 'A better place to work'. A small allocated budget allowed a dedicated day to showcase the bespoke strategy and the core wellbeing initiatives to staff.

In a spirit of participation and inclusion, all staff were given prolonged breaks to spend time outside participating in a festival-type event where they could sign up for the initiatives, such as motor-cycle maintenance, personal development courses, English and maths lessons (Skills for Life programme), Middle Managers Academy for career development, or take time out to relax and socialise with friends and colleagues. The launch also provided competitive events, a climbing wall, free drinks, food and an ice-cream van to build social connections and foster a sense of a caring environment.

Recognising the person and celebrating their achievements

Conversations on the launch day led to development of additional activities such as the celebration tea, where staff could nominate themselves or others in their team for going the extra mile or contributing to another's sense of wellbeing.

Box 16.3 Linking the wellbeing strategy to the features of practice development

- Collaboration, participation and inclusion
- Facilitation, enable and empower
- Knowing what matters
- Celebrating people and their achievements
- Collective leadership
- Living our values
- Creation of a safe, critical and caring environment
- Change for the good Adapted from Manley 2017 (pp. 133-137)

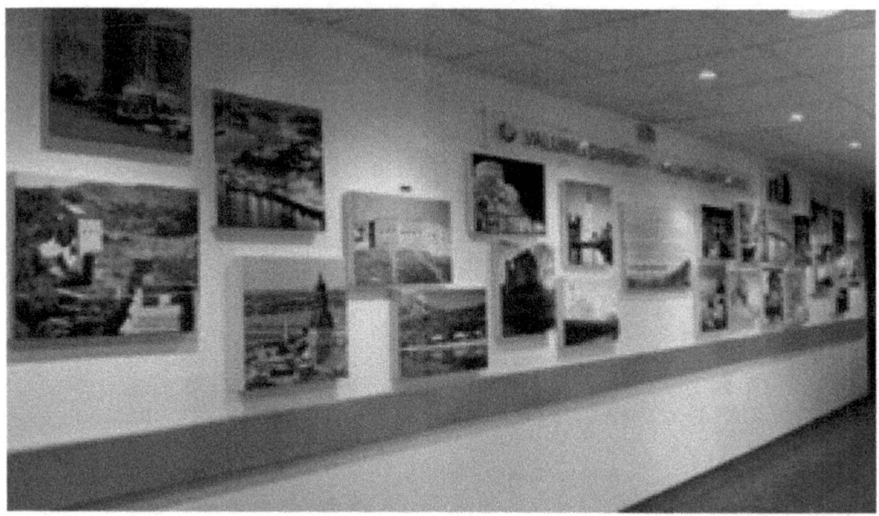

Figure 16.4 The diversity wall

The celebration tea occurred once each month, with celebrants receiving recognition from their manager of their contribution.

Another small but significant activity born out of those conversations was the development of the diversity wall. This was led by HR placing high-quality prints of key landmarks from the employees' own nations at the staff entrance, en route to changing and rest areas (Figure 16.4). The observed reaction was instant, with staff crowding around the images and talking to others about 'home'. One Iranian staff member fell to his knees and held his hand to his heart, pointing to an image, telling us that this was his home. He was very emotional and keen to share stories of his childhood caught up in conflict. He later became a site translator and was proactive in supporting other staff members to participate in 'better place' activities.

Knowing what matters

The survey had revealed that staff wanted access to drinking water throughout the shift other than at break time. The challenge in meeting this basic human need was that as a food-producing company, eating and drinking at the food production workstations were prohibited. However, facilitated conversations between factory staff, engineers and the quality team resulted in an acceptable solution.

Likewise, staff revealed that footwear provided for work was not comfortable and choice was desired. The purchasing manager, in conjunction with occupational health, arranged for self-nominated teams from different production areas to trial a footwear range that met food production standards. This ultimately resulted in employees having choice about workplace footwear. Though these actions were small steps, they helped to build trust by focusing on what mattered to staff.

Enhanced communication opportunities

Language and communication became a powerful theme of the wellbeing strategy. A communication zone was created, incorporating a charter of commitment signed by the senior team and unions. Furthermore, to aid conversations, site translator roles were implemented, along with written briefings and opportunities being offered in a range of languages. The facilitation of communication enabled and empowered staff through 'monthly conversations' in an active commitment to the co-creation of staff wellbeing and the building of cultural transformation.

Access to education

When it became apparent that many of the workforce had low levels of literacy and numeracy, the Skills for Life programme for English speakers was provided collaboratively with a local further education provider and funded by government grant. The voluntary programme offered opportunities for employees to study during work time. The impact was observed through increasing numbers signing up for classes and experienced in casual conversations with employees. Evaluation captured personal benefit:

> *'The maths lessons have helped me a lot at home, I can use what I have learnt when I go shopping and to help pay bills. I am always at my lessons early and if more lessons were available, I would attend them. Today I took an exam and passed.'*
>
> *'Skills for Life is helping me every day at work and private life. It will help me in the future.'*

Living our values

A critical moment early in the programme came when an advisory clinic provided by a local migrant charity had been under way for two hours. The waiting queue was still long and an indigenous employee demanded to know why the migrant staff were being given opportunities that the rest of the staff were not. It was clear that communications about the strategy were not yet right but that some employees now felt able to openly express their needs. An employee assistance programme, which provided confidential advice, counselling and health information, was implemented and received well by staff, evidenced in high utilisation rates across the first year.

The management team undertook both emotional intelligence and mental health first aid training. These programmes were deemed important in ensuring a safe, critical and caring environment and supported open, tolerant conversations about behaviours and absence.

A review at 18 months revealed that while more than half of the workforce were aware of the wellbeing programme, they did not necessarily comprehend that all activities (e.g. provision of water) were aimed at improving subjective wellbeing. Respondents agreed there were opportunities to participate but did not always choose to do so. This was accounted for by a lack of personal relevance, lack of social and psychological availability to commit, or low confidence. However, most employees surveyed agreed that as a result of changes they perceived an increased sense of wellbeing.

The positive relationship between staff wellbeing and organisational benefits was evidenced by the 50% reduction in staff turnover and winning an unexpected award from the local job centre for being considered an employer of choice for the region. Salco was given a prestigious award from the supermarket that it supplied, recognising sustainable practices with ethical commitment to employees; on this alone, the company viewed the wellbeing strategy as a success.

Key insights

As highlighted, wellbeing has nuanced meanings and interpretations. At a corporate level, wellbeing is seen as a policy and series of initiatives or activities linked to adherence to legislation and the reduction of insurance premiums; or a moral obligation under corporate social responsibility activities; or a way to improve productivity and reduce overhead costs (Day and Penney 2017) in an environment where the business, its reputation and its employees thrive.

At the time of writing, the COVID-19 pandemic is reorganising how people work, and in healthcare particularly, employees are being affected by exposure to rapid change, trauma and infection on a scale rarely witnessed (Kisely et al. 2020). Employee wellbeing initiatives matter now more than ever before.

However, prior to the pandemic, employees demanded employers give attention to their wellbeing. In the UK, a generational divide was reported where those under the age of 25 were more likely to demand health and wellbeing benefits (Webber 2018) and particularly attention to their financial and social wellbeing (McQuaid 2019), compared with those over the age of 55. European research (Eurofound 2017) investigating working conditions identified that workplaces recognising and actively addressing needs such as work–life balance for carers and middle-aged workers, and concern for development and learning in older workers, were better able to meet wellbeing needs.

Employees' sense of wellbeing is influenced by a range of issues, and workplace factors such as organisational climate and social support can inhibit or enhance perception of coping, resilience and wellbeing (Lunt et al. 2007). Chari et al. (2018) identified around 150 constructs associated with workplace wellbeing in a review of the literature and reduced them to five themes encompassing the physical environment, policies and culture, the subjective experience of work, and external factors influencing the experience, such as health status and homelife. Their study concluded: 'Defining, promoting, and evaluating worker wellbeing is a complex undertaking requiring partnerships and commitments across not just employers but individuals and communities as well' (Chari et al. 2018, p. 593).

The literature suggests that person-centred practice rather than a generalised approach is more likely to meet the wellbeing needs of employees. Our case studies endorse this, with the insight that improving a sense of wellbeing can be achieved by knowing what matters to workplace communities and collaboratively engaging them in the co-design of change for the collective good.

Workplaces that actively promote learning and development opportunities have been found to have higher worker wellbeing. People who keep learning have satisfaction, optimism, report higher wellbeing and less stress, with a sense of achievement for reaching self-defined targets (Dolan and Fujiwara 2012). Brazilian philosopher Paulo Friere might have argued that this form of education is critical in the empowerment and transformation of the individual, especially where that education is co-constructed in a space that fosters meaningful participation (Magee and Pherali 2019). Likewise, philosopher and social theorist Jurgen Habermas argued that the co-created process of learning provides an opportunity for the learner to authentically come to know self, through critical engagement and reflection (Lovatt 2013). This is particularly important where, as shown in first case study, facilitated self-reflection and learning contribute to the focus of becoming more person-centred (Kinsella 2017). Facilitative leadership inspires and enables others to utilise the workplace as a participatory resource for learning (Akhtar et al. 2016) and self-reflection.

Conclusion

This chapter has outlined the importance of wellbeing within organisations. It illustrated two very different case studies, further demonstrating some founding principles. Practice was embedded as both person- and place-centred, acknowledging the needs and culture of the individual and setting as unique, recognising that culture and having cultural sensitivity are central to working with others.

Having been invited as outsiders into the organisations, working within the culture of those organisations was critical to the successful creation of wellbeing. The case studies highlight the importance of critical evaluations to integrate evidence to inform practice, as well as know what was achieved. The approach to the evidence was blended with conversations and activities to know what matters to workplace communities, leading to co-produced outcomes. Those workplaces were transformed through this co-production and reflexivity, personal voice and choice, and through different styles of learning. A culture that was trusting and safe transformed the workplaces. Employees' meaningful experiences translated beyond their working day into their home lives, and into the lives of others.

References

Akhtar, M., Casha, J., Ronder, J. et al. (2016). Leading the health service into the future: transforming the NHS through transforming ourselves. *International Practice Development Journal* 6 (2): 1–21.

Almeida, S., Bowden, A., Bloomfield, J. et al. (2020). Caring for the carers in a public health district: a case study of a wellbeing initiative to support healthcare professionals. *Journal of Clinical Nursing*. https://doi.org/10.1111/jocn.15398

Balogun, J. and Hailey, V. (2004). *Exploring Strategic Change*. London: Prentice Hall.

Braithwaite, J., Herkes, J., Ludlow, K. et al. (2017). Association between organisational and workplace cultures, and patient outcomes: systematic review. *BMJ Open* 7: e017708. https://doi.org/10.1136/bmjopen-2017-017708

Chari, R., Chia-Chia, C., Sauter, S. et al. (2018). Expanding the paradigm of occupational safety and health: a new framework for worker well-being. *Journal of Occupational and Environmental Medicine* 60 (7): 589–593.

de Chavez, A.C., Backett-Milburn, K., Parry, O. et al. (2005). Understanding and researching wellbeing: its usage in different disciplines and potential for health research and health promotion. *Health Education Journal* 64 (1): 70–87.

Day, A. and Penney, S.A. (2017). Essential elements of organizational initiatives to improve workplace wellbeing. In: *The Routledge Companion to Wellbeing at Work* (eds. C.L. Cooper and M.P. Leiter), 314–331. Abingdon: Routledge.

Dewing, J. and McCormack, B. (2017). Creating flourishing workplaces. In: *Person-centred Practice in Nursing and Healthcare: Theory and Practice* (eds. B. McCormack and T. McCance), 150–161. Chichester: Wiley Blackwell.

Diner, E. and Chan, D.Y. (2011). Happy people live longer: subjective well-being contributes to health and longevity. *Applied Psychology, Health and Wellbeing* 3 (1): 1–43.

Dolan, P. and Fujiwara, D. (2012). Valuing Adult Learning: Comparing Wellbeing Valuation to Contingent Valuation. Department for Business, Innovation and Skills. BIS Research Paper Number 85. London: Crown. www.gov.uk/government/publications/valuing-adult-learning-comparing-wellbeing-valuation-and-contingent-valuation (accessed 30 June 2020).

Eurofound. (2017). *Working conditions of workers of different ages: European Working Conditions Survey 2015*. Luxembourg: Publications Office of the European Union. https://www.eurofound.europa.eu/sites/default/files/ef_publication/field_ef_document/ef1747en.pdf (accessed 30 June 2020).

Gaffney, M. (2012). *Flourishing: How to Achieve a Deeper Sense of Well-being, Meaning and Purpose – Even When Facing Adversity*. London: Penguin.

Health and Safety Executive (2000). What are the Management Standards? www.hse.gov.uk/stress/standards/ (accessed 30 June 2020).

International Labour Organization (2015). Decent work. www.ilo.org/global/topics/decent-work/lang--en/index.htm (accessed 30 June 2020).

Keyes, C.L.M. and Annas, J. (2009). Feeling good and functioning well: distinctive concepts in ancient philosophy and contemporary science. *The Journal of Positive Psychology* 4 (3):197–201.

Kinsella, N. (2017). A journey through the use of critical creative reflection to explore self in a PhD study. *International Practice Development Journal* 7 (2): 1–15.

Kisely, S., Warren, N., McMahon, L. et al. (2020). Occurrence, prevention, and management of the psychological effects of emerging virus outbreaks on healthcare workers: rapid review and meta-analysis. *BMJ* 369: m1642. https://doi.org/10.1136/bmj.m1642

Lovatt, T. (2013). Jurgen Habermas: education's reluctant hero. In: *Social Theory and Education Research: Understanding Foucault, Habermas, Bourdieu and Derrida* (ed. M. Murphy), 69–83. Abingdon: Routledge.

Lunt, J., Fox, D., Bowen, J. et al. (2007). Applying the biopsychosocial approach to managing risks of contemporary occupational health conditions: scoping review. HSL/2007/24. www.hse.gov.uk/research/hsl_pdf/2007/hsl0724.pdf (accessed 30 June 2020).

Maben, J., Adams, M., Peccei, R. et al. (2012). 'Poppets and parcels': the links between staff experience of work and acutely ill older people's experience of hospital care. *International Journal of Older People Nursing* 7: 83–94.

Magee, A. and Pherali, T. (2019). Paulo Freire and critical consciousness in conflict-affected contexts. *Education and Conflict Review* 2: 44–48. https://discovery.ucl.ac.uk/id/eprint/10081479/ (accessed 22 October 2020).

Manley, K. (2017). An overview of practice development. In: *Person-centred Practice in Nursing and Healthcare: Theory and Practice* (eds. B. McCormack and T. McCance), 133–137. Chichester: Wiley Blackwell.

McQuaid, D. (2019). UK employees see social wellbeing as a top priority. *HR Review* September2019.www.hrreview.co.uk/hr-news/uk-employees-see-social-wellbeing-as-top-form-of-support-they-can-recieve/120654 (accessed 30 June 2020).

Ogbonnaya, C. and Daniels, K. (2017). Good work, wellbeing and changes in performance outcomes: illustrating the effects of good people management practices with an analysis of the National Health Service. What works centre for wellbeing. www.whatworkswellbeing.org/wp-content/uploads/2020/01/Good-people-management-NHS-Dec2018.pdf (accessed 30 June 2020).

Phillip, R. (2010). Guest editorial: making sense of wellbeing. *Perspectives in Public Health* 130 (2): 58.

Ryan, R.M. and Deci, E.L. (2001). On happiness and human potentials: a review of research on hedonic and eudaimonic well-being. *Annual Review of Psychology* 52: 141–166.

Ryff, C.D. and Singer, B.H. (2006). Know thyself and become what you are: a eudaimonic approach to psychological well-being. Journal of Happiness Studies*: An Interdisciplinary Forum on Subjective Well-Being* 9 (1): 13–39.

Steptoe, A., Deaton, A. and Stone, A.A. (2015). Subjective wellbeing, health and ageing. *The Lancet* 385 (9968): 640–648.

Titchen, A., McCormack, B., Wilson, V. et al. (2011). Human flourishing through body, creative imagination and reflection. *International Practice Development Journal* 1 (1): 1-1–1-18.

United Nations Development Programme. (2015). Sustainable Development Goals. www.undp.org/content/undp/en/home/sustainable-development-goals.html (accessed 30 June 2020).

Waddell, G. and Burton, K. (2006). *Is Work Good for Your Health and Wellbeing?* London: The Stationery Office.

Webber, A. (2018). Younger staff want employers to put more emphasis on health and wellbeing. *Occupational Health and Wellbeing*. www.personneltoday.com/hr/employers-more-emphasis-on-younger-workers-wellbeing (accessed 30 June 2020).

Wiseman, J. and Brasher, K. (2008). Community wellbeing in an unwell world: trends, challenges, and possibilities. *Journal of Public Health Policy* 29 (3): 353–366.

17. *Flourishing People, Families and Communities*

Carolyn Jackson, Valerie Wilson, Tanya McCance, and Albara Alomari

This chapter focuses on the principles and methods practice developers can use in a range of different contexts to facilitate people, families and communities to become more involved in the planning, design, governance and delivery of health and social care services. First, it explores the concept of human flourishing and its relationship to wellbeing. Drawing on principles of community engagement and community development it highlights the key enablers and attributes required when working with citizens and communities and integrates these with core principles of practice development (PD). In the final part of the chapter, two case studies demonstrate how participatory research methods can help to shape services that meet family and community needs at local and international levels to promote community flourishing.

What is community flourishing?

In healthcare, practice developers argue that human flourishing is a powerful indicator and outcome of an effective workplace culture (McCormack and Titchen 2006; Titchen and McCormack 2010), one that integrates and achieves person-centredness, patient safety and effectiveness to enable all to flourish. The focus is on enabling supportive, helpful relationships based on mutual trust and understanding that empower others to grow and develop, as well as sharing collective knowledge (McCormack and Titchen 2006).

International Practice Development in Health and Social Care, Second Edition.
Edited by Kim Manley, Valerie Wilson, and Christine Øye.

> *'Human flourishing focuses on maximising individuals' achievement of their potential for growth and development as they change the circumstances and relations of their lives at individual, group, community and societal levels. People are helped to flourish (i.e. grow, develop, thrive) during the change experience in addition to an intended outcome of wellbeing for the beneficiaries of the work.'* (Heron and Reason 1997 in Titchen et al. 2011, p. 1)

More broadly, positive psychologists identify flourishing as a *construct* which refers to the experience of a life going well and represents a combination of *feeling good* and *functioning effectively* (Huppert and So 2013). Attributes include living within an optimal range of human functioning (Fredrickson and Losada 2005), presence of mental health, and high levels of emotional, psychological and social wellbeing (Keyes 2015). Flourishing has also been described as a *state* that requires a combination of *hedonic*[1] and *eudaimonic*[2] facets of wellbeing (Huppert and So 2013; Keyes 2002). Four dominant models of flourishing exist (Keyes 2002; Huppert 2009; Diener et al. 2010; Seligman 2012), which include characteristics of positive relationships, engagement and meaning. Keyes' (2002) model has a strong focus on social wellbeing and characteristics of positive emotion, autonomy and personal growth, while Huppert's (2009) model focuses on individual traits such as vitality, resilience, competence, optimism and emotional stability, as well as positive emotion. Seligman's (2011) Theory of Wellbeing notes five elements of a flourishing state, explained by the PERMA acronym:

- **P**ositive emotion and happiness elicited by feelings of pleasure such as warmth, comfort or pleasure.
- **E**ngagement, the act of being interested and involved in an activity or circumstances.
- Positive **R**elationships – mutually beneficial and regular exchanges among individuals.
- **M**eaning in life attained by finding belonging within communities and serving something bigger than the self (Seligman and Royzman 2003).
- **A**ccomplishment – actively realising one's values and acting upon them (Raibley 2012).

It is clear from these definitions that the concept of wellbeing is central to human flourishing. Coburn and Gormally (2015, p. 252) have identified seven elements of wellbeing that help individuals and communities to flourish (Table 17.1).

Seligman (2002) recognises the need for social relationships as they contribute to a larger sense of purpose and accomplishment. The neighbourhood community is one form of social environment that has demonstrated profound effects on individual wellbeing and happiness (McMillan 2011). Community is not only a social structure, it also holds a psychosocial influence on individuals that live,

---

[1] Positive emotional states, e.g. happiness and vitality.

[2] Positive functioning, e.g. purpose in life, competence and social connections.

Table 17.1 Seven elements of wellbeing (Coburn and Gormally 2015, p. 252)

Positive examples of which include:	Identified elements of well-being	Negative examples of which include:
Feeling good, high spirits, balanced, positive state of mind, lack of stress.	**Feeling good**	Feeling bad or in low spirits, unbalanced, negative state of mind, stressed and anxious
Happiness, smiling, contentment, social harmony, sunshine, love, light, weather.	**Social and emotional aspects**	Being unhappy, unsmiling, discontented, social discord, dull, grey, hate, bad weather
Friends, family, colleagues, community, caring, support, inclusion	**Relationships with others**	Lack of friends, no close or regular family connection, absence of community, uncaring, no support, exclusion
Healthy body, good health, service provision (fitness and health)	**Being physically well**	Illness, poor health, lack of service provision
Financial, personal safety, being comfortable, feeling warm and secure.	**Being safe and secure**	Poverty, feeling unsafe or uncomfortable, feeling cold and insecure
Being valued, self-worth, confidence, dignity, being respected	**Achieving self-esteem**	Not valued, low self-worth, lacking confidence, indignity, disrespect
Quality of life, continual journey to improvement, needs being met, a thriving environment.	**Achieving potential**	Poor ideas on quality of life, apathy and lack of fulfilment, needs unmet, giving up, a depressing environment

work and participate in it (Hustedde 2008) and may be impacted by perceptions of individual wellbeing and happiness (Block 2008). Community is also built through *placemaking,* that is the connection observed between happiness, wellbeing and sense of community (Ellery et al. 2017).

> *'[Places] shape the way we live our lives, feel about ourselves and the relationships we have with others. Moreover, places – not least because of their history, character and physical form – contribute significantly to personal and societal wellbeing. [. . .] Most of us have immense affection for the places where we live: they might be places where we grew up, live or work now; where we have family and other relationships; and places are full of memories, stories and our lived experiences.'* (British Academy for the Humanities and Social Sciences 2017, pp. 1–2)

Fulfilling a sense of community (SoC), Seligman (2012) argues, may be a critical extension that is necessary for true flourishing. Sense of community is a term that describes the social connections, mutual concerns and values that exist within a community and the places we live (Perkins et al. 2002), and a feeling that members have of belonging, that members matter to one another and to the group, and a shared faith that members' needs will be met through their commitment to be together (cited in McMillan 2011). Acknowledging how important a sense of community and belonging is to community wellbeing, the next section explores the value of community engagement and development approaches, linking these with PD principles.

Facilitating community engagement and development using practice development principles

There is a wide variety of person- and community-centred approaches to enable people to flourish in the workplace or in the communities in which they live, but they are united by a common purpose. Community development as an approach to change has a set of core values and principles. It promotes social inclusion through an active process of people participation or active citizenship. Since most forms of exclusion are based on lack of power and influence, which are paternalistic or oppressive, participative approaches help communities to learn how power relationships operate and impact, and to develop the opportunity to deal with their problems.

> *'Active citizenship is not based on the idea of do-gooding or benevolent philanthropy but ideas of mutuality and reciprocity which are the "glue" that binds people together and underpins the very idea of society.'* (Scottish Community Development Centre 2019)

Empowering people and communities to be at the heart of health and wellbeing focusing on what is important to them, capturing their opinions and ideas to facilitate the commissioning of better services is much more preferable to 'unlocking the practical skills and capacities of people who receive services' (NESTA 2012, p. 5). Most importantly when working with communities it is about people and their potential, not the problems they have or the challenges they experience; they are the solution (Sanders et al. 2015). Being able to understand that everyone has talents, strengths and passions, and that they have the right to be heard and a contribution to make, is essential. For these things to be realised, people need safe places free from judgement and pressure, where their confidence and self-esteem can grow and supportive relationships can flourish. These trusting reciprocal relationships must be enabled to develop on people's own terms, with local people setting the agenda and determining the pace at which they engage and how they engage. Arguably, local people exercising this choice and control enables people to become part of community life rather than part of a prescriptive project or intervention. In this kind of environment, local people from different backgrounds with a range of experiences and challenges in their lives can engage with one another, develop trust, understanding and empathy, learn how to deal with problems and take preventative action through collaboration. In turn, people participation in public affairs achieves not only best practice and effectiveness of public services but a better understanding of needs and issues, clarity of understanding in terms of who benefits from and who is excluded from services, and a better way of targeting scarce resources. It can also lead to more innovative ways of meeting community needs in partnership, to develop, administer and benefit the operation of services.

While community development work is an organic process, there are some important PD principles that underpin community engagement and development work:

i. Taking a *values and voice-based approach* (NESTA 2012) as an effective way of capturing the voice of patients, consumers, carers and the wider community (Sanders et al. 2015).
ii. *Working collaboratively* using person-centred, collaborative, inclusive and participative ways of working (CIP principles) with all key stakeholders tapping into the voice-based assets of the community which help to keep true to the voice of local people and staff (National Voices 2013). Working in this way requires authentic engagement from the start to bring everyone together and has multiple components, is ongoing and multifaceted, and is reflective of the needs of both individuals and communities (Sanders et al. 2015).
iii. *Learning about the community*, creating psychologically safe spaces free from judgement that are open to all and engage the most vulnerable, making explicit *core values* and *ways of working in a shared governance model.*
iv. *Being evidence based* by building on the insights and intelligence gathered from the community, research with patient participation groups or local community interest groups to inform discussions (Sanders et al. 2015).
v. *Being continuous and iterative* by engaging in cycles of refinement of collaborative work and member sense checking work to validate the principles and emerging themes and issues that impact on the communities and citizens involved (Sanders et al. 2015).

In summary, these enablers, attributes and principles can be conveyed along a continuum of citizen and community flourishing shown in Figure 17.1.

Empowering citizens and communities to flourish through participatory research methods

> *'Transformational research is qualitative research that promotes transformation as both end and means of research. So, in addition to knowledge creation, there is a concern with transformation of ourselves as researchers and, if they so wish, transformation of co-researchers, participants and other stakeholders . . . [T]ransformational research can lead to human flourishing, in creative, spiritual and ethical senses, of both recipients of the research and those undertaking it.'* (Titchen and Armstrong 2007, p. 151).

Practice developers are in a unique position to develop flourishing communities by focusing on what matters most to citizens. A transformative research paradigm

CORE VALUES
Equality and anti-discrimination
Social justice and human rights
Collective action
Collective empowerment
Working and learning together

CITIZEN FLOURISHING IN WORKPLACES — Focused on citizens' individual and collective experiences

FLOURISHING IN COMMUNITIES — Focused on community needs and aspirations

ATTRIBUTES
Using participatory methods to maximise engagement
Groups working collaboratively to co-create strategies and solutions
Drawing on best available evidence
Focusing on people's strengths, skills and abilities
Being systematic using methods that are robust
Collaborative Activities that are continuous and iterative
Reflective learning and peer review

Figure 17.1 Continuum of community flourishing

(Mertens 2007) seeks to change the roles that citizens have traditionally held in research so that previously marginalised citizens can have a voice in shaping health and social care services to meet their needs. Examples of research approaches that enable community empowerment include appreciative inquiry, which begins with a respect for all voices, drawing on the principles of co-design, working locally and engaging in iterative cycles of appreciative inquiry and participative collection action. Realist evaluation methodology is also useful in understanding which community engagement initiatives are effective in improving communities' health outcomes and the sustainability of healthcare systems. This section presents two case studies to illustrate what strategies work best to involve families and communities in research that promotes improved outcomes for consumers.

Case study 1 Family involvement in practice improvement through action research in a hospital setting (Alomari et al. 2017)

This study demonstrates a powerful critical approach to practice improvement by involving parents as advocates for their children in medication management in a hospital setting. The study addressed the importance of family-centred care, the centrality of the role of families in care delivery, and patient and carer involvement in safety. The researchers identified a real and urgent need to develop strategies and processes that engage families, enable collaboration, foster openness, and create a supportive space for critical thinking and reflection, in order to reduce the risks associated with medication administration for vulnerable children. The central intent of the project was to promote the active engagement of families and nurses in the medication management of pre-school-age children with complex health needs, during and after hospitalisation, to:

1. Identify the barriers and facilitators to safe medication practice.
2. Develop targeted interventions supporting family involvement in the medication safety agenda.
3. Implement and evaluate targeted interventions to improve medication safety.

Action research (AR) was chosen to enable the facilitation of practice improvement in a particular setting and the active involvement of families in the research. AR is a democratic process, aimed at both taking action and creating knowledge or theory about the action. Initial findings indicated that while parents had limited insight into medication administration practices, they felt both a strong sense of advocacy and responsibility for their child and 'expertise' that as parents they knew best how to care for their child, including how to manage medicines. Parents identified that they wanted to be more involved in developing a shared plan of care for their child and a need to be more involved in medication administration at the bedside. They felt this would improve medication safety and promote more opportunity for interaction between parents and staff.

This led to the nurses and families working together to develop four targeted interventions that were implemented and evaluated:

1. Four mobile medication administration trolleys with computers visible to parents at the bedside during medication rounds.
2. Additional questions regarding parental involvement in the medication admissions form. This aimed to increase parent engagement at the bedside.
3. Nurse-led quality and safety monthly meetings.
4. Updated organisational medication policy to place more emphasis on engaging families and patients in the medication process.

The interventions enabled nurses to work collaboratively with families more actively in the medication process and to establish a positive relationship that improved the safety of medication administration, resulting in a reduction of medication administration errors by 54.7%. The inclusiveness and active engagement of nurses and families in the research resulted in raised awareness of medication practices (rituals and routines) that might impact on care. The families and nurses were supported to look at the issues through engagement and learning through participation in action research and this enabled them to become more self-aware (enlightened). The research approach therefore was influential in helping both families and nurses to learn how to engage others and how to work with what matters to people. The nurses became empowered to engage families to improve practice, believing that change could occur after reflecting on their existing practice culture. With support from the action research team, nurses and families were free to act and lead (emancipated), to implement and evaluate the effectiveness of the interventions they developed.

The study provides compelling evidence of dynamic collaboration and the creation of an enabling culture for the families and nurses to enable everyone to flourish. This study took an innovative approach by engaging families as researchers in the whole research process – from reviewing already collected data to implementing changes in practice. AR can reach an intersubjective agreement between researcher, families and nurses, a mutual understanding of a situation, consensus about the action plan, and a sense of what people achieve when they do so together. The engagement in this study gave the families an opportunity to learn and understand more about the barriers and facilitators of their medication practice. Using a mixed methods approach to collect the data provided the researcher and the nurses with a comprehensive picture of the medication practice situation. The action research team were able to reflect on the findings, which increased their awareness of the taken-for-granted assumptions they had about practice and about the importance of improving the medication process on their ward (enlightenment).

Case study 2 Enabling flourishing of people in healthcare settings through measurable indicators – an international collaborative community of research practice (McCance et al. 2020)

The focus of this international collaborative community is on improving the care experience for key beneficiaries, including patients, their families and staff, across different clinical specialties, spanning the United Kingdom, Europe and Australia. Data pertaining to the patient experience forms a key part of developing effective workplace cultures in healthcare. In determining a positive patient experience, greater emphasis has been placed on quantifiable indicators. Case study 2 is a programme of research led by Ulster University that showcases outcomes focusing on developing nursing practice and improvements to support healthcare communities to flourish through implementing eight person-centred key performance indicators (KPIs). The underpinning research comprises: (i) the original study, which engaged nurses, midwives and consumers and led to the identification of the KPIs that were appropriate and relevant for nursing and midwifery practice and an accompanying measurement framework (McCance et al. 2012); and (ii) a series of implementation studies (see Table 17.2) that tested the KPIs in a range of clinical settings across the UK, Europe and Australia (McCance and Wilson 2015; McCance et al. 2020).

These eight indicators are considered novel in that they (i) do not conform to the majority of other nursing metrics generally reported in the literature; (ii) are strategically aligned to work on the patient experience; and (iii) measure person-centred practice, as evidenced by their alignment to the Person-centred Nursing Framework (McCormack and McCance 2019) illustrated in Figure 17.2.

Development and implementation of a suite of measurement tools to evidence the person-centred KPIs was conducted with nursing staff and senior nursing executives across three participating organisations involving nine practice settings across the United Kingdom and the Republic of Ireland (McCance et al. 2015). The findings revealed the high value placed on the evidence generated from the implementation of the KPIs as reflected in the following themes: measuring what matters; evidencing the patient experience; engaging staff; a focus for improving practice; and articulating and demonstrating the positive contribution of nursing and midwifery. The implementation of the KPIs and the measurement tools was effective in generating evidence of the patient experience, privileging the patient voice, and offering feedback to nurses and midwives to inform the development of person-centred cultures and support improvements that enable patients and staff to flourish.

Table 17.2 KPI studies

1	*Paediatric International Nursing Study (PINS)* Involved acute paediatric inpatients from 12 organisations.	Northern Ireland, England, Ireland, Denmark and Australia
2	*Implementing and **M**easuring **P**erson-centredness using an **APP** for **K**nowledge **T**ransfer (**iMPAKT**)* The development and feasibility testing of a technological solution to facilitate the collection of data described in the measurement framework.	Northern Ireland and Australia
3	*Use of person-centred nursing KPIs in supporting nurses to lead on the development of person-centred practice in a community context.* A collaborative implementation study using the KPIs in community nursing.	Northern Ireland and Scotland
4	*Co-producing and Implementing Person-centredness in Cancer Nursing (CIP-CAN).* Explore the impact of a co-produced implementation project using the person-centred nursing KPIs to support the development of person-centred care across ambulatory chemotherapy units.	Northern Ireland

1) The Paediatric International Nursing Study saw the KPIs implemented across services provided to sick children. It involved specialist children's hospitals and paediatric wards in general acute care hospitals in Australia (six sites across three states) and Europe (six sites across four countries), totalling 12 organisations (McCance and Wilson 2015). A driving force in this work was to provide consumer data directly to nursing staff, which they could then use to enhance care. Evidence generated across all the participating sites revealed that this process created positivity, assisted staff in identifying ways in which they could support active engagement of families in care, and improved staff morale. The data generated clearly showed that the KPIs provided useful consumer-driven information for nursing staff in terms of what needed to be considered to improve the care experience: 'The KPIs were very specific and it was very easy to pinpoint to what you needed to improve.' One nurse discussing the biggest success of PINS in her ward indicated: 'I think ours has been the consumer – allowing the parents more of an input, and it has also alleviated some of their distress and concerns that they get. Quite a lot of our kids come in for a minimum of two weeks, so at least. . . they feel more empowered to be able to have it, to speak up and say what they want, and know that it's going to be acted on. It's not just going to be left on deaf ears.' In another ward they implemented a parent education programme to ensure

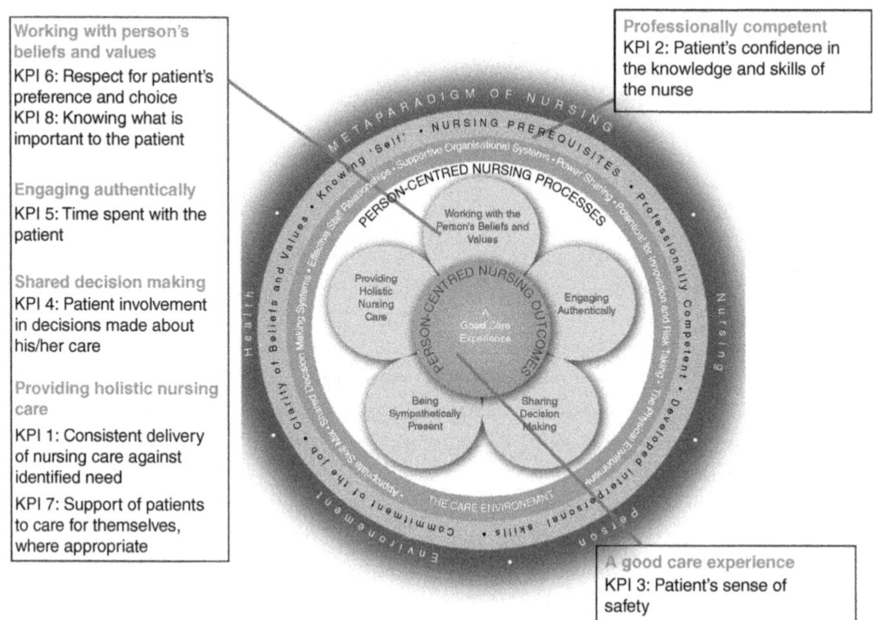

Figure 17.2 Key performance indicators mapped to the Person-centred Nursing Framework Adapted from McCormack and McCance 2019

parents felt able to care for their child with a Thomas splint after discharge home. Although this may seem a simple idea, it was evident that parents did not feel confident and often experienced inconsistent messages which left them feeling uncertain and disempowered on discharge. The education programme assisted parents not only with knowledge and skills but also with the ability to problem solve for their child in the community, thereby ensuring parents and their child could both cope and flourish once back at home.

All nursing participants commented favourably on the feedback they received in relation to their practice, as it focused them 'on areas of quality improvement' and offered an opportunity to benchmark their practice internationally (McCance et al. 2016). More than 60 improvements were undertaken during the study, focused on different areas of practice, such as ward orientation for families, documentation, and improvements in bedside handover where involvement of the consumer and the information they had to offer about their child was considered key to the handover process.

2) There was recognition during PINS that collection and management of KPI data could be enhanced through a technological solution and also assist in creating a wider body of collaborative work. Subsequently an app was developed, implemented and evaluated across two healthcare organisations already committed to the person-centred KPIs and their use in practice. Eleven participating sites used the iMPAKT app, five in Northern Ireland and six in Wollongong, Australia. The sites covered clinical settings such as cancer care, midwifery and the acute

medical short stay unit. The majority of nurses described the app as easy to use, and the generated report on the app provided them with evidence directly from consumers and highlighted their performance in supporting consumers in the healthcare setting. This in turn increased staff morale: '. . . we can also use the iMPAKT app as a starting point to help us with showing the positive things that we are doing' (McCance et al. 2020). The Australian sites continue to use the iMPAKT app and have implemented significant practice change and improved experiences for consumers through initiatives implemented between cycles of data collection which are now being embedded.
3) The KPIs have now been implemented within a community nursing context involving four teams from the South Eastern Health and Social Care Trust (SET) and three teams from NHS Lothian in Scotland. The community nurses reported that working with this data allowed staff to discuss what is happening within the team, enabling them to evaluate their practices through a person-centred lens. It made their work visible and provided feedback where clear actions could be taken forward as a result. This feasibility study supported the transferability of the KPIs within a community context.
4) The positive impact of the KPIs on staff morale and on consumer improvements when implementation was co-produced across ambulatory chemotherapy units in Northern Ireland has been further endorsed. The KPIs were also successful in improving practice and focused on, for example, enhancing the experience of waiting/treatment times, thereby supporting consumers to feel comfortable and cared for. Shaping services across organisations was also evidenced, with one example demonstrating a regional change in the electronic record developed for use across the chemotherapy units in Northern Ireland impacting on KPI8 – nurses' understanding of what is important to the patient and their family.

This programme of work is clearly showing how the KPIs are shaping person-centred cultures internationally with improvements in care delivery, work practices and staff morale, and through providing support to consumers at home, in the community and in hospital. This impact has been achieved through using data that privileges the person's voice, enabling all to flourish and engaging, motivating and inspiring nurses to act on this in partnership.

Conclusion

This chapter has highlighted ways in which practice developers can support the development of flourishing communities by focusing on what matters to them through community development work and participatory research methods and measures. Key to this are a number of important principles:

i. having the skills to co-create a clear purpose, vision and values with people;
ii. working appreciatively from a position of strength rather than focusing on weaknesses or problems;

iii. treating citizens as equals, acknowledging individual circumstances and experiences;
iv. having a methodological approach driven by what citizens want rather than a prescription of what is needed;
v. facilitating a collaborative approach between all sectors and local communities to develop strong partnerships with local ownership, collective leadership and action;
vi. having a strong sense of strategic priorities for local growth and development underpinned by metrics and benchmarks for measuring impact (Local Government Association 2019; Inspiring Scotland 2019; Van Asselt et al. 2015);
vii. drawing on a range of different types of knowledge and evidence to support decision-making in different contexts and the strategies that are effective in transforming practice (Manley and Titchen 2011).

References

Alomari, A., Wilson, V., Solman, A. et al. (2017). Pediatric nurses' perceptions of medication safety and medication error: a mixed methods study. *Comprehensive Child and Adolescent Nursing* 41 (2): 94–110.

Block, P. (2008). *Community: The Structure of Belonging*. San Francisco, CA: Berrett-Koehler Publishers.

British Academy for the Humanities and Social Sciences. (2017). Where we live now: making the case for place-based policy. https://www.thebritishacademy.ac.uk/sites/default/files/Where-we-live-now-making-case-for-place-based-policy.pdf

Coburn, A. and Gormally, S. (2015). Youth work in schools. In: *Youth work: Histories, Policy and Contexts* (ed. S. Bright), 252. London: Palgrave Macmillan.

Diener, E., Wirtz, D., Tov, W. et al. (2010). New well-being measures: short scales to assess flourishing and positive and negative feelings. *Social Indicators Research* 97:143–156.

Ellery, J., Ellery, P., MacKenzie, A. et al. (2017). Placemaking: an engaged approach to community well-being. *Journal of Family and Consumer Sciences* 109 (2): 7–13.

Fredrickson, B.L. and Losada, M.F. (2005). Positive affect and the complex dynamics of human flourishing. *American Psychologist* 60 (7): 678–686.

Heron, J. and Reason, P. (1997). A participatory inquiry paradigm. *Qualitative Inquiry* 3 (3): 274–294.

Huppert, F. (2009). Psychological well-being: evidence regarding its causes and consequences. *Applied Psychology: Health and Well-Being* 1 (2):137–64.

Huppert, F.A. and So, T.T.C. (2013). Flourishing across Europe: application of a new conceptual framework for defining well-being. *Social Indicators Research* 110 (3): 837–861.

Hustedde, R.J. (2008). Seven theories for seven community developers. In: *An Introduction to Community Development* (eds. R. Phillips and H. Pittman), 20–37. New York;: Routledge.

Inspiring Scotland (2019). Link up: local people building flourishing communities. https://www.inspiringscotland.org.uk/publication/link-flourishing-communities. (accessed 30 March 2020).

Keyes, C. (2002). The mental health continuum: from languishing to flourishing in life. *Journal of Health and Social Behavior* 43 (2): 207–222.

Keyes, C. (2015). Human flourishing and salutogenetics. *Genetics of Psychological Well-Being: The Role of Heritability and Genetics in Positive Psychology*. Chapter 1. DOI: 10.1093/acprof:oso/9780199686674.003.0001

Local Government Association. (2019). Building Cohesive Communities. An LGA Guide. March. https://local.gov.uk/sites/default/files/documents/10.31%20Community%20cohesion%20guidance_04.2.pdf. (accessed 4 April 2020).

Manley, K. and Titchen, A. (2011). *Being and Becoming a Consultant Nurse: Towards Greater Effectiveness through a Programme of Support*. London: RCN.

McCance, T. and Wilson, V. (2015). Using person-centred key performance indicators to improve paediatric services: an international venture. *International Practice Development Journal* 5 (Supplement): 8-1–8-7. DOI: 10.19043/ipdj.5SP.010

McCance, T., Hastings, J. and Dowler, H. (2015). Evaluating the use of key performance indicators to evidence the patient experience. *Journal of Clinical Nursing* 24: 3084–3094.

McCance, T., Lynch, B., Boomer, C. et al. (2020). Implementing and measuring person-centredness using an APP for knowledge transfer: the iMPAKT app. *International Journal for Quality in Health Care* 32 (4): 251–258.

McCance, T.V., Telford, L., Wilson, J. et al. (2012). Identifying key performance indicators for nursing and midwifery care using a consensus approach. *Journal of Clinical Nursing* 21 (7–8): 1145–1154.

McCance, T., Wilson, V. and Kornman, K. (2016). Paediatric International Nursing Study: using person-centred key performance indicators to benchmark children's services. *Journal of Clinical Nursing* 25 (13–14): 2018–2027.

McCormack, B. and McCance, T. (2019). Person-centred Nursing Framework. https://www.ulster.ac.uk/nursingframework (accessed 29 July 2020).

McCormack, B. and Titchen, A. (2006). Critical creativity: melding, exploding, blending. *Educational Action Research: an International Journal* 14 (2): 239–266.

McMillan, D.W. (2011). Sense of community, a theory not a value: a response to Nowell and Boyd. *Journal of Community Psychology* 39 (5): 507–519. https://doi.org/10.1002/jcop.20439.

Mertens, D. (2007). Transformative paradigm: mixed methods and social justice. *Journal of Mixed Methods Research* 1 (3): 212–225.

National Voices. (2013). A narrative for person-centred coordinated care. https://www.nationalvoices.org.uk/sites/default/files/public/publications/narrative-for-person-centred-coordinated-care.pdf (accessed 1 May 2020).

NESTA (2012). Asset based approaches in a health and wellbeing context. https://www.nesta.org.uk/feature/realising-value-resource-centre/asset-based-approaches-in-a-health-and-wellbeing-context/. (accessed 1 May 2020).

Perkins, D.D., Hughey, J. and Speer, P.W. (2002). Community psychology perspectives on social capital theory and community development practice. *Community Development* 33 (1): 33–52.

Raibley, J.R. (2012). Happiness is not well-being. *Journal of Happiness Studies* 13 (6): 1105–1129.

Sanders, K., Omar, B. and Webster, J. (2015). Working collaboratively to develop a patient experience definition and strategy to inform clinical commissioning. *International Practice Development Journal* 5 (2) [2]. https://doi.org/10.19043/ipdj.52.002

Scottish Community Development Centre (2019). What is community development? https://www.scdc.org.uk/who/what-is-community-development. (accessed 2 May 2020).

Seligman, M.E. (2002). *Authentic Happiness: Using the New Positive Psychology to Realize Your Potential for Lasting Fulfillment*. New York;: Free Press.

Seligman, M.E. (2011). *Flourish: A Visionary New Understanding of Happiness and Well-being* (1st Free Press hardcover edition). New York;: Free Press.

Seligman, M.E.P. (2012). *Flourish: A Visionary New Understanding of Happiness and Well-being*. New York;: Simon & Schuster.

Seligman, M.E. and Royzman, E. (2003). Happiness: The Three Traditional Theories. Unpublished manuscript. https://www.authentichappiness.sas.upenn.edu/newsletters/authentichappiness/happiness (accessed 5 April 2020).

Titchen, A. and Armstrong, H. (2007). Re-directing the vision: dancing with light and shadows. In: *Being Critical and Creative in Qualitative Research* (eds. J. Higgs et al.), 151–163. Sydney: Hampden Press.

Titchen, A. and McCormack, B. (2010). Dancing with stones: critical creativity as methodology for human flourishing. *Educational Action Research* 18 (4): 531–554.

Titchen, A., McCormack, B., Wilson, V. et al. (2011). Human flourishing through body, creative imagination and reflection. *International Practice Development Journal* 1 (1) [1] https://www.fons.org/library/journal/volume1-issue1/article1

Van Asselt, D., Buchanan, A. and Peterson, S. (2015). Enablers and barriers of social inclusion for young adults with intellectual disability: a multidimensional view. *Journal of Intellectual & Developmental Disability* 40 (1): 37–48.

18. *Practice Development – Towards Co-Creation, Innovation and Systems Transformation to Foster Person-Centred Care*

Christine Øye, Valerie Wilson, and Kim Manley

Introduction

Our aims in this closing chapter are to recognise the achievements of practice development (PD), drawing on the examples presented in this book, so that its contribution can be more widely understood, used and appreciated. Also, to provide key ideas and direction for those practitioners, researchers and educators who will continue to build upon the same values and commitment to the emancipatory intent of PD. Finally, we will draw on insights and identified priorities of the International Practice Development Collaborative as collective leaders in the field, with their expertise in using PD across many different settings.

It is more than a decade since the first edition of this PD book was published (Manley et al. 2008) and this edition reflects subsequent developments in the field. The tradition of PD is not unaffected by developments in health and social care (HSC) practices, sciences and policies. For instance, the PD community has both influenced and been influenced by a stronger emphasis on person-centred care, user participation, stakeholder involvement, co-creation and co-production of knowledge, interprofessional learning, and not least theoretical perspectives about systems. All of these aspects have been touched upon by authors throughout this book and form the basis of this chapter.

International Practice Development in Health and Social Care, Second Edition.
Edited by Kim Manley, Valerie Wilson, and Christine Øye.

Societal challenges for a new decade

Societal challenges in health and social care, e.g. Covid-19, aging population, racism, bring to the fore the need to foster approaches that enhance problem-solving capacity at all levels of society and across different communities. PD has been and will continue to be one of several participatory research and improvement approaches that address different societal challenges by actively engaging with the people affected locally (even if the challenge is relevant worldwide, e.g. COVID-19). This strength complements other improvement approaches, supports increased self-awareness (enlightenment), results in empowerment that enables taken-for-granted assumptions and power structures to be challenged, all of which lead to change that is more likely to be embedded and sustained and is associated with the term radical transformation. One such example of local social change focusing on people and communities that addresses key health and social care challenges is given in Box 18.1.

While the example in Box 18.1 is not labelled as a PD initiative, many of its features characterise PD, namely a focus on what matters to people, a strengths-based approach; enabling empowerment; social contexts where healthcare challenges exist; people working together; and a systematic approach to evaluation involving all stakeholders.

Practice development and person-centred care

Person-centred care has grown stronger in all areas across the PD community from the perspectives of practice (e.g. Manley et al. 2019) (see Chapter 17), theory (e.g. Øye et al. 2020) (see Chapter 9), methods (Wilson et al. 2020), research (Mekki et al. 2017) and education (Manley et al. 2018) (see Chapter 6). Person-centred care has been a central value to PD since its beginning and it is gratifying to see this value has impacted positively on worldwide health and social care policy and governance (WHO 2019). Person-centredness has increasingly gained focus in health and social care delivery at all levels and is recognised as integral to high-quality care and therapy (Santana et al. 2018; Wilberforce et al. 2017). New fields of practice are now being developed, such as person-centred medicine (Van Staden 2020) and person-centred communication (Motschnig and Ladislav 2014).

Person-centred approaches are part of a movement that puts the person first, emphasising the whole person in contrast to biomedical models that focus on the disease and symptoms rather than the person. Therefore, in the tradition of person-centredness, it is the person's experience (of illness) and their expressed needs and preferences that always overrule the perspective of disease. Working with what matters to people and their experiences of care is a key element of PD (see Chapter 17) and also a criterion in high-quality care interrelated with other quality elements such as safety (Manley et al. 2019) and effectiveness where successful evidence implementation depends on blending aspects of the person with other types of evidence.

Box 18.1 Using social prescribing to promote community resilience and wellbeing (Howarth et al. 2020)

Salford community voluntary services (CVS) and Salford Primary Care Together developed a 'Wellbeing Matters' (WBM) programme, using social prescribing to promote resilience and wellbeing in the locality through an asset-based, non-medical approach. The system encourages people to take an active role in their health, live as well as possible with health conditions, and feel in control, valued, motivated and supported. A transformational leadership approach was adopted by Salford CVS to ensure that key partners from local social enterprise, local business, the local authority and community groups were included in the development, design and implementation of the Wellbeing Matters programme. The two main goals were to:

- help reduce inappropriate demand on costly areas of health provision in Salford;
- contribute to improving the health and wider wellbeing of Salford residents through the use of person- and community-centred approaches, including the creation of an overarching social prescribing model for Salford.

The model is predicated on collaboration with existing community assets – through inclusion of five local social enterprises across Salford – which were designated 'Anchor organisations'. Each Anchor organisation recruited a 'community connector' to asset map the community and undertake wellbeing conversations with people referred in the community to determine 'what matters to them' as opposed to 'what is the matter with them' (Reed et al 2019). The mixed methods evaluation by the University of Salford captured objective data from an elemental social prescribing digital platform and subjective data from focus groups and interviews with beneficiaries, GPs and the community connectors – 95% would recommend the service to another and 95% indicated an overall positive experience. The positive feedback from clinicians, staff and beneficiaries indicates the success of the WBM programme and the life-changing impact on people's lives. One GP remarked:

> *'I just think it's [the Wellbeing Matters programme] a great thing, I think it's very much needed with how society and community living is in 2019, . . . I see social prescribing just being part of primary care. . . [the carer] found the service invaluable. . . [she was approached] in a very person-centred and compassionate way, and it has enabled her to access social and educational options now she has more free time.'*

Other professionals, such as social workers, expressed similar views:

> *'I've seen some amazing transitions with people who are [engaged with WBM]. . . hopefully they will turn into long-term things in terms of their lifestyles changing. . . but if nothing else, giving them a sense of purpose through volunteering is great, and that's something which should be really celebrated.'*

The evaluation highlighted positive findings across the system, with benefits noted in beneficiary case studies, GP feedback and across the wider community sector. Equally, benefits have been observed through community and population outcomes through increased community connection, improved confidence and physical activity in relevant cases.

Chapter 2 highlighted how people with stomas can be helped to have an influential role in developing services that are important to them and how to help people with mental health challenges to have a more powerful voice. Chapter 3 showed the need to enable the voice of women to be central in the transformation of maternity services, but also the potential of PD in enabling this and its strong role in complementing other approaches to quality, safety and improvement. Chapter 4 demonstrated that commissioners and systems need to be on board with person-centred values if person-centred care is to be embedded and sustained to achieve its full potential. Hence the need for commissioners and systems leaders to understand the importance of person-centred approaches and the positive impact on improving health outcomes, as in the example in Box 18.1. Chapter 5 shared three case studies, which addressed different challenges in providing person-centred services for people with dementia.

PD and person-centredness share the intent that the person is central. We (the editors) argue that being person-centred is both a pivotal value and a purpose to PD and that person-centred relationships need to be at the heart of communities (see Chapters 4 and 5). However, creating communities and cultures that enable person-centred approaches to be central requires understanding about person-centred relationships, what they look like, how the values are lived and experienced. This aspiration requires facilitation and leadership skills (see Chapters 10–13) combined with the collaborative, inclusive and participative principles of PD (Chapter 8) to achieve this vision. A key challenge for the future of PD is: How do we ensure that person-centred values inform health and social care policy?

Practice development and user involvement through co-creation

Over the last decade PD's emphasis on user and stakeholder engagement and co-creation of services and their evaluation has been embraced by many others to improve health and social care services democratically (e.g. Greenhalgh et al. 2016) in an empowering way (e.g. Voorberg et al. 2015; Alves 2013) (see Chapters 2–3). Central to user involvement and co-creation are the CIP principles (Chapter 8), which have had a broad influence and have been endorsed by policies on user participation and patients' involvement for better quality of care and safety (van den Berg et al. 2019). The lives of people with illness matters in developing care practices, and slogans such as 'What matters to you' (see Box 18.1) have an impact on health and social care policies and practices. These values are underpinned by trends about how to involve persons who receive care, through perspectives on empowerment, patient rights and citizenship, etc. (e.g. Kontos et al. 2020).

Therefore, people with illness experiences (service users) as well as other stakeholders (such as carers) have increasingly been encouraged to be actively involved in PD projects to ensure that the care and treatment are relevant to the preferences and needs of those with illness experiences. User involvement has not only influenced how care is organised, planned and provided in close collaboration with the ones who receive care, but people with illness experiences are increasingly being invited as co-researchers in planning research, collecting data, analyzing data, writing articles and disseminating results (Eriksen et al. 2012) – see, for example, case study 1 in Chapter 17. Despite involving service users, research shows that challenges due to factors such as tokenism and power relations remain (Ocloo and Matthews 2016) and desired outcomes are not always achieved, e.g. more advanced knowledge or improvements in the quality of research (Malterud and Elvbakken 2019).

Therefore, when involving service users, practice developers need to be more explicit about how, when, in what stages of the process and for what purposes service users are involved. How can the user potentially be a 'game changer', and how can the user also be a co-implementer and evaluator and *not* only an informant, co-designer or co-initiator (Voorberg et al. 2015)? This echoes the challenges of the 1940s when Kurt Lewin (1946) introduced action research as a social experiment, where citizens contributed as informants only in the first stage of the action cycle (reconnaissance) rather than in the innovation, implementation and evaluation stages. PD with its continued emancipatory intent needs to constantly ask how to re-position power relations to include the voices of:

1. people with illness to inform social learning and transformation (Chapter 2)
2. citizens when building sustainable person-centred communities (Chapters 3 and 4)
3. staff and employees in the workplace (Chapter 16).

Practice development and innovation

The PD community has been influenced by developments in innovation practice and theory. For example, Jacobsen (2020) highlights the theoretical premises of innovation in relation to care and policy development, while Simons (2015) was inspired by PD in developing new ways of pain management targeting children at hospital by using appreciative inquiry.

A common understanding of innovation is that it is 'an idea, practice or object that is perceived as new by an individual or other unit of adoption. . . the adoption of an existing idea for the first time by a given organization' (De Vries et al. 2016, p. 152). PD has been operating with and influenced by such a definition, but often the process of innovation starts with a vision based on ideas put forward by staff in the workplace (Dewing et al. 2014). The potential for innovation in PD is also linked to developing workplace cultures where people can flourish, enabling psychological safety for both creativity and critical debate to happen (see Chapter 15).

Responsible innovation is an important aspect of innovation practice, as potentially innovation can conflict with policy on collaborative practice and research for societal benefit (Øye et al. 2019; Stilgoe et al. 2013). The push for innovation to solve societal challenges might put practice developers in a moral dilemma if innovative policies contradict personal moral standards. Researchers and practice developers may feel pressure to get their projects done due to deadlines and funding constraints. Such pressure might tempt them to take ethical 'short cuts' in relation to informed consent, the principle of voluntariness and integrity to get the work completed on time (Øye et al. 2019). In any research, including co-creative research such as PD, it is imperative to follow ethical and PD principles so that participants are informed, involved and feel safe. In times of crisis when working with people experiencing additional stress and uncertainty, greater attention is required in order to avoid persons being unsafe. A key part of PD work as well as being person-centred is paying attention to verbal and non-verbal cues of consent and indicators of feeling stressed, uncertain or unsafe and addressing these as they arise (see Chapter 8 for PD principles). This means keeping in mind what is at stake for different participants (Oeye et al. 2007) and creating a safe and inclusive environment for people to flourish but still respecting those who do not want to participate or may wish to withdraw their participation.

PD as a 'free space' to create visions and knowledge in a 'bottom-up' way might be a contested space between practice developers, stakeholders and top-down policies. An increasing challenge in PD work will not only be to collaborate with stakeholders such as staff, health and social care leaders, service users, carers, etc. but also to collaborate with policymakers to ensure good organisational conditions, since several studies have shown that organisational barriers can hamper PD work (e.g. Øye et al. 2015; Dahl et al. 2018; Manley et al. 2019). Therefore, if PD projects are to succeed ensuring that systems enhance person-centred care and that staff can flourish in the workplace (see Chapter 16), we need to address the question: How can we involve stakeholders with bureaucratic and political backgrounds in PD work?

Practice development and system approaches

The success of innovations often requires people to work together closely in a co-creative way as mentioned above. However, the way to create system conditions for success is still an enigma for PD, although the Venus model based on PD research proposes five skillsets (facilitation, culture change, clinical and systems leadership, improvement and PD including knowledge translation) required by the workforce to achieve sustainable person-centred transformation (Manley and Jackson 2020).

First, success is dependent on how stakeholders themselves create the conditions and capacity to work for a common vision from a bottom-up approach (Alves 2013) across historical boundaries and silos (Manley 2016). Second, success is dependent on existing conditions and readiness to embrace PD work (see Chapter 3). That is, identifying elements in systems that promote or hinder improvement or innovation in PD. Finally, and not least, PD is dependent on identifying analytically the elements in the system that hamper possibilities for problem-solving and change, or identifying the appreciative strategies that work across different contexts. For instance, do the hierarchies and fixed roles in the workplace hinder staff from coming forward with experiences and suggestions that make agreeing values and visions especially demanding.

The roles people play in systems need further understanding since change and learning is a social process where people learn individually and collectively (see Chapter 6). Individuals in the system learn in the context of other individuals, albeit influenced by the socio-organisational context of which they are part. Therefore, successful learning involves sharing assumptions and the consequences of our actions on others as well as strengthening existing identities and roles for renewing confidence and recognising achievements (see Chapter 10).

Achieving change is more than the sum of what individuals know and learn, and as such exists beyond individuals (Berta et al. 2015) (see Chapter 11). People learn as part of systems through playing the roles they have been socialised to play, which are often embedded into people's self-identity and self-esteem and are not easily 'corrected' or improved through the process of facilitated reflection. However, the purpose of facilitation is not to 'correct' or otherwise create new identities or roles, but to develop new insights about individual and whole-systems approaches to health and social care. Chapter 14 identified the need for both systems leadership and facilitation expertise that integrates multiple purposes and embraces complexity. PD has been at the forefront of both areas. A major aim in the years to come is to find theoretical and practical solutions to how PD can work alongside or overcome systems that hamper its work. A key challenge for the future of PD is: How can practice developers further create system conditions to raise the success of their PD work?

PD: *enabling through leadership and facilitation*

While many different improvement approaches aspire to make a difference, it is PD that explains the 'how' improvement happens through leadership and facilitation based on person-centred values, the CIP principles and theoretical insights about the strategies that work. Facilitation as a reflective and practical skill is about helping people understand how they impact on others at the individual, team, organisation and systems levels to influence and support people's participation. Facilitated creative ways of working to overcome barriers for active participation will continue to be the aim and scope of future PD work. Chapter 10 unpacks this vital skillset and Chapter 11 explains its multiple facets.

Facilitation is essential for helping people explore and challenge the roles played as well as ways of working that may have been accepted in the context (Dahl et al. 2018). Therefore, facilitation work encourages people at all levels to see their problems and possible solutions in light of the workplace context and wider health and social care system, including the roles they play, as possibilities to modify or solve rather than just 'put up with' (Berta et al. 2015, p. 6).

Facilitation expertise is an essential skill to be developed as part of organisational and systems responsiveness (see Chapter 14). This organisational skillset has been demonstrated as an enabler to developing safety cultures, quality improvement skills and leadership in frontline teams across healthcare organisations (Manley et al. 2019). An integrated approach to facilitation embracing multiple purposes was identified as a prerequisite to transform whole systems. The international standards subsequently developed through a Delphi study (Martin and Manley 2017) focused on all the facilitation purposes that enable more effective functioning, namely person-centred, safe and effective care, learning, improving, developing, innovation, knowledge translation and inquiry, all embraced by PD. (See Chapters 11 and 14.)

The facilitation skillset is one of five identified in the Venus model mentioned earlier for sustainable systems transformation, in which the measurement and tools of quality improvement are also included. Chapter 3 identified other improvement methodologies used by the chapter authors before discovering PD and acknowledged PD as the missing part of the jigsaw for successful transformation. While many health and social care organisations argue for a single methodology, often meaning quality improvement or lean methodology, the need for eclectic approaches which can complement each other has been argued for (Manley et al. 2017). While each methodology brings its strengths, it is the PD focus on shared values, vision, direction, co-creation with all stakeholders as well as facilitation that is often missing in other approaches.

Leadership, the other enabling approach, is the main way that workplace cultures can change at any level. Chapter 12 showed this through person-centred and relationship-based approaches to leadership that support PD values, ways of working and cultures where people can flourish. The vital role of leadership in PD is endorsed in this book through according it three chapters: relation-based leadership (Chapter 12), effective team leadership (Chapter 13) and systems leadership (Chapter 14). A key challenge for the future of PD is: How do we ensure the centrality of facilitation and leadership remain as enabling factors that supports PD work at the micro, meso and macro levels?

Practice development beyond methods and a new global manifesto for PD

A challenge in the next decade will be to further build reflective, analytic and practice capacity to depict, identify and solve challenges in local health and social care services for people to flourish. New societal challenges will arise, which will still put pressure on those who provide and experience care in health and social services, and therefore it will still be necessary to invent and re-invent creative, joyful and inspiring spaces for people to grow and flourish (see Chapters 15–17). PD communities can be such a space, where skilled facilitators can enhance learning for persons to give, receive and co-create person-centred care practices for those both providing and experiencing care.

Box 18.2 Revised PD principles derived from a global manifesto (Chapter 8)

PD is fundamentally about **person-centred practice** that promotes **safe and effective workplace cultures** where all can **flourish.**
PD uses **collaborative, inclusive and participatory** (CIP) approaches.
PD blends **creativity** with learning, freeing people's hearts, minds and souls to achieve new ways of thinking, doing and being.
PD utilises **active work-based learning** to facilitate individual, practice, cultural (*and system*) transformation.
PD is a **facilitated** process that seeks to promote **critically informed action.**
PD uses inclusive **evaluation** to integrate **evidence** from process and outcomes of **transformation.**
PD focuses on **supportive relationships** across individuals, teams and systems to stimulate effective change.
PD is a **complex methodology** that uses a variety of evidence to inform transformation for individuals, teams and systems.

The revised PD principles developed collaboratively with members of the IPDC (see Chapter 8) mark a new era also epitomised in its title as a *new global manifesto.* These principles have benefited from 12 years (since they were first published) of global experience using, explaining, facilitating and researching PD at many different levels across varied contexts. It is therefore fitting to highlight them again here as these will be our guiding lights for the next generation (see Box 18.2). A key challenge for the future of PD is: In what ways can we both advocate for and use the PD principles to support our work and those we work with in transforming health and social care?

New directions through the International Practice Development Collaborative (IPDC)

Members of the IPDC (past and present) have made a significant contribution to advancing PD methods, theory, practice and capacity building over the last 30 years or more. They have also contributed to many chapters in this book. As we came to the end of this latest edition it seemed only appropriate to ask IPDC members to reflect upon what has been achieved thus far and what the future focus of PD should be. A synthesised response to the questions we asked each member organisation is captured below.

Q1 Who are the up-and-coming practice developers in your area?

There was a broad range of roles captured in response to this question. They included direct care staff, those undertaking courses in PD (foundational and advanced IPDC schools), authors who contribute to the *International Practice*

Development Journal (*IPDJ*), and those in leadership roles such as nursing unit managers and executive directors. While it was acknowledged that many of these come from a nursing/midwifery background, we are starting to see the spread of practice developers across health and social care professions. There was also an emphasis on those in academic roles such as those engaging in curriculum development and delivery, lecturers/practitioners, researchers using action or participatory approaches, and those undertaking research degrees at masters and PhD level. There has also been an increase in the number of networking/support/capacity-building groups at local, state, national and international levels. These groups are ensuring that we are creating a PD alumni.

Q2 What professions (and consumers) do you currently engage in PD work?

PD has been led by nurses (and midwives), however there have been great strides in engaging with other health and social care staff (e.g. anaesthetists, physicians, occupational therapists, social workers, dieticians, porters, cleaners, administrative staff), volunteers, service users (e.g. mental health consumers, paediatrics and maternity), academics, researchers, decision-makers (e.g. chief nurses, advisory groups, funding bodies, charities), commissioners and policymakers. Key to this have been strategic partnerships within health and social care organisations (e.g. safety and quality units), across HSC organisations (e.g. prison health service) and between HSC and universities (e.g. lecturer/practitioner role in academic practice units). While great progress has been made, the challenge to include service users across the breadth of PD remains.

Q3 What areas of PD should we be focusing on in the coming years?

There are several areas of focus highlighted for the coming years to ensure PD can become more mainstream and is embedded and sustained in health and social care practice. This includes the ongoing issue of demonstrating the impact of PD and systematically evaluating what we do to ensure we have outcomes at the micro, meso and macro levels that support the continuing development of person-centred workplace cultures. Another aspect of this is ensuring we are disseminating our findings more broadly and making explicit the connection between PD and person-centred practice. There needs to be an articulation of PD alongside other methodologies and approaches such as quality improvement and the ways in which PD can inform workplace strategy. We need to ensure that we use the CIP principle and co-design approaches to engage across the range of health and social care staff and service users. The role of technology is changing rapidly and we need to harness this as we progress the PD agenda and the opportunities this provides PD. There is a continued need to build capacity and remain connected to our PD alumni. This would be further enhanced by ensuring that those coming into our profession have opportunities to engage with PD through their undergraduate programmes.

Q4 What is one thing you would like to celebrate in relation to PD?

After 30-plus years, PD is still alive and kicking and is engaging and working with people across disciplines and consumers (e.g. engaging consumer peer workers in mental health). We need to recognise how far we have come and take the time to acknowledge and celebrate our achievements. Things we can be thankful for include the ongoing support and sponsorship for PD programmes, initiatives, research and capacity building (e.g. five-day foundational programmes, the biennial international Enhancing Practice conference). We can evidence PD and the transformation of people and systems that come with it within policies, embedded within practice and undergraduate teaching. PD tools have been translated into different languages as we spread the work across the world. The following quotes from four IPDC members provide different aspects of PD celebration.

> *'Keep broadcasting the (PD) messages honestly and humbly.'*

> *'Right now the world is shouting at us to hear the voices of those usually discounted or intentionally ignored. PD provides a framework to assist us to seek and hear from other people. CIP principles actively encourage a person to seek out others' opinions, thoughts and needs. PD calls us to acknowledge the replies and asks us to respond.'*

> *'One of the most significant celebratory points is the ongoing and unsolicited reports of how an introduction to PD has made a difference to people's lives as we see every day how PD contributes to people's experiences of themselves, their care, their colleagues and their communities.'*

> *'I like how the world looks because of PD and how it has shaped and influenced how we care for our communities.'*

Conclusion

This final chapter sets out to signpost the essences of this book as an invaluable resource for all practitioners of health and social care practice, community development, research, education and leadership who are committed to developing person-centred cultures where everyone can flourish. While there is much to be learnt from the experiences shared and the insights developed through ongoing research and inquiry, there remain questions to be answered and explored for further establishment of PD as an approach that is essential for successful and sustained transformation of our health and social care systems and communities across the world. We leave you with our own key message as editors:

Hold on to the values that guide how we work together as people.
Even though living them is challenged every day.

Hold on to seeing the light in others, kindling their sparks and keeping those lights glowing.

Even though there are many times when the lights are nearly extinguished from forces that want to diminish them.

Hold on to a constellation of connected stars across the world with one voice as collective leaders – to make a difference through person-centred cultures that enable everyone to flourish.

References

Alves, H. (2013). Co-creative and innovation in public services. *The Service Industries and Journal* 33: 7–8, 671–682. DOI: 10.1080/02642069.2013.740468

Berta, W., Cranley, L., Dearing, J.W., Dogherty, E.J., Squires, J.E. and Estabrooks, C.A. (2015). Why (we think) facilitation works: insights from organizational learning theory. *Implementation Science* 10: 141. DOI: 10.1186/s13012-015-0323-0

Dahl, H., Dewing, J., Mekki, T.E., Haaland, A. and Øye, C. (2018). Facilitation of a workplace learning intervention in a fluctuating context: an ethnographic, participatory research project in a nursing home in Norway. *International Practice Development Journal* 8 (2): 1–17, doi.org/10.19043/ipdj.82.004

De Vries, H., Bekkers, V. and Tummers, L. (2016). Innovation in the public sector: a systematic review and future research agenda. *Public Administration* 94 (1): 146–166. DOI: 10.1111/padm12209

Dewing, J., McCormack, B. and Titchen, A. (2014). *Practice Development Workbook for Nursing, Health and Social care Teams*. Oxford: Wiley Blackwell.

Eriksen, K.A., Sundfør, B. and Karlsson, B. (2012). Recognition as a valued human being: perspectives of mental health service users. *Nursing Ethics* 19: 357–368.

Greenhalgh, T., Jackson, C., Shaw, S. and Janamian, T. (2016). Achieving research impact through co-creation in community-based health services: literature review and case study. *The Milbank Quarterly* 94 (2): 392–429.

Howarth, M., Gibbons, A., Witkam, R., Page, B. and Poole, D. (2020) *Evaluation of the Salford Wellbeing Matters Programme: interim findings*. Unpublished.

Jacobsen, F.F. (2020). Innovation in persons. An analysis of two prominent academic narratives. *International Practice Development Journal* 10: 2, 1–10. https://www.fons.org/Resources/Documents/Journal/Vol10Suppl/IPDJ_10Suppl_002.pdf

Kontos, P., Grigorovich, A. and Colobong, R. (2020). Towards a critical understanding of creativity and dementia: new directions for practice change *International Journal of Practice Development* 10 (Suppl) [3]. https://doi.org/10.19043/ipdj.10Suppl.003

Lewin, K. (1946). Action research and minority problems. *Journal of Social Issues* 2 4: 34–46. https://doi.org/10.1111/j.1540-4560.1946.tb02295.x

Malterud, K. and Elvbakken, K.T. (2019). Patients participating as co-researchers in health research: a systematic review of outcomes and experiences. *Scandinavian Journal of Public Health*: 1–12. DOI: 10.1177/1403494819863514

Manley, K. (2016). An overview of practice development. In: *Person-Centred Practice in Nursing and Health Care Theory and Practice, 2nd Edition*, (eds. B. McCormack and T. McCance), 133–149. Chichester: Wiley Blackwell.

Manley, K., Buscher, A., Jackson, C., Stehling, H. and O'Connor, S. (2017). Overcoming synecdoche: why practice development and quality improvement approaches should be better integrated. Commentary response to Lavery, G. (2016). Quality improvement – rival or ally of practice development? Critical commentary, *International Practice Development Journal* 6 (1): 15. www.fons.org/library/journal/volume6-issue1/article15

Manley, K. and Jackson, C. (2020). The Venus model for integrating practitioner-led workforce transformation and complex change across the health care system. *Journal of Evaluation in Clinical Practice – International Journal of Public Health Policy and Health Services Research*, 20 January. https://doi.org/10.1111/jep.13377

Manley, K., Jackson, C. and McKenzie, C. (2019). Microsystems culture change – a refined theory for developing person centred, safe and effective workplaces based on strategies that embed a safety culture. *International Journal of Practice Development* 9 2: Article 4. https://doi.org/10.19043/ipdj.92.004

Manley, K., Martin, A., Jackson, C. and Wright, T. (2016). Using systems thinking to identify workforce enablers for a whole systems approach to urgent and emergency care delivery: a multiple case study. *BMC Health Services Research* 16: 368. https://doi.org/10.1186/s12913-016-1616-y

Manley, K., Martin, A., Jackson, C. and Wright, T. (2018). *A realist synthesis of effective continuing professional development (CPD): a case study of healthcare practitioners. Nurse Education Today* 69: 134–141. https://doi.org/10.1016/j.nedt.2018.07.010

Manley, K., McCormack, B. and Wilson, V. (2008). *International Practice Development in Nursing and Healthcare*. Oxford: Blackwell Publishing.

Martin, A. and Manley, K. (2017). Developing standards for an integrated approach to workplace facilitation for interprofessional teams in health and social care contexts: a Delphi study. *Journal of Interprofessional Care* 32 (1): 41–51.

Mekki, T.E., Øye, C., Kristensen, B.B., Dahl, H., Håland, A., Nordin, K.M.A., Strandos, M., Terum, T.M., Ydstebø, A.-E. and McCormack, B. (2017). The impact of context and facilitation on an education intervention to reduce restraint and agitation in nursing homes. *Journal of Advanced Nursing* 10.1111/jan.13340

Motschnig, R. and Ladislav, N. (2014). *Person-Centred Communication: Theory, Skills And Practice*. Berkshire: Open University Press, McGraw-Hill Education.

Ocloo, J. and Matthews, R. (2016). From tokenism to empowerment: progressing patient and public involvement in healthcare improvement. *BMJ Qual Saf.* 25 (8): 626–632. DOI: 10.1136/bmjqs-2015-004839

Oeye, C., Bjelland, A.K. and Skorpen, A. (2007). Doing participant observation in a psychiatric hospital – research ethics resumed. *Social Science & Medicine* 65 (11): 2296–2306.

Øye, C., Thorkildsen, K.M. and Synnes, O. (2020). Critical perspectives on person, care and aging: unmasking their interconnections. *International Practice Development Journal*, https://doi.org/10.19043/ipdj.10Suppl.001

Øye, S., Mekki, T.E., Skår, R., Dahl, H., Førland, O. and Jacobsen, F.F. (2015). Evidence molded by contact with staff culture and patient milieu: an analysis of the social process of knowledge utilization in nursing homes. *Vocation and Learning* 8: 319–334, DOI: 10.1007/s12186-015-9135-2

Øye, C., Sørensen, N.Ø., Dahl, H. and Glasdam, S. (2019). Tight ties in collaborative health research puts research ethics on trial? A discussion on autonomy, confidentiality, and integrity in qualitative research. *Qualitative Health Research* 29 (8): 1227 –1235. DOI: 10.1177/1049732318822294

Reed, S., Göpfert, A., Wood, S., Allwood, D. and Warburton, W. (2019). *Building healthier communities: the role of the NHS as an anchor institution*. London: The Health Foundation.

Santana, M.J., Manalili, K., Jolley, R.J., Zelinsky, S., Quan, H. and Lu, M. (2018). How to practice person-centred care: a conceptional framework. *Health Expectations* 21: 429–440. DOI: 10.1111/hex.12640

Simons, J. (2015). A proposed model of the effective management of children's pain. *Pain Management Nursing* 16 (4): 570–578. DOI: https://doi.org/10.1016/j.pmn.2014.10.008

Stilgoe, J., Owen, R. and Macnaghten, P. (2013). Developing a framework for responsible innovation. *Research Policy* 42: 1568–1580. Doi.org/10.1016/j.respol.2013.05.008

van den Berg, A., Dewar, B., Smits, C. and Jukema, J.S. (2019). Experiences of older adults and undergraduate students in co-creating age-friendly services in an educational living lab. *International Practice Development Journal* 9 2, Article 2. https://doi.org/10.19043/ipdj.92.002

Van Staden, W. (2020). Six differences between person-centred medicine and patient-centred medicine. International College of Person Centred Medicine (ICPCM). Newsletter, February. https://personcenteredmedicine.org/doc/newsletter-feb-2020.pdf (accessed 29 July 2020).

Voorberg, W.H., Bekkers, V.J. and Tummers, L.G. (2015). A systematic review of co-creation and co-production: embarking on the social innovation journey. *Journal of Public Management Review* 17 9: 1333–1357. https://doi.org/10.1080/14719037.2014.930505

Wilberforce, M., Challis, D., Davies, L., Kelly, M.P., Roberts, C. and Clarkson, P. (2017). Person-centredness in the community of older people: a literature-based concept synthesis. *International Journal of Social Welfare* 16: 86–98.

WHO (2019). Handbook. Guidance on person-centred assessment and pathways in primary care. https://apps.who.int/iris/bitstream/handle/10665/326843/WHO-FWC-ALC-19.1-eng.pdf?sequence=17&isAllowed=y

Wilson, V., Dewing J., Cardiff, S., Mekki, T.E., Øye, C. and McCance, T. (2020). A person-centred observational tool: devising the Workplace Culture Critical Analysis Tool®. *International Practice Development Journal* 10 1, Article 3. https://doi.org/10.19043/ipdj.101.003

Index

Aboriginal and Torres Strait Islander communities, 60
ACER. *See* Achieving and Celebrating Excellence Recognition scheme
Achieving and Celebrating Excellence Recognition scheme (ACER), 176–78, 180
Action research (AR), 243–44
Action research team, 123
Active citizenship, 240
Active learning, 9, 26, 68–69, 109, 119, 136
  work-based, 32, 67f, 79, 105t, 110f, 112
Adaptability, 153
ADI. *See* Alzheimer's Disease International
Ageing, 52
Ageism, 52, 59–60
Aging
  population, 252
Alzheimer's Disease International (ADI), 53
Approach (reward) response, 30–31
AR. *See* Action research
Assertiveness, humble, 147–57
Asset-based approach, 221
Associate, in leadership, 161–62
Assumptions, 128–29, 198
Attitude, person-centred, 57
Authenticity, 14, 133, 159, 165, 182
Autonomy, 156, 238
Awareness
  ethical, 97
  of self, 141, 252
  story writing and, 121

Baart's theory of presencing, 163
Backer, Chris, 126f
Balance, 152
  in leadership, 163
Baldie, Deborah, 128–29
Best practice, in maternity care, 26
Better Births Illawarra, 34–35
Bicultural concepts, 126f, 126
Bicultural perspective, 125–27, 126f
Bicultural principles, 126f
Blossom, Faye, 126f
Brain, changes in, 41
BUDset tool, 35
Burgess, Jean Michel, 126f

Cancer Taskforce Recommendations, 40
Cardiff's action research study, 162, 167
Cause, commitment to, 34
CCIs. *See* Claims, concerns and issues
Cellular Pathology Service, 176
Change, 209t, 214–15. *See also* Contextual readiness
  achievement of, 257

International Practice Development in Health and Social Care, Second Edition.
Edited by Kim Manley, Valerie Wilson, and Christine Øye.

Change (*cont'd*)
approach to, 32
barriers to, 31, 156
catalyst for, 123, 139
disruptive, 181
effective, 113
facilitation and, 148
focus on, 183b
influences that affect, 30
observed, 94
opportunity for, 31
organisational, 148, 155
plans for, 96
practice-drive realisation of, 99
process, 31
promotion of, 33
qualitative, 113
quantitative, 113
resistance to, 174
sustained, 30
system-level, 34
transformative, 148
after trauma, 180–82
values-based, 99, 178–79
vision for, 178–79
CHIME. *See* Connectedness, hope and optimism about future, identity, meaning in life, and empowerment
Chronic conditions, 14
Ciaran's eureka, 27–29
CIP. *See* Collaboration, inclusion, and participation principle
CIP-CAN. *See* Co-producing and Implementing Person-centredness in Cancer Nursing
Citizenship, active, 240
Claims, concerns and issues (CCIs), 53–54, 100, 103t, 175–76, 179, 211
Clinical deterioration, 120
Clinical leadership, 27
for frontline culture change, 184
background, 173–75
case studies, 175–82
discussion, 182–83, 183b, 184f
paradoxes of, 184f
transformative, 173
Clinical Leadership Programme (CLP), 175–77, 182, 183b, 184
Clinical management, 27
Clinical outcomes, 14
Clinical partnering, 198
Clinical policy, 15
Clinician education, 15
CLP. *See* Clinical Leadership Programme
Co-creation, 251, 254–55
Co-design, 67, 68f
Coercion, 14
Cognitive decline, 41
Collaboration, 22–23, 28, 43, 92, 94, 109, 159
diversity in, 197t
in facilitation process, 150–51
in healthcare practices, systems leadership and, 187–98, 188t, 190f, 192t, 193t, 194t, 195f, 197t
key learning from, 197t
in nursing curriculum, 66
in PD, 27
process, 197
system-level, 151–52
Collaboration, inclusion, and participation (CIP) principle, 8, 67, 108t, 110f, 111, 111b, 170, 223, 257, 258b, 261
in communities, 241
Collaborative community, international, 244
Collaborative inquiry, 206
guiding lights through
changes that make differences, 214–15
collective leadership, 207, 208t, 210–11
learning environments, 212–14
shared values, 211–12
Collective action, 155
Collective crisis, 97

Collective leadership, 207, 208t, 210–11, 262
Collective ownership, 33–34
Communication, 15, 89, 252
  barriers, 90
  improvement in, 94
  language and, 231
  in leadership, 163
  virtual, 3
Communities
  CIP and, 241
  collaborative, 2, 244
  development of, 237, 240
  engagement in, 237, 240–42
  ephemeral, 42
  evidence based, 241
  human flourishing in, 237–48, 239t, 242f, 245t, 246f
  PD in, 251
  sense of, 239–40
  as social environment, 238
  sustainable, 41
Community voluntary services (CVS), 253b
Conceptual framework, 67, 67f
Confidence, 15, 133
Connectedness, 19, 21, 160–62, 161f
Connectedness, hope and optimism about future, identity, meaning in life, and empowerment (CHIME), 19
Constructivist learning theory, 67f
Consultant practice, 195f
Contextualization, 162–63, 182
Contextual readiness, 29–30
Continuing professional development (CPD)
  knowledge translation and, 78t, 81–82
  outcomes of, 83
  transformation and, 77t–79t, 79–81
  workplace and, 73, 77b, 77t–79t, 79–83
Continuity of care, 34
Controlled surrender, 156
Conversations, 32, 121
Coordination reform, 151
Co-producing and Implementing Person-centredness in Cancer Nursing (CIP-CAN), 245t
Co-production, 34–35
Council of Deans network, 104
COVID-19, 2–3, 61, 191, 232, 252
CPD. *See* Continuing professional development
Creative thinking, 32, 106t, 107t, 108t, 110f
Crisis
  collective, 97
  PD theory and, 122–24
  response, 3
  situational, 123
Critical creativity, 120, 139
Critical-emancipatory scholarship, 119
Critical ethnographer, 87–89
Critical ethnography
  action cycle, 89f
  benefits of, 90
  case studies, 88–94, 89f, 91f
  culture change-oriented work and, 90
  design, 92, 94
  embedded research and, 87–88
  emotions with, 91
  as facilitator approach, 89
  healthcare culture and, 89f
  hidden practices and, 94–96
  internal-external partnership in, 95–96
  PD and, 94–96
  positionality in, 96
Critically informed action, 108t, 113
Critical reflection, 69, 127
  PD theory and, 120–22
  research, 132
Critical reflection log (CRL), 189
Critical social science (CSS), 119, 121–24
Critical theory, 119
Critical thinking skills, 66, 69, 108t
CRL. *See* Critical reflection log
CSS. *See* Critical social science
Cultural transformation, 99, 112

Cultural Workforce Development
Team, 126f
Culture, 10
barriers, 96
change, 9, 93, 139, 173, 184
as commonality, 153–55
compliance-based, 174
experience of, 2
facilitation and, 153–55
frontline change in, 173–84, 183b, 184f
healthcare, 86–97, 89f, 91f
healthful, 61
of inquiry, 79
leadership and, 173–84, 183b, 184f
organisational, 43, 92, 97
person-centred, 159
shift, 92
team-learning, 74t
toxic, 175
workplace, 2–4, 6, 32, 86, 154, 157, 164
development of, 205–7, 208t–9t, 210–17
Curriculum
for Foundation PD School, 99–100
person-centred, 66–69, 67f, 68f
CVS. *See* Community voluntary services

DDDA. *See* Dementia and Driving Decision Aid booklet
DDO. *See* Deliberately Developmental Organisation
Decision-making, 15, 33, 66, 81, 121, 133
Delegation, 14
Deliberately Developmental Organisation (DDO), 181
Delphi study, 258
Dementia, 41–42, 52, 54–60, 62. *See also* Person-centred care
COVID-19 and, 61
Dementia and Driving Decision Aid (DDDA) booklet, 54–56, 61
Department of Health (DOH), 60
Dewey, John, 141
Dialogue, internal, 132
Director of Nursing (DON), 222
Discipline silos, 174
Dissemination, of well-being, 225–29, 226f, 227f, 228b
Diversity, 126, 150, 197
DNQP. *See* German Network for Quality Development in Nursing
DOH. *See* Department of Health
DON. *See* Director of Nursing

East Kent Training Hub, 70
Education
case study models, 67–73, 67f, 68f, 74t–76t, 77b, 77t–79t
professional, 17–18, 23, 66–69, 67f, 68f, 231
Emancipatory change, 87
Emancipatory practice development (ePD), 119, 122, 136, 136b
Embedded research, 4, 7, 94, 96
Emotional intelligence, 232
Emotional touchpoints interviews, 180
Empathy, 18
Empowerment, 1, 155, 252
CHIME, 19
of citizens, 241–47, 242f, 245t, 246f
of communities, 240–47, 242f, 245t, 246f
of consumer, 21–22, 40
promotion of, 15
workforce, 174
Enablers
individual, 201
qualities of, 201
system, interdependent partners, and organisations, 202
Engagement, 30–31
authentic, 159
community, 242
robust, 34
Engagement principles, 28
Enhancing Practice conference, 261
Enlightenment, 252
Environment

creative and critical learning, 209t
dynamic, 159
high-support, 121
for learning, 212–14
safe, 43, 198, 209t
social, 238
ePD. *See* Emancipatory practice development
Essentials of Care Framework, 91
Essentials of Care Programme, 4, 6, 89, 103t
Esther Model, 44–47
Ethical awareness, 97
Ethics, 40, 197t, 223
Ethno-cultural diversity, 150
Eudaimonic well-being, 221, 238
Evaluation, 18, 100, 108t, 113, 164
Evidence
accurate, 34
in PD, 2, 114, 114b, 196
research, 27–28
Evidence based communities, 241
Evoke cards, 20
Experience, lived, 16, 19
Expertise, 197t
Expression, creative, 112
External-internal partnership model, 95–96

Facilitated learning, 187–90, 188t, 190f
Facilitation, 9, 23, 31–33, 92, 94, 112, 119
advanced, 140–43, 142b, 142f, 143b, 144f
learning outcomes, 141b
take-home message, 144
approach to, 156–57
authentic, 133
capability, 189
change and, 148
collaboration in, 150–51
context and, 135
in cross-sectorial group, 151–52
development, 136, 138
elements of, 133
embodiment of, 135
evaluation of, 143, 144f
expertise, 258
external, 132f, 134
fluidity in, 135
impact of, 141b
internal, 132f
interprofessional, 72
multilayered, 148
outcomes, 142b
participation processes in
case examples, 149–52
complexity of, 152–53
culture, 153–55
meaningful, 152–53
PD and, 5–6, 257–58
among peers, 150–51
person-centred approach to, 131, 136, 137f
process of, 149–52
programme, 143b
relationality in, 131
relationships, 147
research, 145
research themes and sub-themes, 132, 132f
skills, 108t, 109, 112b, 113, 131, 135, 258
strategies, 71
theories, 134–35, 140
transformational, 131, 132f, 135, 139, 145
translation of, 109
understanding of, 100
unpacking and development of
advanced, 140–44, 141b, 142b, 142f, 143b, 144f
overview of, 131–39, 132f, 136b, 137f, 139b
Facilitation activity plan (FAP), 189
Facilitation evaluation plan (FEP), 189
Facilitator development action plan (FDAP), 189
Facilitator training model, 190f
Faculty of Multiprofessional Learning in Maternity, 28

FAP. *See* Facilitation activity plan
Fay, Bryan, 3, 122–23, 126f, 129
FDAP. *See* Facilitator development action plan
Feedback, 92, 94, 104
  anonymous, 180
  constructive, 32
  data-sourced, 88
  for IMAGINE programme, 225
  key themes from, 101t–3t
  PD revision, 101t–3t
  positive, 73
  revision, 101t–3t
  for Skills for Life programme, 232
FEP. *See* Facilitation evaluation plan
Financial barriers, 15
'Five Year Forward View,' 42
Foundation of Nursing Studies (FoNS) newsletter, 100, 101t, 104
Foundation PD School, 99–100
Fourth Generation Evaluation, 6
Future
  hope and optimism for, 19
  person-centred practitioners, 83

Gatekeeping, professional, 15
German Network for Quality Development in Nursing (DNQP), 56–57
'Good Enough Evaluation', 7
Group-based programmes, 16
Growth, 238
  local, 248
  strategies for, 179–80
Guiding lights study, 164–67

Habermas, Jurgen, 233
Health and social care (HSC), 251
  demands on, 40
  inclusive, 80
  organisations, 260
  PD transformation
    developments since 2008, 4–7
    interprofessional collaboration, shared values and, 3–4
    key concepts and structure of, 8–10
    relevance to contemporary health, social care, and crisis, 2–3
    scene for, 1
    values and, 7–8
  systems, 262
Healthcare delivery
  improvement, 86–97, 89f, 91f
  inclusive approaches to, 15
  paternalistic approach of, 40
  quality and safety in, 21
Healthcare system
  complexities of, 190
  historical boundaries in, 191
Health Education and Training Institute (HETI), 187–89
Healthful culture, 61
Health LEADS Australia, 188
Health literacy, 15
Health outcomes, 66
Health services, 14, 23–24
Health services collaboration
  approaches to
    facilitators' experiences in, 20–21
    flexibility and collaboration in, 16
    inclusive, 15–16
    IOIG, 16–18
    knowledge building/sharing within, 17
    participant experiences in, 20
    patient centred, 16
    professional education, 17–18
    recovery courses, 19–21
    relational aspects and, 18
  power hierarchies in, 21
  between professional providers and service users., 14–24
Hedonic wellbeing, 221, 238
Hegemony, 120–21
Helplessness, 90, 94
Heterogeneity, 95

HETI. *See* Health Education and Training Institute
Hierarchical relationships, 174, 207, 257
Holistic facilitation models, 128
Holistic safety, 4
Homogeneity, 154
Hospital admissions, 44
HSC. *See* Health and social care
Human flourishing, 108t, 109, 111, 173, 221
as a construct, 238
in healthcare settings, 244–47, 245t, 246f
models of, 238
in people, families, and communities, 237–48, 239t, 242f, 245t, 246f
principles and methods practice for, 237
well-being and, 237
workplace culture and, 237
Human function, 238
Humanness, 2
Humble assertiveness, 147–57
Huppert's model of flourishing, 238

Identity, 19
Illawarra Ostomy Information Group (IOIG), 16–18
Illawarra Shoalhaven Local Health District (ISLHD), 222
IMAGINE programme, 222–25, 223t, 224f
Imagining Potential Across Complex Teams (ImPACT), 101t
Implementing and Measuring Person-centredness using an APP for Knowledge Transfer (iMPAKT), 245t, 246–47
Improvement
continuous, 28
drivers, 216
qualitative measures of, 31–32
quantitative measures of, 31
Inclusion, 1, 109
Inclusivity, 27–28
Indigenous workforce, 125, 126
Individual patient allocation (IPA) model, 91
Innovation
PD and, 255–56
processes, 6, 114, 148
specialist, 34
Interdisciplinary team, 149, 183, 183b
International Practice Development Collaborative (IPDC), 10, 99, 119, 140, 141b
in health and social care, 104f
member organisation, 101t–3t
new directions through, 259
International Practice Development Journal (IPDJ), 3, 259–60
Interprofessional collaboration, shared values and, 3–4
Interprofessional learning, 65
Interprofessional practice, 4
IOIG. *See* Illawarra Ostomy Information Group
IPA. *See* Individual patient allocation model
IPDC. *See* International Practice Development Collaborative
IPDJ. *See* International Practice Development Journal
ISLHD. *See* Illawarra Shoalhaven Local Health District

Kent and Medway Medical School, 45
Kent's Design and Learning Centre, 44
Keyes's model of flourishing, 238
Key performance descriptors (KPDs), 189
Key performance indicators (KPIs), 244–45, 247
in Person-centred Nursing Framework, 246f
for person-centred practice, 82
Knowledge. *See also* Continuing professional development
building of, 17
collective, 237

Knowledge (*cont'd*)
  co-production of, 86
  development, 16
  interdisciplinary, 167
  professional, 16
  sharing of, 17, 81
  transformation, 149
  translation, 2, 4
  up-to-date, 47, 78t
Knowledge continuum, 6
KPDs. *See* Key performance descriptors
KPIs. *See* Key performance indicators

Language, 103t, 127
  accessible, 104, 109
  communication and, 231
  person-centred, 145
Leadership, 30
  adaptive, 174
  associate, 161–62
  authentic, 182
  balance in, 163
  challenges, 184
  clinical, 27, 164, 173–84, 183b, 184f, 192t
  collective, 47–48, 166, 195, 207, 208t, 210–11, 262
  communication in, 163
  in communities, 164
  connectedness and, 160–62, 161f
  crisis, 180
  culture and, 173–84, 183b, 184f
  designated, 191
  development, 6, 167–70
  distributed, 191
  in education, 164
  in environment of care, 164
  facilitative, 197t, 233
  flexible, 160
  guiding lights of, 164–67
  in health, 168
  hierarchical, 211
  in interprofessional teams, 164
  NSW Health Leadership Programme, 188, 188t
  older people and, 196–97, 197t
  in organisations, 164
  PD through, 257–58
  person-centred, 159, 167
  in person-centred care, 162f
  qualities, 167
  relational, 160–62, 160–64, 161f, 162f
  relationships, 9, 159–70, 161f, 162f
  skills, 83, 96, 197t, 201
  in social care, 164
  strengthening of, 164–67
  of systems, collaborative health-care practices and, 187–98, 188t, 190f, 192t, 193t, 194t, 195f, 197t
  transformational, 31, 34, 174, 183b
  transformative, 34
  during the unpredictable, 166
  workplace culture and, 167–70
Leadership Masterclass, 44
Learner autonomy, 156
Learning
  active work-based, 32, 67f, 79, 105t, 110f, 112
  appreciative, 121
  approaches, 168–69
  collaborative, 67
  continuous, 28
  culture, 70, 74t, 212–14
  environment, 20, 71–73
  facilitator guided, 67f
  personal commitment to, 69
  person-centred, 74t
  reflective, 79
  student-led, 67
  systematic, 194t
  translation of, 169
  work-based, 112, 112b
  in workplace, 183b
Lens of facilitation theme, 138
Lewin, Kurt, 255

Listening, 165
Long Term Plan, 44

Management, clinical, 27
Manipulation, 133
Marie Curie charity, 136, 136b, 139
Marriott, Lin, 126f
Maternity care, 26–27, 29
McCance, Tanya, 5
McCormack, Brendan, 5
MDT. *See* Multidisciplinary team
Medical anthropology, 92–93
Medicine, person-centred, 252
Meditation, 223t
Mental health, 19, 103t, 149
 first aid training, 232
Mentorship, 137f, 181
Methodology
 approach, 248
 complex, 110f
 realist evaluation, 242
MGP. *See* Midwifery Group Practice
Micro-cultures, 216
Micro-systems, 105t, 113, 113b, 206
Midwife, 3, 31
Midwifery Group Practice (MGP), 34
Mindfulness, 223, 223t
Multicare research project, 150
Multidisciplinary developmental frameworks, 75t
Multidisciplinary leaders, 197t
Multidisciplinary team (MDT), 91
Multiprofessional leadership programme, 47
Multiprofessional learning, 27, 43
Multiprofessional team training, 28
Mutuality, 240

National Health and Medical Research Council (NHMRC), 61
National Health Service (NHS), 42
Neuroplasticity, 41
Neuroscience, 31
New South Wales (NSW), 100, 187, 223
NGOs. *See* Non-governmental organisations
NHMRC. *See* National Health and Medical Research Council
NHS. *See* National Health Service
'The NHS Long Term Plan' (2019), 42
Non-governmental organisations (NGOs), 62
NSW. *See* New South Wales
NSW Health Leadership Programme, 188, 188t
Nursing curriculum, 65–67
Nursing home, 56–58

Oakden Report, 180
Occupational health, 230–31
Occupational therapist (OT), 54
Older people, 252
 leadership and, 196–97, 197t
 needs of, 52
 person-centred care for, 52–62
Opportunities, 21, 34
Oppression, 120
Organisational culture, 97
OT. *See* Occupational therapist
Outreach efforts, 15
Ownership, 197
 local, 248
 sense of, 151, 155
 shared, 194t

Paediatric International Nursing Study (PINS), 245–46
Pain management, 56
Palliative care, 136
Pandemic, global, 1–2, 5, 191, 232, 252
Participant observation, 93
Participation, 139b, 152–53, 155
Participative approach, 27
Partnership, 14–15
Patient, 16
 assessment, 120

Patient (*cont'd*)
experience, 194t
feedback, 15
perception, 15
safety, 237
satisfaction, 14
support, 15
voice of, 31
PBL. *See* Place-based learning
PCNs. *See* Primary care networks
PCPF. *See* Person-Centred Practice Framework
PCTC. *See* Person-Centred Training and Curriculum Scoping Group
PD. *See* Practice development
PDFs. *See* Practice development facilitators
Peer consulting, 43
Peer networking, 15
Peet, Jacqueline, 122
PERMA elements, 238
Person-centred care
approach for, 41
attitude for, 57
challenges of, 40
framework of, 61
improvement of, 86
interaction and communication in, 57
international, cross-setting and interdisciplinary learning in, 60–61
knowledge required for, 81
leader development in, 42–44
leadership in, 162f
in nursing school, 46
for older people, 52–62
PD and, 251–62, 253b, 254, 259b
philosophy, 83
practice, 111
safe, 149
support of, 44–45
sustainable community design and practice, 39–48
TIC and, 60
Person-centred leadership framework, 162–64, 162f
Person-centredness
care, 7, 23–24, 26, 31, 48
communities, 9, 39–48
core principles of, 66
cultures, 5, 262
frameworks, 4
PD theory and, 122–24
practice, 3
relationships, 45
research, 4
systems, 9
Person-centred Nursing Framework, 244, 246f
Person-centred practice, 67f, 82, 188t
Person-Centred Practice Framework (PCPF), 66, 69, 124, 136, 140, 142
Person-Centred Training and Curriculum (PCTC) Scoping Group, 48
Philanthropy, benevolent, 240
PINS. *See* Paediatric International Nursing Study
Place-based learning (PBL), 65, 83
attributes of, 74t–76t
benefits of, 71, 71b
consequences of, 74t–76t
enablers in, 74t–76t
facilitation strategies, 71
implementation and impact framework of, 74t–76t
learning environment for, 71–72
outcomes, 72–73, 74t–76t
population needs in, 69–71, 70b, 71b
primary care demands in, 69–71, 70b, 71b
retention and recruitment with, 73
shared purpose of, 70, 70b, 74t–76t
values of, 74t
Placemaking, in community, 239
Policymakers, 198
Positionality, 96–97

Power, 139
  imbalance, 152
  role of, 129
  structures of, 120
Practice developers, 259–60
Practice development (PD). *See also* Continuing professional development; Person-centredness
  accessibility of, 109, 115
  in aged care services, 62
  brainstorming for, 142f
  celebration of, 261
  CIP and, 111, 111b
  co-creation and, 254–55
  collaboration in, 27
  concept analysis, 6
  in constant renewal, 114–15
  contemporary patient/provider partnership models in, 15
  contextual readiness and, 29–30
  co-production and, 33–35
  core principles of
    comparison of 2008 and 2020, 110–15, 110f, 111b, 112b, 113b, 114b
    critical review of, 101t–3t
    emergent themes, 104, 109–10, 110f
    process revision of, 100, 101t–3t, 104, 104f
    simplified, 115
    stepped approach to, 115
  critical ethnography and, 86–97, 89f, 91f
  education models of, 65–83, 67f, 68f, 74t–76t, 77b, 77t–79t
  effectiveness of, 116
  engagement and, 30–31
  evaluation of, 113b
  evidence base through, 2, 114, 114b, 196
  facilitation, 5–6, 31–33, 86, 131–45, 132f, 136b, 137f, 139b, 141b, 142b, 142f, 143b, 144f
  to foster person-centred care, 251–62, 253b, 259b
  foundations of, 8, 110f, 115
  future challenges of, 254, 257–61
  as global manifesto, 114–15
  global manifesto for, 258–59
  implementation, 31
  inclusivity in, 27
  innovation and, 255–56
  interdisciplinary implementation of, 52
  international, 119
  interprofessional collaboration, shared values and, 3–4
  through leadership and facilitation, 257–58
  in maternity care, 26
  methodology, 4, 29, 33–36, 100, 109, 114b, 115, 120
  beyond methods, 258–59, 259b
  models, 15
  outcome-focused, 100, 115
  outcomes of, 110f
  participative approach in, 27
  person-centred care and, 252, 254
  person-centred practice and, 3, 5
  philosophy, 35, 65–83, 67f, 68f, 74t–76t, 77b, 77t–79t
  political roots of, 119
  positionality in, 96
  principles of, 29
    emergent themes of, 104, 105t–8t, 109–10, 110f
    ordering of, 109–10, 110f
    review timelines for, 104f
    stepped approach to, 109–10, 110f
  processes of, 110f, 112, 115
  professional engagement in, 260
  relevance of, 1, 111b
    to contemporary health, social care, and crisis, 2–3
  research, 2, 120
  revised principles of, 3, 105t–8t, 110b, 111b, 112b, 258b
  as self-discovery, 99

Practice development (PD) (*cont'd*)
stages of, 115
system approaches for, 256–57
systems leadership and, 187–98, 188t, 190f, 192t, 193t, 194t, 195f, 197t
theory
in action, 125–27, 126f
bicultural perspective and, 125–27, 126f
commentary, 128–29
crisis and, 122–24
critical reflection and, 120–22
CSS and, 122–24
future of, 127–28
origins of, 119–20
person-centredness and, 122–24
research and, 122–24
webinar, 119
tools for, 29
tradition of, 4
transformational, 27, 32, 114b, 115
translation of, 109
USD of, 103t
user involvement and, 254–55
values and impact, 65–83, 67f, 68f, 74t–76t, 77b, 77t–79t
visuals of, 115
wheel, 91–92, 91f
whole-system integration and, 5
at work, 233
Practice development facilitators (PDFs) programme, 136–38, 136b
Practice improvement
AR in, 243–44
family involvement in, 242
Practitioners, 2, 47–48
'Praxis model', 7
Presencing, 163
Pressure injury, prevention of, 56
Primary care networks (PCNs), 74t
mnemonic for, 70, 70b
system and, 75t
values of, 70, 70b
Problem-solving, 33, 43
Productive Ward programme, 31–32
Professional development, 55, 80
Professional growth, 69
Professional networking, 197t
Programme success, indicators of, 23
Psycho-emotional support, 16
Purpose, 32, 43

QI. *See* Quality improvement
Qualitative improvement (QI), 31–32
Quality improvement (QI), 6, 28, 33, 100, 183, 183b
Quality of care, 40
Quality of life measures, 45

RACGP. *See* Royal Australian College of General Practitioners
Racism, 252
Randomised control trial (RCT), 41
Realist evaluation methodology, 242
Reciprocity, 14, 240
"Recognising and Developing Effective Workplace Cultures" (Webster), 217
Recovery
courses, 23
framework, 19
Recovery Colleges, 19
Recruitment, 30
Reflection, 121, 123–24, 128, 145, 168, 170
"Reflections on theory in practice development" (Stephenson), 118
Reflexive inquiry, 88
Reflexivity, 113, 162
Registered nurse (RN), 121
Relational connectedness, 160–62, 161f
Relational leadership, 160–62, 161f
Relational transparency, 174
Relationship-based approaches, 5
Relationship goods, 40
Relationships, 105t
collegial, 30

on continuum, 160
with dementia, 57
guiding light study in, 164–67
hierarchical, 174
internal, 210
leadership and, 159–70, 161f, 162f
person-centred, 46, 48
social, 238
with staff, 212
supportive, 110f, 114, 237
therapeutic, 40, 48
'Releasing Time to Care,' 31
Research, 15
action-oriented approaches for, 4, 123, 242
AR, 243–44
in collaborative community, 244
context-based, 6
critical reflection, 132
embedded, 4, 7, 86–97, 89f, 91f, 94, 96
evidence, 27–28
funding for, 73
for IMAGINE programme, 225
of KPIs, 244, 245t
Multicare project, 150
participatory, 6
PD theory and, 122–24
person-centredness, 4
practice-based, 2
qualitative, 241
student, 124
study, 65
themes and sub-themes, 132, 132f
traditional, 7
transformational, 241
of well-being, 221
Resource utilisation, 33–34
Responsibility, diffusion of, 90, 94
RN. *See* Registered nurse
Role modelling, 32, 210
Royal Australian College of General Practitioners (RACGP), 55
Royal College of Psychiatrists, 48
Royal Commission into Aged Care Quality and Safety, 60

Safety, 4, 26, 160, 174
Safety Culture Quality Improvement Realist Evaluation (SCQIRE) project, 206, 212, 214
Salco company, 228
SCARF© model, 30–31
SCQIRE project. *See* Safety Culture Quality Improvement Realist Evaluation project
Self-awareness, 141, 252
Self-determination, 160
Self-management, 16
Self-worth, 165
Seligman's Theory of Wellbeing, PERMA elements, 238
Sense of community (SoC), 239–40
Senses, in assessment, 162
Sensory information, 162
Service contextual readiness, 29–30
Service improvement, 15, 33
Service redesign, 31
Service users, 255
'Seven out of ten miss out,' 35
Shared decision-making, 66
Shared governance model, 241
Skills for Life programme, 231–32
SLTT. *See* Speech and Language Therapy Team
SoC. *See* Sense of community
Social care, 39, 252, 253b
Social cognitive neuroscience, 31
Social domains, 31
Social justice, 80
Social media, 164
Social norms, 2, 205
Social science theory, 9, 122, 129
Society, challenges in, 252
Socio-demographics, 52
Speech and Language Therapy Team (SLTT), 178

Stance, as position, 163–64
Stephenson, Loraine, 118
Stigmas, 15, 21
Stomal Therapy Nurses (STNs), 17, 23
Story writing, for awareness, 121
Substance abuse, 19, 149
Sustainability, of well-being, 225–29, 226f, 227f, 228b
Sustainable person-centered communities, 39–48, 197
Systematic evaluation, 100
System enablers, 192, 193t, 195
Systems leadership
  attributes of, 201
  collaborative healthcare practices and, 187–98, 188t, 190f, 192t, 193t, 194t, 195f, 197t
  complex healthcare systems and, 190–91
  consequences, 201
  development and management of, 187–90, 188t, 190f, 193t, 203
  facilitative, 196–97, 197t
  functions of, 193
  outcomes, 194t
  PD and, 187
  transformation, 191–95, 192t, 193t, 194t, 195f
Systems transformation, 6, 251–62, 253b, 259b

TADA. *See* Taiwanese Alzheimer's Disease Association
Taipei Medical University (TMU), 55
Taiwanese Alzheimer's Disease Association (TADA), 54–56
Team
  based model, 91
  performance, 212
  training, 27
Teamwork, 150
  effective, 211
  model, 123
  multidisciplinary, 43
  during pandemic, 2
Technological innovations, 3, 92
Telemedicine, 3
Theoretical perspectives, 9
Theoretical underpinnings, 137f
TIC. *See* Trauma-informed care
TMU. *See* Taipei Medical University
Tokenism, 15
Transformation
  bottom-up, 216
  cultural, 99, 112
  from ground up, 176–77
  large-scale, 191
  sustained, 197
  true, 32
  workforce strategies for, 192t
Transformational leadership, 31, 34, 174, 183b
Transformational research, 241
Transformation Programme, 33
Transformative leadership, 34
Transformative work, person-centred, 221
Trauma, 58, 180–82
Trauma-informed care (TIC), 59, 61
  benefits of, 60
  person-centred care and, 60
Treaty of Waitangi, 125

UN. *See* United Nations
Unique selling point (USP), 103t
United Nations (UN), 52
University of Wollongong (UOW), 54–56, 223
USP. *See* Unique selling point

Values, 7–8, 114, 182, 262
  shared, 2, 82, 208t, 211–12
  voice-based approach and, 241
Venus model of PD, 256
Vulnerability, 162

WBM program. *See* Wellbeing Matters programme
Webster, Jonathan, 217
Well-being
beliefs about, 228
elements of, 239t
eudaimonic, 221, 238
hedonic, 221, 238
human flourishing and, 237
IMAGINE programme, 222–25, 223t, 224f
importance of, 228b
within organisations, 233
as priority, 1, 229
research of, 221
sense of, 224
staff, 7
as transformative work, 221
Wellness Wednesdays, 223, 227
at work
communication opportunities, 231
dissemination and sustainability of, 225–29, 226f, 227f, 228b
diversity, 230f
education access, 231
evaluation of, 233
flourishing at, 221
importance of, 228b, 230–31
initiatives for, 232
key insights, 232–33
PD approach to, 233
recognition and achievement, 229–30, 230f
significance of, 222–25, 223t, 224f
strategies of, 228b, 229, 229b
understanding of, 220
values and, 231–32
Wellbeing Matters (WBM) programme, 253b
Wellness Wednesdays, 223, 227
WHO. *See* World Health Organization
Whole-system approach, integrated, 5
Workforce
availability, 40
empowered, 174
enablers, 192t
ethno-cultural diversity among, 150
indigenous, 125
systems leadership and, 191–95, 192t, 193t, 194t, 195f
transformation, 46, 192t
Workplace
barriers in, 95
behaviour at, 222
changes in, 87
CPD in, 81
enablers, 206
environment, 74t
health and social care, 220
hierarchies, 95
improvement, 92
oppressive, 119
relationships, 174
as resource for learning, developing, and improving, 65–83, 67f, 68f, 74t–76t, 77b, 77t–79t
transformation, 4, 27
unsafe, 87
well-being at, 220–33, 223t, 224f, 226f, 227f, 228b, 229b, 230f
Workplace culture, 32, 88, 93–95, 105t, 111, 119, 154–57, 164
change in, 205
collaborative inquiry, 206–7, 208t–9t, 210–15
CPD and, 78t–79t, 82–83
development of, 205–7, 208t–9t, 210–17
in future, 215–16
guiding lights and, 207, 208t–9t, 210–15
within health and social care organisations, 205
human flourishing and, 237
importance of, 205–6
improvement drivers for, 215

Workplace culture (*cont'd*)
indicators of, 237
leadership and, 167–70
outcomes of, 215
positive, 6, 33
prerequisites to, 2
safe and effective, 3
SCQIRE project, 206
transformation of, 78t–79t
unchallenged, 205
Workshops, 137f
face-to-face, 55–56
person-centred, 196
train the trainer, 56
World Health Organization (WHO), 5, 52